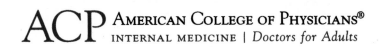

ACP American College of Physicians®
INTERNAL MEDICINE | *Doctors for Adults*

MKSAP®16

Medical Knowledge Self-Assessment Program®

Gastroenterology and Hepatology

Welcome to the Gastroenterology and Hepatology section of MKSAP 16!

We present an authoritative review of gastroesophageal reflux disease, peptic ulcer disease, dyspepsia, *Helicobacter pylori* infection, gastrointestinal complications of NSAIDs, gastrointestinal bleeding, gastric adenocarcinoma, pancreatitis, colorectal cancer, diarrhea, constipation, and other clinical challenges. All of these topics are uniquely focused on the needs of generalists and subspecialists *outside* of gastroenterology and hepatology.

The publication of the 16th edition of Medical Knowledge Self-Assessment Program heralds a significant event, culminating 2 years of effort by dozens of leading subspecialists across the United States. Our authoring committees have strived to help internists succeed in Maintenance of Certification, right up to preparing for the MOC examination, and to get residents ready for the certifying examination. MKSAP 16 also helps you update your medical knowledge and elevates standards of self-learning by allowing you to assess your knowledge with 1,200 all-new multiple-choice questions, including 96 in Gastroenterology and Hepatology.

MKSAP began more than 40 years ago. The American Board of Internal Medicine's examination blueprint and gaps between actual and preferred practices inform creation of the content. The questions, refined through rigorous face-to-face meetings, are among the best in medicine. A psychometric analysis of the items sharpens our educational focus on weaknesses in practice. To meet diverse learning styles, we offer MKSAP 16 online and in downloadable apps for tablets, laptops, and phones. We are also introducing the following:

High-Value Care Recommendations: The Gastroenterology and Hepatology section starts with several recommendations based on the important concept of health care value (balancing clinical benefit with costs and harms) to address the needs of trainees, practicing physicians, and patients. These recommendations are part of a major initiative that has been undertaken by the American College of Physicians, in collaboration with other organizations.

Content for Hospitalists: This material, highlighted in blue and labeled with the familiar hospital icon (🏥), directly addresses the learning needs of the increasing number of physicians who work in the hospital setting. MKSAP 16 Digital will allow you to customize quizzes based on hospitalist-only questions to help you prepare for the Hospital Medicine Maintenance of Certification Examination.

We hope you enjoy and benefit from MKSAP 16. Please feel free to send us any comments to mksap_editors@acponline.org or visit us at the MKSAP Resource Site (mksap.acponline.org) to find out how we can help you study, earn CME, accumulate MOC points, and stay up to date. I know I speak on behalf of ACP staff members and our authoring committees when I say we are honored to have attracted your interest and participation.

Sincerely,

Patrick Alguire, MD, FACP
Editor-in-Chief
Senior Vice President
Medical Education Division
American College of Physicians

Gastroenterology and Hepatology

Committee

Amy S. Oxentenko, MD, FACP, Editor[1]
Assistant Professor of Medicine
Division of Gastroenterology and Hepatology
Mayo Clinic
Rochester, Minnesota

Thomas Fekete, MD, FACP, Associate Editor[1]
Professor of Medicine
Section of Infectious Diseases
Temple University Medical School
Philadelphia, Pennsylvania

Timothy B. Gardner, MD[2]
Assistant Professor of Medicine
Section of Gastroenterology and Hepatology
Dartmouth-Hitchcock Medical Center
Lebanon, New Hampshire

Michael D. Leise, MD[2]
Assistant Professor of Medicine
Division of Gastroenterology and Hepatology
Mayo Clinic
Rochester, Minnesota

Paul J. Limburg, MD, MPH[2]
Professor of Medicine
Division of Gastroenterology and Hepatology
Mayo Clinic
Rochester, Minnesota

Roman Perri, MD[1]
Assistant Professor of Medicine
Division of Gastroenterology, Hepatology, and Nutrition
Vanderbilt University Medical Center
Nashville, Tennessee

Ganapathy Prasad, MD, MSc[2]
Associate Professor of Medicine
Division of Gastroenterology and Hepatology
Mayo Clinic
Rochester, Minnesota

Corey A. Siegel, MD[2]
Assistant Professor of Medicine
Section of Gastroenterology and Hepatology
Dartmouth-Hitchcock Medical Center
Lebanon, New Hampshire

Jayant (Jay) Talwalkar, MD, MPH[2]
Associate Professor of Medicine
Division of Gastroenterology and Hepatology
Mayo Clinic
Rochester, Minnesota

Editor-in-Chief

Patrick C. Alguire, MD, FACP[1]
Senior Vice President, Medical Education
American College of Physicians
Philadelphia, Pennsylvania

Deputy Editor-in-Chief

Philip A. Masters, MD, FACP[1]
Senior Medical Associate for Content Development
American College of Physicians
Philadelphia, Pennsylvania

Senior Medical Associate for Content Development

Cynthia D. Smith, MD, FACP[2]
American College of Physicians
Philadelphia, Pennsylvania

Gastroenterology and Hepatology Clinical Editor

Mary Jane Barchman, MD, FACP[2]

Gastroenterology and Hepatology Reviewers

Robert D. Arbeit, MD[2]
Amindra Arora, MD[1]
Arnold Asp, MD, FACP[1]
Dawn E. DeWitt, MD, FACP[2]
Douglas Einstadter, MD, MPH, FACP[1]
Rabeh Elzuway, MD[1]
Richard M. Hoffman, MD, MPH, FACP[2]
Richard H. Moseley, MD, FACP[1]
Michael Vaezi, MD[1]

Gastroenterology and Hepatology Reviewers Representing the American Society for Clinical Pharmacology & Therapeutics

John Thomas Callaghan, MD, PhD[2]
Fracisco J. Leyva, MD[1]

Gastroenterology and Hepatology ACP Editorial Staff

Katie Idell[1], Senior Staff Editor
Sean McKinney[1], Director, Self-Assessment Programs
Margaret Wells[1], Managing Editor
Linnea Donnarumma[1], Assistant Editor

ACP Principal Staff

Patrick C. Alguire, MD, FACP[1]
Senior Vice President, Medical Education

D. Theresa Kanya, MBA[1]
Vice President, Medical Education

Sean McKinney[1]
Director, Self-Assessment Programs

Margaret Wells[1]
Managing Editor

Valerie Dangovetsky[1]
Program Administrator

Becky Krumm[1]
Senior Staff Editor

Ellen McDonald, PhD[1]
Senior Staff Editor

Katie Idell[1]
Senior Staff Editor

Randy Hendrickson[1]
Production Administrator/Editor

Megan Zborowski[1]
Staff Editor

Linnea Donnarumma[1]
Assistant Editor

John Haefele[1]
Assistant Editor

Developed by the American College of Physicians

---

1. Has no relationships with any entity producing, marketing, re-selling, or distributing health care goods or services consumed by, or used on, patients.

2. Has disclosed relationships with entities producing, marketing, re-selling, or distributing health care goods or services consumed by, or used on, patients. See below.

Conflicts of Interest

The following committee members, reviewers, and ACP staff members have disclosed relationships with commercial companies:

Robert D. Arbeit, MD
Employment
Idera Pharmaceuticals, Inc.

Mary Jane Barchman, MD, FACP
Speakers Bureau
Novartis
Honoraria
National Board of Medical Examiners

John Thomas Callaghan, MD, PhD
Employment
Eli Lilly and Company Retiree
Stock Options/Holdings
Eli Lilly, Abbott, Isis
Consultantship
Marcaida, Biogen Idec

Dawn E. DeWitt, MD
Honoraria
Sanofi-Aventis, NovoNordisk
Speakers Bureau
Sanofi-Aventis, NovoNordisk

Timothy B. Gardner, MD
Consultantship
Boston Scientific
Research Grants/Contracts
ChiRhoClin, Inc.

Richard M. Hoffman, MD, FACP
Employment
Foundation for Informed Medical Decision Making
Royalties
UpToDate

Michael D. Leise, MD
Research Grants/Contracts
Bristol Myers-Squibb: Virology M.D. Fellows Research Program Grant

Paul J. Limburg, MD, MPH
Consultantship
Genomic Health, Inc.
Research Grants/Contracts
Olympus America, Beneo-Orafti Group, Bayer Healthcare, Fujinon, Inc., Boston Scientific, AstraZeneca
Honoraria
American School of Oncology
Royalties
Exact Sciences

Ganapathy Prasad, MD, MSc
Research Grants/Contracts
AstraZeneca, Fujinon, Takeda Pharmaceuticals, Given
Imaging, NIH, American College of Gastroenterology

Corey A. Siegel, MD
Consultantship
Abbott, Elan Pharmaceuticals, Warner-Chilcott, Allos
Pharmaceuticals, Janssen
Honoraria
Abbott, UCB, Merck
Research Grants/Contracts
Abbott, UCB, Warner-Chilcott, Salix
Other
Risk Prediction Model (Patent Holder)

Cynthia D. Smith, MD, FACP
Stock Options/Holdings
Merck and Company

Jayant (Jay) Talwalkar, MD, MPH
Research Grants/Contracts
Salix Pharmaceuticals, Merck, Bristol-Myers Squibb
Other
AASLD (Chair, Practice Guidelines Committee)

Acknowledgments

The American College of Physicians (ACP) gratefully
acknowledges the special contributions to the development
and production of the 16th edition of the Medical
Knowledge Self-Assessment Program® (MKSAP® 16)
made by the following people:

Graphic Services: Michael Ripca (Technical Administrator/
Graphic Designer) and Willie-Fetchko Graphic Design
(Graphic Designer).

Production/Systems: Dan Hoffmann (Director, Web Services
& Systems Development), Neil Kohl (Senior Architect), and
Scott Hurd (Senior Systems Analyst/Developer).

MKSAP 16 Digital: Under the direction of Steven Spadt,
Vice President, ACP Digital Products & Services, the digital
version of MKSAP 16 was developed within the ACP's
Digital Product Development Department, led by Brian
Sweigard (Director). Other members of the team included
Sean O'Donnell (Senior Architect), Dan Barron (Senior
Systems Analyst/Developer), Chris Forrest (Senior Software
Developer/Design Lead), Jon Laing (Senior Web Application
Developer), Brad Lord (Senior Web Developer), John
McKnight (Senior Web Developer), and Nate Pershall
(Senior Web Developer).

The College also wishes to acknowledge that many other
persons, too numerous to mention, have contributed to the
production of this program. Without their dedicated efforts,
this program would not have been possible.

Introducing the MKSAP Resource Site (mksap.acponline.org)

The MKSAP Resource Site (mksap.acponline.org) is a con-
tinually updated site that provides links to MKSAP 16
online answer sheets for print subscribers; access to MKSAP
16 Digital, Board Basics® 3, and MKSAP 16 Updates; the
latest details on Continuing Medical Education (CME) and
Maintenance of Certification (MOC) in the United States,
Canada, and Australia; errata; and other new information.

ABIM Maintenance of Certification

Check the MKSAP Resource Site (mksap.acponline.org) for
the latest information on how MKSAP tests can be used to
apply to the American Board of Internal Medicine for
Maintenance of Certification (MOC) points.

RCPSC Maintenance of Certification

In Canada, MKSAP 16 is an Accredited Self-Assessment
Program (Section 3) as defined by the Maintenance of
Certification Program of The Royal College of Physicians &
Surgeons of Canada (RCPSC) and approved by the
Canadian Society of Internal Medicine on December 9,
2011. Approval of this and other Part A sections of MKSAP
16 extends from July 31, 2012, until July 31, 2015.
Approval of Part B sections of MKSAP 16 extends from
December 31, 2012, to December 31, 2015. Fellows of the
Royal College may earn three credits per hour for partici-
pating in MKSAP 16 under Section 3. MKSAP 16 will
enable Fellows to earn up to 75% of their required 400
credits during the 5-year MOC cycle. A Fellow can achieve
this 75% level by earning 100 of the maximum of 174
AMA PRA Category 1 Credits™ available in MKSAP 16.
MKSAP 16 also meets multiple CanMEDS Roles for
RCPSC MOC, including that of Medical Expert,
Communicator, Collaborator, Manager, Health Advocate,
Scholar, and Professional. For information on how to apply
MKSAP 16 CME credits to RCPSC MOC, visit the
MKSAP Resource Site at mksap.acponline.org.

The Royal Australasian College of Physicians CPD Program

In Australia, MKSAP 16 is a Category 3 program that may
be used by Fellows of The Royal College of Physicians
(RACP) to meet mandatory CPD points. Two CPD credits
are awarded for each of the 174 *AMA PRA Category 1
Credits*™ available in MKSAP 16. More information about
using MKSAP 16 for this purpose is available at the
MKSAP Resource Site at mksap.acponline.org and at
www.racp.edu.au. CPD credits earned through
MKSAP 16 should be reported at the MyCPD site at
www.racp.edu.au/mycpd.

Continuing Medical Education

The American College of Physicians is accredited by the Accreditation Council for Continuing Medical Education (ACCME) to provide continuing medical education for physicians.

The American College of Physicians designates this enduring material, MKSAP 16, for a maximum of 174 *AMA PRA Category 1 Credits*™. Physicians should claim only the credit commensurate with the extent of their participation in the activity.

Up to 14 *AMA PRA Category 1 Credits*™ are available from July 31, 2012, to July 31, 2015, for the MKSAP 16 Gastroenterology and Hepatology section.

Learning Objectives

The learning objectives of MKSAP 16 are to:
- Close gaps between actual care in your practice and preferred standards of care, based on best evidence
- Diagnose disease states that are less common and sometimes overlooked and confusing
- Improve management of comorbid conditions that can complicate patient care
- Determine when to refer patients for surgery or care by subspecialists
- Pass the ABIM Certification Examination
- Pass the ABIM Maintenance of Certification Examination

Target Audience

- General internists and primary care physicians
- Subspecialists who need to remain up-to-date in internal medicine
- Residents preparing for the certifying examination in internal medicine
- Physicians preparing for maintenance of certification in internal medicine (recertification)

Earn "Same-Day" CME Credits Online

For the first time, print subscribers can enter their answers online to earn CME credits in 24 hours or less. You can submit your answers using online answer sheets that are provided at mksap.acponline.org, where a record of your MKSAP 16 credits will be available. To earn CME credits, you need to answer all of the questions in a test and earn a score of at least 50% correct (number of correct answers divided by the total number of questions). Take any of the following approaches:

1. Use the printed answer sheet at the back of this book to record your answers. Go to mksap.acponline.org, access the appropriate online answer sheet, transcribe your answers, and submit your test for same-day CME credits. There is no additional fee for this service.

2. Go to mksap.acponline.org, access the appropriate online answer sheet, directly enter your answers, and submit your test for same-day CME credits. There is no additional fee for this service.

3. Pay a $10 processing fee per answer sheet and submit the printed answer sheet at the back of this book by mail or fax, as instructed on the answer sheet. Make sure you calculate your score and fax the answer sheet to 215-351-2799 or mail the answer sheet to Member and Customer Service, American College of Physicians, 190 N. Independence Mall West, Philadelphia, PA 19106-1572, using the courtesy envelope provided in your MKSAP 16 slipcase. You will need your 10-digit order number and 8-digit ACP ID number, which are printed on your packing slip. Please allow 4 to 6 weeks for your score report to be emailed back to you. Be sure to include your email address for a response.

If you do not have a 10-digit order number and 8-digit ACP ID number or if you need help creating a username and password to access the MKSAP 16 online answer sheets, go to mksap.acponline.org or email custserv@acponline.org.

Disclosure Policy

It is the policy of the American College of Physicians (ACP) to ensure balance, independence, objectivity, and scientific rigor in all of its educational activities. To this end, and consistent with the policies of the ACP and the Accreditation Council for Continuing Medical Education (ACCME), contributors to all ACP continuing medical education activities are required to disclose all relevant financial relationships with any entity producing, marketing, reselling, or distributing health care goods or services consumed by, or used on, patients. Contributors are required to use generic names in the discussion of therapeutic options and are required to identify any unapproved, off-label, or investigative use of commercial products or devices. Where a trade name is used, all available trade names for the same product type are also included. If trade-name products manufactured by companies with whom contributors have relationships are discussed, contributors are asked to provide evidence-based citations in support of the discussion. The information is reviewed by the committee responsible for producing this text. If necessary, adjustments to topics or contributors' roles in content development are made to balance the discussion. Further, all readers of this text are asked to evaluate the content for evidence of commercial bias and send any relevant comments to mksap_editors@acponline.org so that future decisions about content and contributors can be made in light of this information.

Resolution of Conflicts

To resolve all conflicts of interest and influences of vested interests, the ACP precluded members of the content-creation committee from deciding on any content issues that involved generic or trade-name products associated with proprietary entities with which these committee members had relationships. In addition, content was based on best evidence and updated clinical care guidelines, when such evidence and guidelines were available. Contributors' disclosure information can be found with the list of contributors' names and those of ACP principal staff listed in the beginning of this book.

Hospital-Based Medicine

For the convenience of subscribers who provide care in hospital settings, content that is specific to the hospital setting has been highlighted in blue. Hospital icons (▣) highlight where the hospital-only content begins, continues over more than one page, and ends.

Educational Disclaimer

The editors and publisher of MKSAP 16 recognize that the development of new material offers many opportunities for error. Despite our best efforts, some errors may persist in print. Drug dosage schedules are, we believe, accurate and in accordance with current standards. Readers are advised, however, to ensure that the recommended dosages in MKSAP 16 concur with the information provided in the product information material. This is especially important in cases of new, infrequently used, or highly toxic drugs. Application of the information in MKSAP 16 remains the professional responsibility of the practitioner.

The primary purpose of MKSAP 16 is educational. Information presented, as well as publications, technologies, products, and/or services discussed, is intended to inform subscribers about the knowledge, techniques, and experiences of the contributors. A diversity of professional opinion exists, and the views of the contributors are their own and not those of the ACP. Inclusion of any material in the program does not constitute endorsement or recommendation by the ACP. The ACP does not warrant the safety, reliability, accuracy, completeness, or usefulness of and disclaims any and all liability for damages and claims that may result from the use of information, publications, technologies, products, and/or services discussed in this program.

Publisher's Information

Unauthorized Use of This Book Is Against the Law

MKSAP 16 ISBN: 978-1-938245-00-8
(Gastroenterology and Hepatology) ISBN: 978-1-938245-03-9

Printed in the United States of America.

For order information in the U.S. or Canada call 800-523-1546, extension 2600. All other countries call 215-351-2600. Fax inquiries to 215-351-2799 or email to custserv@acponline.org.

Errata and Norm Tables

Errata for MKSAP 16 will be available through the MKSAP Resource Site at mksap.acponline.org as new information becomes known to the editors.

MKSAP 16 Performance Interpretation Guidelines with Norm Tables, available July 31, 2013, will reflect the knowledge of physicians who have completed the self-assessment tests before the program was published. These physicians took the tests without being able to refer to the syllabus, answers, and critiques. For your convenience, the tables are available in a printable PDF file through the MKSAP Resource Site at mksap.acponline.org.

Table of Contents

Gastroenterology and Hepatology High-Value Care Recommendations

The American College of Physicians, in collaboration with multiple other organizations, is embarking on a national initiative to promote awareness about the importance of stewardship of health care resources. The goals are to improve health care outcomes by providing care of proven benefit and reducing costs by avoiding unnecessary and even harmful interventions. The initiative comprises several programs that integrate the important concept of health care value (balancing clinical benefit with costs and harms) for a given intervention into various educational materials to address the needs of trainees, practicing physicians, and patients.

To integrate discussion of high-value, cost-conscious care into MKSAP 16, we have created recommendations based on the medical knowledge content that we feel meet the below definition of high-value care and bring us closer to our goal of improving patient outcomes while conserving finite resources.

High-Value Care Recommendation: A recommendation to choose diagnostic and management strategies for patients in specific clinical situations that balance clinical benefit with cost and harms with the goal of improving patient outcomes.

Below are the High-Value Care Recommendations for the Gastroenterology and Hepatology section of MKSAP 16.

- Use a trial of proton pump inhibitor therapy rather than endoscopy for patients with suspected gastroesophageal reflux disease without alarm symptoms (see Item 15 and Item 69).

- Do not perform repeat endoscopy to confirm ulcer healing for uncomplicated duodenal ulcers unless the patient remains symptomatic despite treatment.

- For patients who have a history or high risk of ulcer disease, use standard-dose proton pump inhibitors as first-line therapy for prophylaxis of NSAID-related ulcers because they are as effective as high-dose proton pump inhibitors (see Item 43).

- Do not routinely perform stool studies (fecal leukocytes, stool culture, ova and parasites, *Clostridium difficile* toxin assay) for patients with acute diarrhea, because the vast majority of patients will have a self-limited viral gastroenteritis that responds to supportive care (see Item 4).

- Do not repeat colonoscopy within 5 years of an index colonoscopy in asymptomatic patients with low-risk adenomas (1 to 2 adenomas, <1 cm, tubular morphology, and low-grade dysplasia).

- Patients with a small number of hyperplastic polyps should be screened according to general population guidelines (every 10 years).

- The best serologic test to screen for celiac disease is the tissue transglutaminase (tTG) IgA antibody, but the sensitivity (69%-93%) and specificity (96%-100%) vary significantly among laboratories (see Item 10).

- Caution should be used when ordering tests for serologic and genetic markers for diagnosis of inflammatory bowel disease, because a false-positive result can lead to unnecessary testing and higher insurance premiums, and false negatives can lead to neglect of a proper evaluation.

- Observation, not cholecystectomy, is recommended for adult patients with asymptomatic gallstones (see Item 42).

Disorders of the Esophagus

Symptoms of Esophageal Disorders

Dysphagia

Dysphagia is defined as difficulty in swallowing. Patients typically describe a sensation of obstruction or difficulty passing food and/or liquid through the mouth, pharynx, or esophagus. Oropharyngeal or transfer dysphagia is characterized by difficulty in the initial phase of swallowing, in which the bolus is formed in the mouth and is transferred from the mouth through the pharynx to the esophagus. Esophageal dysphagia is characterized by difficulty in passage of the bolus through the esophagus. Defining the area of involvement (oropharyngeal or esophageal) often affects assessment, differential diagnosis, and treatment options. Causes of dysphagia are described in **Table 1**.

Oropharyngeal Dysphagia

Causes of oropharyngeal dysphagia may be either neuromuscular or anatomic. Patients may have associated symptoms that

TABLE 1. Causes of Dysphagia	
Condition	**Diagnostic Clues**
Oropharyngeal Dysphagia	
Structural disorders	
Cervical osteophytes	High dysphagia
Cricoid webs	High dysphagia
Pharyngoesophageal (Zenker) diverticulum	Presents with aspiration, neck mass, and regurgitation of foul-smelling food
Thyromegaly	
Neurologic/myogenic disorders	
Amyotrophic lateral sclerosis	Presents with upper and lower motor neuron signs; fasciculations
Central nervous system tumor	
Stroke	Neurologic deficits
Muscular dystrophy	Proximal muscle weakness
Myasthenia gravis	Weakness with repetitive activity
Parkinson disease	Bradykinesia, tremor
Dementia	
Sjögren syndrome	Dry mouth, dry eyes
Esophageal Dysphagia	
Structural disorders	
Dysphagia lusoria (vascular dysphagia)	
Epiphrenic/traction diverticulum	
Esophageal strictures	Intermittent dysphagia, especially for solid food; history of reflux
Eosinophilic esophagitis	Rings, strictures
Esophageal webs or rings	Usually incidental finding; may be associated with iron deficiency anemia
Neoplasms	Rapidly progressive dysphagia for solids then liquids; anorexia; weight loss
Motility disorders	
Achalasia	Concomitant liquid and solid dysphagia; chest pain
Diffuse esophageal spasm	Chest pain
Scleroderma	Tight skin, telangiectasias

provide clues to the underlying diagnosis, such as coughing (caused by aspiration), nasal regurgitation (caused by dysfunction of the soft palate in neurologic disorders), or other neurologic symptoms such as dysphonia, diplopia, and muscular weakness. Recurrent pneumonia may signal chronic aspiration. The diagnostic test of choice is videofluoroscopy (also referred to as a modified barium swallow), in which the oropharyngeal phase of swallowing is assessed with foods of different consistencies. Any indication of an intraluminal structural cause should prompt additional endoscopic evaluation. The management of functional disorders should include dietary and postural measures to improve swallowing and reduce the risk of aspiration; consultation with a speech pathologist can be helpful in this regard.

Esophageal Dysphagia

Patients with esophageal dysphagia often report a sensation of food "sticking" in the esophagus. Esophageal dysphagia tends to occur after the initiation of the swallow. The sensation of dysphagia at the lower portion of the esophagus (particularly near the gastroesophageal junction) may accurately reflect a lower-esophageal pathology; however, the sensation of dysphagia at the upper portion of the esophagus (especially near the upper sternum) has poor specificity. Esophageal dysphagia often has an intraluminal cause, such as strictures, Schatzki rings, or masses (**Figure 1**). Progressive solid-food dysphagia may indicate a mechanical cause of obstruction; concomitant liquid and solid dysphagia may indicate a motility disorder such as achalasia. Associated symptoms such as reflux (indicating a possible peptic stricture), chest pain (indicating achalasia or diffuse esophageal spasm), or weight loss (concerning for malignancy) may help in narrowing the differential diagnosis. The diagnostic test of choice for esophageal dysphagia is upper endoscopy, which can be both diagnostic (allowing biopsy and visualization of the mucosa) and therapeutic (allowing dilation to be performed if indicated). Management depends on the underlying cause detected during evaluation, as described in later sections.

Reflux

Typical symptoms of reflux are heartburn and acid regurgitation. Heartburn (or pyrosis) is defined as retrosternal burning pain or discomfort that is improved by therapy with antacids. Regurgitation occurs when a bitter- or sour-tasting fluid comes up into the throat or mouth. Almost 20% of the U.S. population experiences heartburn and/or regurgitation at least once per week. These symptoms are approximately 70% to 80% sensitive and specific for gastroesophageal reflux disease (GERD), as assessed by upper endoscopy or ambulatory pH studies. However, symptom severity does not correlate well with the severity of reflux. Factors that may precipitate or worsen reflux are listed in **Table 2**. For diagnosis and treatment of reflux, see Gastroesophageal Reflux Disease.

Chest Pain

Chest pain caused by esophageal disorders can be difficult to distinguish from cardiac chest pain because of the anatomic proximity and common innervation of the esophagus and the

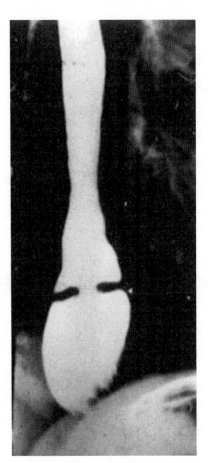

FIGURE 1. Barium esophagography showing a Schatzki ring

TABLE 2.	Factors Associated with Reflux
Category	**Factor**
Lifestyle	Cigarette smoking
Eating habits	Eating large meals Eating late at night
Foods and beverages	Alcohol Chocolate Citrus fruits and juices Coffee Fatty and fried foods Onions Peppermint
Medications	Anticholinergic agents Aspirin and other NSAIDs Calcium channel blockers Nitrates Progesterone
Body position	Bending over, exercising (both result in increased intra-abdominal pressure)

heart. Esophageal chest pain is often prolonged, nonexertional, and associated with other esophageal symptoms such as dysphagia, odynophagia, or reflux. The most common cause of noncardiac chest pain is untreated GERD, followed by motility disorders. Owing to the potentially life-threatening consequences of untreated cardiac chest pain, a comprehensive cardiac evaluation must be performed and cardiac causes must be ruled out before attributing chest pain to an esophageal cause. An empiric trial of a proton pump inhibitor (PPI) can be diagnostic after cardiac causes have been ruled out. If the symptoms do not respond to medical therapy, upper endoscopy followed by ambulatory pH monitoring and/or esophageal manometry is indicated. **H**

Odynophagia

Odynophagia, or painful swallowing, is often a symptom of esophageal ulceration, which is usually caused by infectious esophagitis or pill-induced esophagitis. Upper endoscopy is the best test for odynophagia.

Globus Sensation

Globus sensation is the awareness of a lump or tightness in the throat that is unrelated to meals or swallowing. Although the sensation is uncomfortable, it is usually related to emotional distress, is transient, and has no long-term sequelae. Rarely, globus sensation occurs in the setting of GERD.

KEY POINTS

- Dysphagia, heartburn, acid regurgitation, chest pain, odynophagia, and globus sensation are common symptoms of esophageal disorders.
- The diagnostic test of choice for oropharyngeal dysphagia is videofluoroscopy.
- The diagnostic test of choice for esophageal dysphagia is upper endoscopy.
- Cardiac causes must be ruled out before attributing chest pain to an esophageal cause.

Nonmalignant Disorders of the Esophagus

Esophageal Motility Disorders

The esophagus is a muscular tube that extends from the upper esophageal sphincter to the lower esophageal sphincter. The upper third of the esophagus is composed of striated muscle, whereas the lower two thirds are composed of smooth muscle; innervation of the esophagus is via the vagus nerve. Between meals, both sphincters are tonically contracted and closed. At the initiation of a swallow, both upper and lower esophageal sphincters relax and a peristaltic wave progresses distally, propelling the food bolus into the stomach (**Figure 2**). Dysregulation of this function can lead to

dysphagia, aspiration, and chest pain. Motility disorders are classified as hypertonic (spastic) or hypotonic.

Hypertonic Motility Disorders

Achalasia and Pseudoachalasia

Achalasia is characterized by failure of esophageal peristalsis and failure of the lower esophageal sphincter to relax with swallowing. It is a rare disorder (annual incidence of 1 in 100,000), is usually diagnosed between the ages of 25 and 60 years, and has no gender predominance. Achalasia is thought to be caused by degeneration of the myenteric plexus, which results in loss of inhibitory neurons in the lower esophageal sphincter; this causes the lower esophageal sphincter to remain tonically contracted.

The functional obstruction of the distal esophagus leads to dysphagia, chest pain, regurgitation of fermented retained food, and weight loss. The presenting symptom in a minority of patients is chest pain, which is due to simultaneous esophageal wall contraction. Patients may be wrongly diagnosed with reflux owing to regurgitation of retained foods, but symptoms of achalasia do not respond to empiric trials of conventional antireflux medications such as PPIs and H$_2$ blockers.

Plain chest radiographs may show a dilated esophagus with an air/fluid level. Barium radiography (barium swallow) is the primary screening test for achalasia; it usually reveals esophageal dilation with the classic "bird's beak" appearance distally and the to-and-fro movement of barium (loss of peristalsis) (**Figure 3**). Manometry is required to confirm the diagnosis and reveals esophageal aperistalsis and incomplete (or absence of) relaxation of the lower esophageal sphincter with wet swallows (**Figure 4**). Upper endoscopy is often performed to exclude mechanical obstruction of the esophagus in the region of the lower sphincter, particularly if there is concern for underlying malignancy (indicated by shorter duration of symptoms and weight loss that is rapid and out of proportion). If obstruction is caused by a malignant lesion, the disorder is called pseudoachalasia.

Treatments for achalasia are directed at lowering the resting pressure of the lower esophageal sphincter. The choice of therapy frequently depends on the expertise available at a given medical setting, as well as the age and medical status of the patient. Surgical release of the lower esophageal sphincter by myotomy can now be performed laparoscopically through the abdomen and is considered first-line therapy. It is often complicated by secondary GERD; antireflux procedures such as Nissen fundoplication are now routinely performed following myotomy to reduce the risk of GERD. Other therapies for achalasia are available for patients who are not good surgical candidates, but these tend to be less effective than surgical therapy and have less durable results. Endoscopic pneumatic balloon dilatation provides symptomatic improvement of achalasia in most patients but is associated with an approximate 5% risk of esophageal perforation; results are not

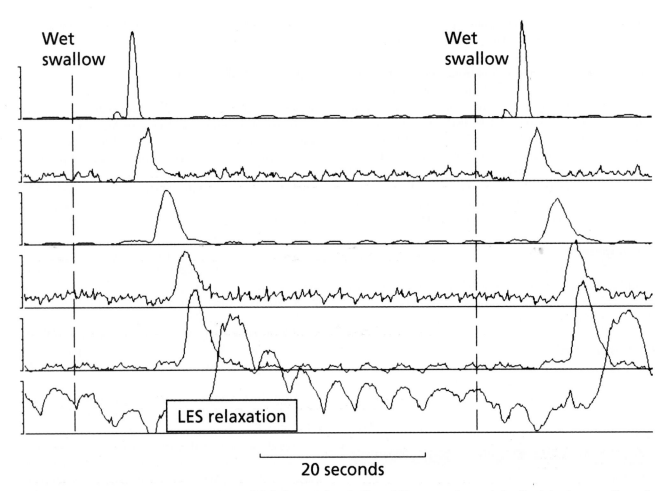

Wet swallow

Wet swallow

LES relaxation

20 seconds

FIGURE 2. Normal esophageal manometric tracing, in which the lower esophageal sphincter (LES) pressure relaxes to the baseline during the wet swallow, and peristaltic waves are seen. (The scale for the esophageal leads is 100 mm Hg.)

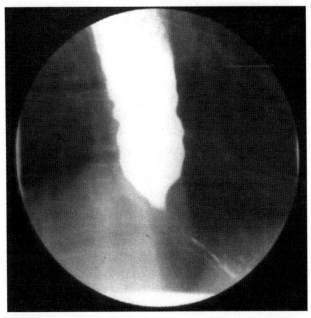

FIGURE 3. Barium radiography (swallow) with the typical "bird's beak" appearance of the distal esophagus in a patient with achalasia

permanent, and most patients need repeat dilatations. Injection of botulinum toxin into the lower esophageal sphincter may provide symptomatic relief, but the effect is usually temporary (lasting 6-9 months); this therapy is now rarely first line in patients with acceptable risk for dilatation or surgery. Smooth-muscle relaxants such as nitrates and calcium channel blockers may provide temporary relief for some patients but are not recommended owing to inconsistent effectiveness and potential for other systemic side effects.

Diffuse Esophageal Spasm and Nutcracker Esophagus
Many hypertonic motility disorders of varying severity have been defined manometrically. Diffuse esophageal spasm is a motility disorder that is less well defined than achalasia. It is usually characterized by dysphagia or chest pain. Manometry shows intermittent, high-amplitude (>30 mm Hg), simultaneous, nonperistaltic contractions in response to swallowing. Diagnosis is made by clinical presentation, typical findings on barium swallow, and/or manometry following exclusion of other disorders, especially cardiac disease and GERD. Findings of a "corkscrew esophagus" (caused by multiple

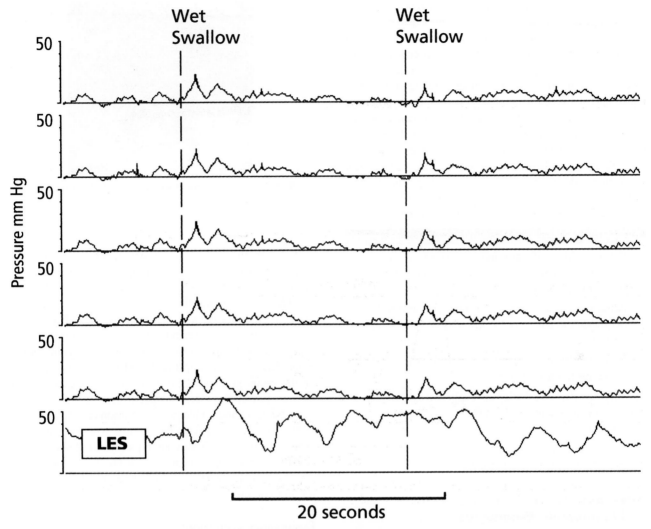

FIGURE 4. Esophageal manometric tracing in a patient with achalasia, in which the elevated lower esophageal sphincter (LES) pressure does not relax during the wet swallow. In addition, there is no esophageal body peristalsis (the waves seen are superimposable). The vertical scale is set in increments of 10 mm Hg (to a maximum of 50 mm Hg).

simultaneous contractions) on barium swallow are typical of diffuse esophageal spasm. In a small number of patients, diffuse esophageal spasm may progress to achalasia.

Nutcracker esophagus refers to a manometric finding of average distal esophageal pressures during peristalsis of greater than 220 mm Hg. Nutcracker esophagus may not be associated with specific esophageal symptoms.

Because these disorders are not usually progressive or life threatening, treatment is symptomatic. Calcium channel blockers are recommended as first-line treatment for diffuse esophageal spasm. Medications such as trazodone and imipramine have been shown in small studies to alleviate pain associated with these disorders; it is presumed that these medications work by modulating visceral sensory perception. Botulinum toxin injections may be considered when these other therapies are unsuccessful.

Hypotonic Motility Disorders
Esophageal hypomotility is less common than hypermotility. Symptoms include dysphagia, slower transit times, and increased risk for pill-induced erosions. On manometry, most hypomotility syndromes show low-amplitude contractions with a substantial proportion of nonperistaltic contractions, known as ineffective esophageal motility. Hypomotility syndromes occur most frequently in the setting of GERD.

Causes of esophageal hypomotility include medications (such as narcotics) and systemic diseases (particularly scleroderma). Patients with scleroderma may present with aperistalsis on manometry; this is distinguished from achalasia by the manometric finding of a hypotensive lower esophageal sphincter (in achalasia, the lower esophageal sphincter is hypertensive). This can lead to severe esophageal reflux and complications, such as esophagitis and strictures, caused by a combination of reduced lower esophageal sphincter pressure and esophageal aperistalsis that leads to poor acid clearance. Such patients do not always have reflux, and symptom onset may occur years after recognition of the connective tissue disorder, presumably owing to esophageal hyposensitivity along with hypomotility. The combination of manometrically determined aperistalsis of the esophageal body and a hypotensive lower esophageal sphincter is called "scleroderma esophagus"; however, less than half of patients with these manometric abnormalities have evidence of connective tissue disease. Treatment is largely aimed at controlling acid reflux, which may reduce stricturing. Surgical therapy (fundoplication) is not an option because of the esophageal aperistalsis that would lead to severe dysphagia after fundoplication.

KEY POINTS

- Patients with esophageal motility disorders usually present with dysphagia to solids and liquids, aspiration, or chest pain.

- Achalasia is characterized by failure of esophageal peristalsis and failure of the lower esophageal sphincter to relax with swallowing.

- Barium radiography (barium swallow) is the primary screening test for achalasia.

- Surgical release of the lower esophageal sphincter by laparoscopic myotomy is first-line therapy for achalasia.

- Esophageal manometry helps to classify hypertonic motility disorders of the esophagus.

Infectious, Pill-Induced, and Eosinophilic Esophagitis

Infectious Esophagitis

Infectious esophagitis is typically caused by *Candida albicans*, herpes simplex virus (HSV), and cytomegalovirus (CMV). Other organisms that can cause esophagitis are human papillomavirus, *Trypanosoma cruzi*, *Mycobacterium tuberculosis*, and *Treponema pallidum*. These infections typically occur in patients who are immunosuppressed owing to medications (such as corticosteroids, azathioprine, or tumor necrosis factor-α inhibitors) or congenital or acquired immunodeficiencies. Use of swallowed aerosolized corticosteroids may put an immunocompetent patient at risk for some of these infections.

C. albicans is the most common cause of infectious esophagitis in immunocompetent patients and is often associated with oropharyngeal candidiasis. It often presents with dysphagia, odynophagia, and curdy white esophageal plaques seen on upper endoscopy (**Figure 5**). CMV tends to cause isolated esophageal ulcers, while HSV usually causes multiple superficial ulcers. Definitive diagnosis can be established with brushings (for *Candida*) or biopsies from either the ulcer base (for CMV) or the edges (for HSV). Treatment is

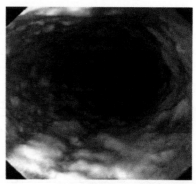

FIGURE 5. Upper endoscopy showing white adherent plaques suggestive of *Candida* esophagitis

directed at the cause: antifungal agents for *Candida* esophagitis, acyclovir for HSV, and ganciclovir for CMV.

Pill-Induced Esophagitis

Pill-induced esophagitis is characterized by odynophagia, dysphagia, and sometimes retrosternal chest pain. Pills typically cause local injury at sites of anatomic narrowing of the esophagus, such as the aortic arch, gastroesophageal junction, or the esophageal indentation caused by an enlarged left atrium. Tetracycline, iron sulfate, bisphosphonates, potassium, NSAIDs, and quinidine are common causative medications. Diagnosis is suspected by medication review and is confirmed by endoscopy. Treatment typically includes temporary cessation of the culprit medication or taking the medication with a large bolus of water and avoiding a recumbent posture for 30 to 60 minutes after ingestion.

Eosinophilic Esophagitis

Eosinophilic esophagitis is characterized by eosinophilic infiltration of the esophageal mucosa. It typically presents in adults with solid-food dysphagia and food impaction. The presentation in children is nonspecific; symptoms vary from vomiting and abdominal pain to failure to thrive. The incidence of eosinophilic esophagitis is thought to be increasing, and it seems to parallel the increasing incidence of allergic disease and asthma. Asthma and systemic and seasonal allergies have significant prevalence in adults with eosinophilic esophagitis. Population prevalence in adults is as high as 54 per 100,000 in the United States. There is a strong male predominance.

Eosinophilic esophagitis is diagnosed by the finding of greater than 15 eosinophils/hpf on esophageal endoscopic biopsy and by exclusion of GERD. GERD must be excluded because it can also cause esophageal eosinophilic infiltration. This can be done either with ambulatory pH monitoring before beginning treatment or with lack of response to a therapeutic trial of a PPI twice a day for 6 weeks. Endoscopy often reveals characteristic findings such as rings, longitudinal furrows, and sometimes strictures. Treatment is usually begun with swallowed aerosolized corticosteroids. This is usually successful; however, the disease often recurs and retreatment is often needed. Patients with refractory disease may need a combination of esophageal dilation, systemic corticosteroids, or a food elimination diet, which has been shown to be successful in children.

KEY POINTS

- *Candida albicans* is the most common cause of infectious esophagitis, and it presents with dysphagia and curdy white esophageal plaques seen on endoscopy.
- Pill-induced esophagitis is characterized by odynophagia, dysphagia, and sometimes retrosternal chest pain and is often caused by tetracycline, iron sulfate, bisphosphonates, potassium, NSAIDs, or quinidine.
- Eosinophilic esophagitis is diagnosed by endoscopic biopsy after gastroesophageal reflux disease has been excluded; it can be treated with swallowed aerosolized corticosteroids.
- The incidence of eosinophilic esophagitis is thought to be increasing and seems to parallel the increasing incidence of allergic disease and asthma.

Gastroesophageal Reflux Disease

GERD occurs when the reflux of stomach contents causes symptoms or complications that are troublesome for the patient. Symptoms of GERD (most commonly heartburn and regurgitation) are very common in the United States and the Western world. Prevalence is lower in Asia but is reported to be increasing. Complications of GERD are esophagitis, bleeding, stricture, Barrett esophagus, and adenocarcinoma.

The esophagus is protected from excessive exposure to gastric contents by several defense mechanisms: (1) physical barriers to reflux (elevated resting tone of the lower esophageal sphincter and external pressure from the diaphragmatic crura), (2) esophageal acid clearance (mediated by peristalsis and alkaline salivary secretions), and (3) epithelial defenses (epithelial tight junctions and hydrogen ion extruding pumps in the squamous epithelium).

Mild GERD appears to be caused by an excessive number of transient lower esophageal sphincter relaxations, which are non–swallow-related relaxations of the lower esophageal sphincter. More severe GERD appears to be caused by disruption of the normal gastroesophageal junction anatomy, in which reduced resting lower esophageal sphincter pressures and weakening of the diaphragmatic crural pressure lead to hiatal hernia formation.

GERD may be exacerbated by diseases such as xerostomia (which decreases salivary secretions), scleroderma (which is associated with reduced lower esophageal sphincter pressures), and gastroparesis (which delays clearance of gastric contents). Drugs may also be implicated, because they can reduce lower esophageal sphincter pressures or lessen salivary secretions. Nicotine can induce lower esophageal sphincter relaxations. Obesity can lead to reflux by increasing the frequency of transient lower esophageal sphincter relaxations, by increasing intragastric pressure and the gastroesophageal pressure gradient, and by hiatal hernia formation.

Diagnosis

GERD is diagnosed by symptoms, endoscopy, or ambulatory pH monitoring. The presence of heartburn, regurgitation, or both is enough to diagnose GERD if symptoms are of sufficient severity and frequency to be troublesome for the patient. A favorable response to empiric therapy with PPIs is supportive evidence for a diagnosis of GERD and is a reasonable first step in a patient without alarm symptoms.

When empiric therapy is not effective, endoscopy may be helpful to confirm GERD or explore alternative diagnoses. Endoscopy is indicated as a first step in patients with alarm symptoms (dysphagia, anemia, vomiting, or weight loss); these symptoms are suggestive of complications from mucosal injury. Esophagitis is seen in less than 40% of patients with GERD, and other complications are seen in less than 15%. Severity of reflux symptoms does not correlate well with the severity of mucosal damage seen on endoscopy.

Ambulatory pH monitoring is usually performed in patients who do not respond to antireflux medications and who have a negative upper endoscopy to make a definitive diagnosis, especially in those being considered for surgery. Conventional ambulatory pH monitoring is performed by inserting a pH catheter transnasally into the esophagus, allowing distal esophageal pH measurement over 24 hours and the correlation of reported symptoms. An alternative, "tubeless" ambulatory pH technique uses a sensor that is deployed in the distal esophagus and wirelessly transmits pH data over a 48-hour period. This technique may be more comfortable for the patient and may be more accurate than conventional techniques. Ambulatory pH impedance is a newer technique used to identify both acid and nonacid reflux by measuring a drop in the electric impedance (or resistance) of the esophagus that results from reflux of liquid contents into the esophagus from the stomach. It is often combined with pH monitoring so that refluxate detected by impedance can be classified as acid or nonacid.

Treatment

An algorithm outlining the management of GERD is presented in **Figure 6**.

Lifestyle Modifications

Smoking cessation and weight loss are uniformly suggested given their physiologic relationship to worsening GERD and other adverse consequences. Lifestyle modifications that may improve GERD include avoidance of triggering foods,

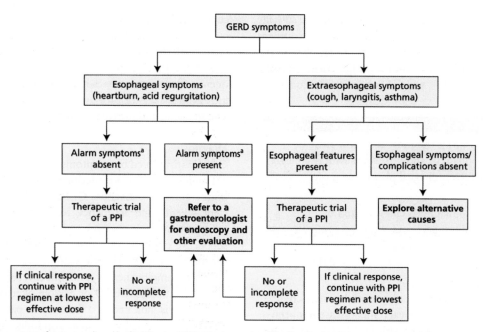

FIGURE 6. Management of gastroesophageal reflux disease. GERD = gastroesophageal reflux disease; PPI = proton pump inhibitor.

[a]Alarm symptoms = dysphagia, anemia, weight loss, and vomiting.

postural changes (such as elevating the head of the bed), and dietary precautions (eating smaller, more frequent meals and eating at least 4 hours before bedtime). However, the evidence supporting these modifications is weak; these lifestyle modifications should be reserved for patients in whom particular foods or behaviors are clearly associated with worsening symptoms.

Medications

Antisecretory drugs are recommended and are cost effective as initial therapy for GERD without alarm symptoms (which would necessitate endoscopic evaluation). PPIs have been shown to be superior to H₂ blockers or placebo in relieving symptoms of GERD and healing esophagitis. H₂ blockers may be used in patients who are intolerant of or allergic to PPIs. Tachyphylaxis may occur with H₂ blockers.

There are no convincing data to suggest that one PPI is superior to another in the treatment of uncomplicated GERD. Therapy is usually initiated at once a day and can be escalated to twice a day if symptom control is incomplete. Genetic variation in rates of drug metabolism, including PPIs, may decrease effectiveness in some populations (especially white patients), providing a rationale for twice-daily dosing for some patients. Before drug dose escalation, adherence and correct administration (30 to 45 minutes before a meal) should be confirmed. When adequate symptom relief is obtained, it is reasonable to decrease to the lowest effective dose or even stop therapy in patients without evidence of mucosal damage. In patients who have esophagitis on upper endoscopy, PPI dosing may be decreased after 8 to 12 weeks;

however, indefinite PPI therapy is often recommended because the rate of esophagitis relapse is high following PPI cessation. Prokinetic medications such as metoclopramide have no role in the therapy of GERD.

The most common immediate side effects of PPIs are headache, diarrhea, abdominal pain, and constipation. Switching to a different PPI or reducing the dose is usually sufficient to reduce or eliminate these adverse effects. PPIs have been used to treat GERD for almost three decades and are one of the safest classes of medications. However, some data suggest that prolonged PPI therapy may increase susceptibility to gastrointestinal infections (particularly *Clostridium difficile*) and pneumonia. The absolute increase in risk is small. Conflicting data suggest an increased risk of hip fractures (acid inhibition may decrease calcium absorption); this may be more pronounced in patients with other risk factors for fracture. Adequate calcium and vitamin D intake should be recommended to patients on long-term PPI therapy. Increased cardiac events have been reported in patients taking both PPIs and antiplatelet drugs (particularly clopidogrel), but there is conflicting and inconsistent evidence on this interaction.

Antireflux Surgery

Owing to the risks associated with surgery and the excellent results with medications, surgery should be considered only in patients who have refractory reflux (confirmed by pH studies or endoscopy), have PPI intolerance or allergies, or do not wish to take long-term medications. Surgery is effective in the treatment of GERD, and efficacy rates are comparable to those of PPI therapy. Surgical correction of reflux due to poor lower esophageal sphincter tone is performed by wrapping the fundus around the subdiaphragmatic esophagus, forming a collar and changing the angle of the esophagogastric junction. This leads to functional closure of the sphincter. There is a small but significant rate (10% to 15%) of dysphagia, bloating, and diarrhea after successful antireflux surgery. Up to one third of patients need acid suppression therapy 5 to 10 years after surgery to treat recurrent GERD symptoms. Loosening of the surgical wrap may also occur with time, and success rates after reoperation are lower. Results of surgical intervention for GERD are optimized when performed by experienced surgeons in high-volume centers. Surgery has not been shown to decrease the risk of developing adenocarcinoma.

Endoscopic Therapy

Initial enthusiasm for endoscopic management of GERD has largely dissipated. There are three major types of endoscopic interventions: radiofrequency application to the lower esophageal sphincter, endoscopic sewing devices, and injection of polymers into the lower esophageal sphincter. All have been shown to decrease GERD symptoms for the first 6 to 12 months, but none have demonstrated a durable decrease in the use of PPIs, increase of lower esophageal sphincter pressure, or decrease in acid exposure. The American Gastroenterological Association position statement concludes that there are no definite indications for endoscopic therapy for GERD at this time.

Extraesophageal Manifestations

Figure 7 describes the extraesophageal syndromes that have been associated with GERD. Up to one third of patients evaluated for heartburn have extraesophageal reflux symptoms.

Chest Pain

GERD is the most common cause of noncardiac chest pain. After cardiac causes have been excluded by comprehensive cardiac examination (particularly in those with risk factors), an 8- to 10-week trial of PPI therapy is reasonable in patients who do not have alarm symptoms before further testing, such as endoscopy, barium studies, esophageal manometry, or pH studies. **H**

Cough, Laryngitis, and Asthma

Cough, laryngitis, and asthma are associated with GERD, but the causal relationship between GERD and these syndromes is tenuous and unproved. The data that support antireflux therapy for cough, laryngitis, or asthma in the absence of GERD symptoms are very weak. The current consensus is that empiric PPI therapy should be prescribed for these syndromes only when accompanying GERD symptoms are present. In the absence of GERD symptoms, other causes, such as sinusitis or allergies, should be pursued.

KEY POINTS

- Typical symptoms of gastroesophageal reflux disease are heartburn and regurgitation, and the presence of one or both of these symptoms is enough to make the diagnosis if they are of sufficient severity and frequency to be troublesome for the patient.

- Empiric therapy with a proton pump inhibitor is recommended and is cost effective as initial therapy for gastroesophageal reflux disease without alarm symptoms.

- Patients with suspected gastroesophageal reflux disease whose symptoms do not respond to an empiric trial of proton pump inhibitor therapy should undergo endoscopy to assess for alternative diagnoses.

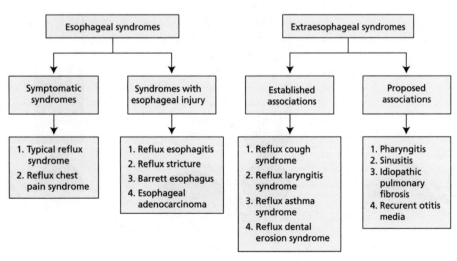

FIGURE 7. Classification of gastroesophageal reflux disease and its subsets

Reprinted with permission from Macmillan Publishers Ltd: American Journal of Gastroenterology. Vakil N, van Zanten SV, Kahrilas P, Dent J, Jones R. The Montreal definition and classification of gastroesophageal reflux disease: a global evidence-based consensus. 101:1900-1920. Copyright 2006.

- Proton pump inhibitors have been shown to be superior to H$_2$ blockers or placebo in relieving symptoms of gastroesophageal reflux disease and healing esophagitis.

- The most common immediate side effects of proton pump inhibitors (PPIs) are headache, diarrhea, abdominal pain, and constipation; switching to a different PPI or reducing the dose is usually sufficient to reduce or eliminate these adverse effects.

Metaplastic and Neoplastic Disorders of the Esophagus

Barrett Esophagus

Barrett esophagus (BE) is a complication of GERD in which the normal squamous epithelium of the distal esophagus is replaced by specialized columnar epithelium (**Figure 8**). The disorder is most common in white patients with long-standing and severe GERD. Patients with BE have more severe esophageal acid reflux than those with nonerosive reflux disease.

BE is a premalignant condition; affected patients have an estimated 30- to 50-fold increased risk of esophageal adenocarcinoma compared with those without BE and an annual incidence of esophageal adenocarcinoma of 0.5%. Approximately 10% of patients with chronic GERD symptoms have BE on endoscopy. Overall survival in patients with BE is comparable to that of age- and gender-matched populations. Adenocarcinoma accounts for less than 10% of the total mortality of patients with BE.

Screening

Screening for BE is currently not recommended by most national gastrointestinal societies, although there is some evidence that outcomes may be improved and that it may be cost effective. Endoscopic assessment for BE in patients with chronic reflux symptoms should be individualized after a discussion with patients on the need for surveillance if BE is detected.

Diagnosis and Management

The diagnosis of BE is suggested by endoscopic findings (**Figure 9**) and is confirmed histologically by the presence of specialized intestinal metaplasia with acid-mucin–containing goblet cells. BE is classified into long-segment BE (greater than 3 cm of columnar-lined esophagus) and short-segment BE (less than 3 cm of columnar-lined esophagus). BE is thought to progress in a stepwise fashion from no dysplasia to low-grade dysplasia to high-grade dysplasia to invasive adenocarcinoma. Surveillance is advisable in patients with BE to detect progression and initiate early therapy. Management of BE largely depends on the grade of dysplasia as determined by histology, which remains the most widely accepted risk-stratification tool for BE. Progression to adenocarcinoma occurs slowly.

Recommendations for the surveillance and management of BE are summarized in **Table 3**. PPIs are used to control symptoms of reflux in patients with BE. There is some evidence from retrospective cohort studies that PPIs may lower the risk of developing high-grade dysplasia, but more evidence from prospective randomized studies is

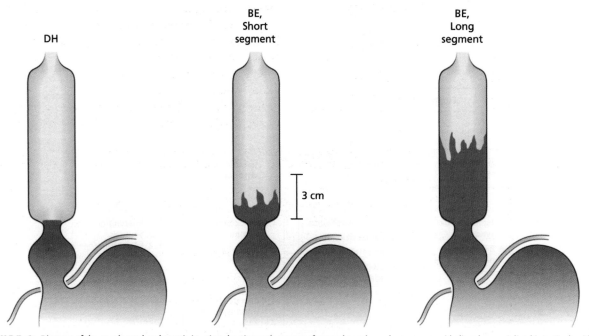

FIGURE 8. Diagram of the esophageal and gastric junction showing replacement of normal esophageal squamous epithelium by specialized intestinal epithelium (shown in red) in Barrett esophagus. BE = Barrett esophagus; DH = diaphragmatic (hiatal) hernia.

Courtesy of Dr. Alan Cameron

needed. Fundoplication has not been shown to reduce the risk of progression. Endoscopic ablative therapies (such as photodynamic therapy and radiofrequency ablation) have been shown to be effective in the management of patients with high-grade dysplasia; cohort studies show comparable outcomes with surgery and endoscopic treatment. Choice of treatment may be influenced by local expertise (endoscopic versus surgical) and patient preference. Cohort study data suggest that patients on aspirin and NSAIDs may have a reduced risk of developing esophageal adenocarcinoma.

KEY POINTS

- Barrett esophagus is a premalignant complication of gastroesophageal reflux disease in which the normal squamous epithelium of the distal esophagus is replaced by specialized columnar epithelium.

- The diagnosis of Barrett esophagus is suggested by endoscopic findings and is confirmed histologically.

- Barrett esophagus is associated with a 30- to 50-fold increased risk of esophageal adenocarcinoma.

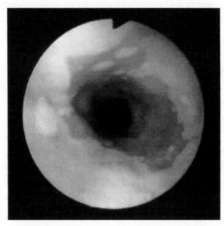

FIGURE 9. Upper endoscopic view of Barrett mucosa, with salmon-colored mucosa representing Barrett mucosa compared with the normal pearl-colored squamous mucosa

Esophageal Carcinoma

Epidemiology

Esophageal carcinoma is the most common malignant tumor of the esophagus. Esophageal carcinoma has two histologic types: squamous cell and adenocarcinoma. The majority of esophageal carcinomas are now adenocarcinomas; this is a significant change over the last 3 decades, as the incidence of squamous cell carcinoma has been decreasing while that of adenocarcinoma has risen by more than 300% in this time period. Outcomes are poor for most patients diagnosed after the onset of symptoms. Of 16,000 new cases of esophageal carcinoma diagnosed in 2009, 14,000 deaths were reported, making esophageal carcinoma the seventh leading cause of death from malignancies in the United States. Five-year survival is less than 20%. Esophageal carcinoma has a substantial male predominance, and onset is typically in the fifth or sixth decade of life.

Risk Factors

Risk factors for squamous cell carcinoma include long-term exposure to alcohol and tobacco, nitrosamine exposure, corrosive injury to the esophagus, dietary deficiencies (zinc, selenium), achalasia, tylosis (keratosis of the palms and soles), and human papillomavirus infection. Risk factors for the development of adenocarcinoma include tobacco use, obesity (especially central obesity), symptomatic GERD, and BE.

Diagnosis and Staging

Progressive solid-food dysphagia is the most common presenting symptom. Associated weight loss (as a consequence of reduced oral intake), anorexia, and anemia (from gastrointestinal bleeding) may be present as well. Despite the association of GERD with adenocarcinoma, many patients do not have frequent or severe reflux symptoms. This may be because of decreased perception of acid reflux in these patients. Endoscopy is usually diagnostic. Squamous cell carcinoma usually affects the proximal esophagus, while adenocarcinoma usually affects the distal esophagus. Staging of the tumor is critical in determining therapy and prognosis.

TABLE 3. Practice Guidelines for Endoscopic Surveillance of Barrett Esophagus

Dysplasia Grade	Recommendation
None	Repeat endoscopy 1 year after diagnosis to detect prevalent dysplasia; if negative for dysplasia, endoscopic surveillance every 3 years
Low-grade	Confirmation by expert pathologist
	Repeat endoscopy 6 months after diagnosis to detect prevalent dysplasia, then endoscopic surveillance yearly
High-grade	Confirmation by expert pathologist
	Endoscopic evaluation for any focal lesion (may indicate more advanced neoplasia): if present, focal lesion(s) should be removed by endoscopic mucosal resection for diagnosis and staging
	Options for further management: esophagectomy, endoscopic ablation, surveillance every 3 months

Reprinted by permission from Macmillan Publishers Ltd: American Journal of Gastroenterology. Wang KK, Sampliner RE; Practice Parameters Committee of the American College of Gastroenterology. Updated guidelines 2008 for the diagnosis, surveillance and therapy of Barrett's esophagus. 103(3):788-797; Copyright 2008.

Staging is typically done with CT (to detect distant metastases), endoscopic ultrasound (for locoregional staging), and PET (to follow up on indeterminate lesions found with other staging modalities). For treatment of esophageal carcinoma, see MKSAP 16 Hematology and Oncology.

KEY POINTS

- Esophageal adenocarcinoma is the most common type of esophageal carcinoma, and its incidence has risen considerably in the last three decades.
- Progressive solid-food dysphagia is the most common presenting symptom of esophageal carcinoma.
- Most cases of esophageal carcinoma are diagnosed at advanced stages (after the onset of symptoms), and 5-year survival is less than 20%.

Disorders of the Stomach and Duodenum

Peptic Ulcer Disease

Peptic ulcer disease (PUD) comprises gastric and duodenal ulcers. PUD is defined endoscopically as a mucosal break greater than 5 mm that is covered with fibrin; it is defined histologically as a defect in the gastrointestinal mucosa that extends through the muscularis mucosa. A mucosal break less than 5 mm is called an erosion. *Helicobacter pylori* infection and NSAIDs cause more than 90% of peptic ulcers. Less common causes of PUD are gastrinoma (Zollinger-Ellison syndrome), Crohn disease, mastocytosis, G-cell hyperplasia, viral infections (such as cytomegalovirus), infiltrative diseases (such as sarcoidosis and amyloidosis), and radiation.

Clinical Features, Diagnosis, and Complications

PUD is asymptomatic in 4% to 20% of patients and is commonly diagnosed because of complications such as bleeding. Symptoms, when present, consist of dyspepsia localized to the epigastrium that has a burning or gnawing quality. Gastric ulcer pain usually occurs shortly after meals and is less likely to be relieved by antacids; duodenal ulcer pain may occur 2 to 5 hours after meals (when fasting or at night) and is relieved by food or antacids. However, these patterns occur inconsistently and lack sensitivity in predicting the presence or absence of PUD.

The diagnosis of PUD is made by upper endoscopy. Barium radiography can be used for patients who cannot undergo endoscopy. Multiple gastric ulcers can occur in up to 20% of patients. The occurrence of multiple ulcers beyond the duodenal bulb along with esophagitis and diarrhea should raise suspicion for a gastrinoma. Benign gastric ulcers cannot always be distinguished from malignant ulcers, but heaped-up, irregular ulcer edges should raise suspicion for gastric cancer.

H. pylori infection and chronic NSAID use are the most frequent underlying causes of PUD. For diagnosis and management of these causes, see *Helicobacter pylori* Infection and Gastrointestinal Complications of NSAIDs.

Complications of PUD include bleeding, penetration, perforation, and obstruction and occur at a rate of 1% to 2% per ulcer per year. Complications may occur more often in patients with a giant (>2-cm) ulcer, ulcers that are within 2 cm of the pylorus, or a prolonged ulcer history. The most common complication of PUD is overt gastrointestinal bleeding, which appears to be decreasing in frequency (see Gastrointestinal Bleeding). Penetration is deep ulceration through the bowel wall without free perforation into the peritoneum; penetration can involve any adjacent structure, but the pancreas is most commonly involved. Penetration can cause pain to become more intense, prolonged, and referred to the back. Perforation occurs when intestinal contents freely flow into the peritoneum. It can arise from the duodenum (60%), antrum (20%), or gastric body (20%) and results in peritoneal signs. Gastric outlet obstruction is encountered least frequently and manifests with early satiety, vomiting, and weight loss. Obstruction results from inflammation, edema, and pylorospasm.

Management

Gastric ulcers should be biopsied to rule out malignancy. Duodenal ulcers carry little to no risk of malignancy and do not require biopsy.

All patients with PUD should be tested for *H. pylori* infection regardless of NSAID use, and testing for eradication of *H. pylori* should be performed after treatment in those with documented infection (see *Helicobacter pylori* Infection). Eradication of *H. pylori* infection heals ulcers and prevents recurrence. Acid suppressants are not required after *H. pylori* treatment for uncomplicated duodenal and gastric ulcers (<1 cm) in asymptomatic patients. However, in clinical practice it is common to continue 4 to 8 weeks of proton pump inhibitor (PPI) therapy for patients with gastric ulcers, as the evidence for sufficiency of *H. pylori* treatment alone is lacking, and gastric ulcers may heal more slowly than duodenal ulcers. Larger *H. pylori*–related ulcers (>1.5 cm) do not heal consistently with *H. pylori* treatment alone, and a PPI should be continued until *H. pylori* eradication testing is performed.

NSAIDs should be discontinued at the time of diagnosis of PUD. If low-dose aspirin is required, it should be restarted when the cardiovascular risk outweighs the risk of bleeding. Clopidogrel alone poses a higher risk for rebleeding than the combination of aspirin and a PPI. After NSAID-related PUD has healed, prophylaxis against recurrent gastric injury should be started if NSAID therapy must be resumed. PPIs are superior to H_2 receptor blockers, misoprostol, and sucralfate for this purpose.

Idiopathic ulcers that are not related to NSAIDs or *H. pylori* are not well characterized, but long-term antisecretory therapy may be considered.

Repeat endoscopy to confirm ulcer healing is not recommended for uncomplicated duodenal ulcers unless the patient remains symptomatic despite treatment. Follow-up endoscopy for gastric ulcers is indicated if the patient remains symptomatic after treatment, the cause is uncertain, gastric ulcer biopsies were not performed during index upper endoscopy, or worrisome endoscopic features were noted.

For management of bleeding ulcers, see Upper Gastrointestinal Bleeding.

Gastric outlet obstruction related to PUD should initially be managed medically with a high-dose intravenous PPI to help with ulcer healing and decrease gastric secretions. A nasogastric tube should be placed for gastric decompression. When medical therapy is ineffective, endoscopic dilation of the pylorus up to 15 mm may be performed for acute ulcers without associated gastric cancer. A minority of patients may require surgical vagotomy with pyloroplasty and/or antrectomy.

Perforation can be managed medically in stable patients less than 70 years of age if the perforation is contained (as shown by a water-soluble contrast study). Upper endoscopy is contraindicated when perforation has occurred. Medical management consists of fluid resuscitation and antibiotics for peritonitis caused by orogastric flora. Most patients with perforation will require surgery. **H**

> **KEY POINTS**
> - *Helicobacter pylori* infection and NSAIDs cause more than 90% of peptic ulcers.
> - Peptic ulcer disease is asymptomatic in 4% to 20% of patients; it is commonly diagnosed because of complications such as bleeding.
> - Patients with peptic ulcer disease should be tested for *Helicobacter pylori* infection and treated if present, and NSAID use should be discontinued.

Dyspepsia

Clinical Manifestations

Dyspepsia is a general term used to describe upper gastrointestinal tract symptoms such as nausea, abdominal pain or discomfort, and reduced appetite. Approximately 70% of patients with dyspepsia have no physiologic explanation for their symptoms; this is known as functional dyspepsia. The pathophysiology of functional dyspepsia is not well understood, but putative factors include delayed gastric emptying, impaired gastric accommodation, *H. pylori* and other infections, visceral hypersensitivity, and psychosocial factors.

According to the Rome III criteria, functional dyspepsia includes one or more of the following: (1) bothersome postprandial fullness, (2) early satiety, (3) epigastric burning, and (4) epigastric pain with lack of structural disease on upper endoscopy. To make the diagnosis, these criteria should be met for 3 months, with symptom onset at least 6 months prior to diagnosis. Predominant heartburn or regurgitation symptoms should be categorized as gastroesophageal reflux disease rather than dyspepsia. Most patients have multiple symptoms; 80% report five or more symptoms that may include bloating, nausea, vomiting, and belching. About one third of patients with functional dyspepsia have symptoms of irritable bowel syndrome, and many also have symptoms of gastroesophageal reflux disease. Patients with functional dyspepsia commonly have other conditions such as headaches, fibromyalgia, back pain, interstitial cystitis, depression, and anxiety. Spontaneous resolution occurs in up to half of patients with dyspepsia, while some have continued symptoms despite multiple medication trials and physician visits.

Management

Management of dyspepsia is described in **Figure 10**. Guidelines recommend upper endoscopy for patients with dyspepsia and alarm features. Alarm features include onset after age 50 years; anemia; dysphagia; odynophagia; vomiting; weight loss; family history of upper gastrointestinal malignancy; personal history of PUD, gastric surgery, or gastrointestinal malignancy; and abdominal mass or lymphadenopathy on examination. For patients younger than 50 years without alarm features, a test-and-treat approach for *H. pylori* is reasonable and cost effective when the patient is from an area where the prevalence of *H. pylori* is high (such as developing countries). However, a PPI is the most appropriate first-line strategy if the patient is from an area where the prevalence of *H. pylori* is low. Endoscopic evaluation should be reserved for those who do not respond to therapy. Cost-effective tests for *H. pylori* include urea breath testing and fecal antigen testing.

> **KEY POINTS**
> - Dyspepsia is a general term used to describe upper gastrointestinal tract symptoms such as nausea, abdominal discomfort, and reduced appetite.
> - For patients with dyspepsia who are younger than 50 years and have no alarm features, a test-and-treat approach for *Helicobacter pylori* is reasonable and cost effective when the patient is from an area with a high prevalence of *H. pylori* infection (such as developing countries); however, a proton pump inhibitor is the most appropriate first-line strategy if the patient is from an area where the prevalence of *H. pylori* is low.

Helicobacter pylori Infection

Clinical Features

H. pylori is a gram-negative flagellated bacterium that burrows into the luminal mucous layer overlying the gastric

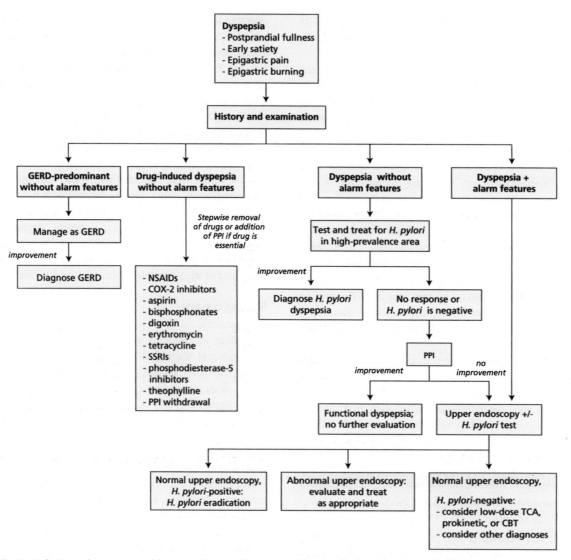

FIGURE 10. Evaluation and management of dyspepsia. CBT = cognitive behavioral therapy; COX-2 = cyclooxygenase-2; GERD = gastroesophageal reflux disease; *H. pylori* = *Helicobacter pylori*; PPI = proton pump inhibitor; SSRI = selective serotonin reuptake inhibitor; TCA = tricyclic antidepressant.

mucosa. It is able to withstand the acidic gastric environment through the production of urease. Infection with *H. pylori* is estimated to affect greater than 50% of the worldwide population and 30% to 40% of the U.S. population. Infection often occurs in early childhood by fecal-oral transmission and is more prevalent in areas of lower socioeconomic status.

Infection with *H. pylori* results in three common phenotypes. The most common manifestation is a mild pangastritis (85%-90%). The majority of patients with this phenotype are asymptomatic and do not develop serious gastrointestinal disease. Approximately 10% to 15% of patients will develop the duodenal ulcer phenotype, which is characterized by an antral-predominant gastritis. In this phenotype, *H. pylori*–related inflammation destroys the antral D cells that produce somatostatin and disrupts the natural inhibitory mechanism of gastric acid secretion. The resulting increase in

acid production contributes to ulcer formation. The gastric cancer phenotype is present in 1% of infected patients and results in a corpus (body)–predominant gastritis with multifocal atrophy and decreased acid production despite high gastrin levels. Gastric cancer is thought to arise through the sequence of *H. pylori*–induced gastritis to atrophy to intestinal metaplasia to dysplasia to carcinoma. A fourth manifestation of *H. pylori* is mucosa-associated lymphoid tissue (MALT) lymphoma, which constitutes 40% of all gastric lymphomas. Histologic evidence of *H. pylori* is present in up to 90% of MALT tumors.

Diagnostic Tests

Diagnostic tests for *H. pylori* are indicated in patients with active PUD, prior PUD without previous treatment for

H. pylori, MALT lymphoma, and persistent dyspepsia without alarm features. *H. pylori* testing is also indicated after endoscopic resection of early gastric cancer.

Noninvasive tests for *H. pylori* include serology (anti–*H. pylori* antibodies), urea breath testing, and fecal antigen testing. Serology is readily available and inexpensive, but its sensitivity (85%) and specificity (79%) are suboptimal. *H. pylori* IgG positivity confirms past exposure to *H. pylori*, but it does not indicate if it was previously treated and eradicated or if it is untreated and still active. Urea breath testing has a sensitivity and specificity greater than 95% but is more costly than antibody testing or fecal antigen testing. Fecal antigen testing is an enzyme immunoassay that has a sensitivity, specificity, and predictive value exceeding 90% before and after treatment. It is fast, accurate, and cost effective and is the test of choice for both initial diagnosis and proof of eradication.

PPIs, H$_2$ blockers, antibiotics, and bismuth decrease the sensitivity of all *H. pylori* tests except serology. PPIs should be stopped 2 weeks before all nonserologic *H. pylori* testing; antibiotics and bismuth should be stopped 4 weeks before; and H$_2$ blockers should be stopped 24 to 48 hours before.

Endoscopic tests for *H. pylori* consist of histology, rapid urease test, and culture. Histology has been considered by some to be the gold standard and has a sensitivity and specificity of 95%, but it is subject to sampling error and is relatively expensive. Rapid urease testing, which is performed on biopsy specimens, has a sensitivity of 88% to 95% and a specificity of 95% to 100%. Culture for *H. pylori* infection is time consuming, costly, and has inferior performance, but it may be helpful to determine resistance patterns in patients whose disease is refractory to treatment. If endoscopy is indicated for evaluation of the patient who is not taking a PPI, H$_2$ blocker, or bismuth, the most cost-effective approach is gastric biopsies with rapid urease testing. If the patient is taking one of these medications, gastric biopsies from the antrum, incisura, and corpus should be obtained for histologic assessment of *H. pylori*, although there is a risk of false-negative results. Patients with recent upper gastrointestinal bleeding also commonly have false-negative results on histology and rapid urease tests. A second test such as serology can be used if there is a high degree of suspicion of *H. pylori* infection in the presence of negative histology results.

Treatment

H. pylori is a type I carcinogen and should be treated when it is diagnosed. First-line treatment is triple therapy with clarithromycin, amoxicillin, and a twice-daily PPI for a 10- to 14-day course. Metronidazole should be substituted for amoxicillin in patients who have penicillin allergy. Alternative first-line regimens are (1) quadruple therapy with tetracycline, metronidazole, bismuth, and a twice-daily PPI and (2) sequential therapy with twice-daily PPI and amoxicillin (days 1-5), and twice-daily PPI with clarithromycin and metronidazole or tinidazole (days 6-10). Owing to increasing failure

rates for triple therapy (>20%) secondary to clarithromycin resistance, which may be geographically specific, consideration of quadruple or sequential treatment may be reasonable dependent on local resistance patterns. Suboptimal eradication rates are common with 7 days of therapy; therefore, a 10- to 14-day course is recommended with any first-line regimen. The cornerstone of second-line therapy is to avoid using antibiotics that have already failed, most importantly clarithromycin. In patients in whom triple therapy is unsuccessful, quadruple therapy is a good choice. Another option is twice-daily PPI, amoxicillin, and metronidazole or tetracycline. In patients in whom first- and second-line therapy are unsuccessful, salvage therapy consists of a PPI twice daily and amoxicillin twice daily plus levofloxacin, rifabutin, or furazolidone daily for 10 days. *H. pylori* culture with antimicrobial susceptibilities and referral to a specialist should be considered prior to initiation of empiric salvage therapy.

Eradication Testing

Eradication testing for *H. pylori* is indicated for patients with PUD, MALT lymphoma, resected early gastric cancer, and persistent dyspepsia despite treatment of *H. pylori*. A urea breath test or fecal antigen test should be performed 4 to 6 weeks after treatment, ensuring avoidance of medication interference as noted previously. Because serologic testing will remain positive, it is not helpful in documenting resolution of *H. pylori*.

KEY POINTS

- Infection with *Helicobacter pylori* is estimated to affect greater than 50% of the worldwide population and 30% to 40% of the U.S. population.
- Diagnostic tests for *Helicobacter pylori* are indicated in patients with active peptic ulcer disease, prior peptic ulcer disease without previous treatment for *H. pylori*, mucosa-associated lymphoid tissue lymphoma, and dyspepsia without alarm features.
- First-line treatment for *Helicobacter pylori* is a 10- to 14-day course of triple therapy with clarithromycin, amoxicillin, and a twice-daily proton pump inhibitor.

Gastrointestinal Complications of NSAIDs

Epidemiology and Risk Factors

NSAIDs cause topical mucosal injury and inhibit prostaglandin synthesis, thereby decreasing mucosal mucus production, bicarbonate secretion, and mucosal blood flow. Ulceration most commonly arises in the stomach and duodenum, but pathognomonic diaphragm-like ulcers can appear throughout the small and large bowel. Up to 25% of chronic NSAID users develop peptic ulcers (many asymptomatic); 2% to 4% have PUD-related bleeding or perforation, which translates into 100,000 hospitalizations and 16,000 deaths annually. Aspirin, the only acetylated NSAID, is associated with a relative risk of 2 to 4 for gastrointestinal bleeding. The term "NSAID" here will exclude aspirin.

Patients at highest risk for NSAID-related gastrointestinal toxicity are those with a history of complicated PUD (designated by bleeding or perforation) or the presence of more than two of the following moderate risk factors: age greater than 65 years; high-dose NSAID therapy; concomitant use of aspirin, anticoagulants, or corticosteroids; or history of an uncomplicated peptic ulcer. Patients with one or two moderate risk factors are considered to have an intermediate risk for NSAID-induced gastrointestinal toxicity; a low-risk patient has none of these risk factors. *H. pylori* infection is an additional risk factor for gastrointestinal complications in the setting of NSAID use.

Prevention of NSAID-Induced Injury

Figure 11 describes recommendations issued by the American College of Gastroenterology for prevention of NSAID-related ulcer complications based on the risk of NSAID-induced gastrointestinal toxicity and the risk of cardiovascular events.

Standard-dose PPIs are effective, have limited side effects, and are first-line therapy for ulcer prophylaxis.

Misoprostol is a synthetic prostaglandin E_1 analogue that replaces the protective prostaglandins that are consumed by prostaglandin-inhibiting therapies such as NSAIDs and decreases gastric parietal cell gastric acid production. It is more effective than H_2 blockers and PPIs in the setting of NSAID use. However, misoprostol has a high rate of side effects (mainly diarrhea [>20%] and cramping), but lower dosing regimens are as effective as PPIs with no more side effects than placebo.

High-dose H_2 blockers are inferior to PPIs and misoprostol and are generally not recommended for preventing NSAID-related gastrointestinal injury.

For patients who require continued NSAID therapy despite a moderate or high gastrointestinal risk, a nonselective NSAID should be used in conjunction with a PPI or misoprostol. An alternative strategy for patients at high risk is to use a cyclooxygenase-2 (COX-2) inhibitor plus a PPI or misoprostol. A Cochrane systematic review concluded that COX-2 inhibitors result in a significant reduction in ulcer complications as compared with nonselective NSAIDs. However, COX-2 inhibitors reduce but do not eliminate the risk of gastrointestinal injury. The gastroprotective effects of COX-2 inhibitors are nullified by the addition of low-dose aspirin, and thus a nonselective NSAID plus a PPI or misoprostol should be used for patients who continue taking aspirin.

COX-2 inhibitors are associated with an excessive and dose-dependent risk of ischemic cardiovascular events, which resulted in an FDA black-box warning for celecoxib. A celecoxib dose of 200 mg/d was not associated with excess cardiovascular risk, but the risk for doses exceeding 200 mg cannot be excluded. Therefore, the lowest possible dose of celecoxib should be used for patients at the highest risk. The safety of long-term celecoxib use is unknown at this time and should be discussed with patients. Other nonselective NSAIDs (with the possible exception of naproxen) carry this same risk. A randomized controlled trial (PRECISION) to evaluate the relative cardiovascular safety of celecoxib, ibuprofen, and naproxen in patients at high risk for cardiovascular events is ongoing. Patients with both high gastrointestinal and cardiovascular risk should avoid COX-2 inhibitors and nonselective NSAIDS.

Enteric-coated NSAIDs and aspirin are not effective in preventing PUD and its complications.

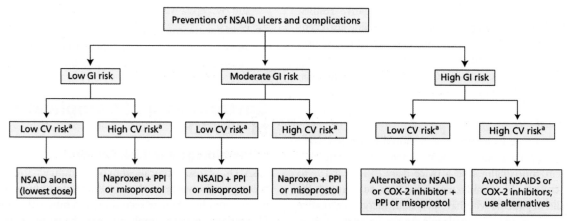

FIGURE 11. Prevention of NSAID ulcers and complications. CV = cardiovascular; COX-2 = cyclooxygenase-2; GI = gastrointestinal; PPI = proton pump inhibitor.

[a]High CV risk = need for aspirin to prevent cardiovascular events.

Data from Lanza F, Chan FK, Quigley EM; Practice Parameters Committee of the American College of Gastroenterology. Guidelines for prevention of NSAID-related ulcer complications. Am J Gastroenterol. 2009;104(3):728-738. [PMID: 19240698]

Evidence suggests that eradication of *H. pylori* may provide additional benefit for patients without a history of PUD who require long-term NSAIDs, but this has not yet been formally recommended. However, patients older than 50 years who require chronic NSAID therapy should be tested for *H. pylori* infection.

For treatment of NSAID-induced injury, see Peptic Ulcer Disease.

KEY POINTS

- Up to 25% of chronic NSAID users develop peptic ulcers; many are asymptomatic.
- Patients at highest risk for NSAID-related gastrointestinal toxicity are those with a history of complicated peptic ulcer disease (designated by bleeding or perforation) or the presence of more than two of the following moderate risk factors: age greater than 65 years; high-dose NSAID therapy; concomitant use of aspirin, anticoagulants, or corticosteroids; or history of an uncomplicated peptic ulcer.
- Standard-dose proton pump inhibitors are effective, have limited side effects, and are first-line therapy for prophylaxis of NSAID-related ulcers.

Gastroparesis

Gastroparesis is defined by symptomatic impaired gastric emptying in the absence of mechanical obstruction. The most common causes include diabetes mellitus and gastric surgery, but it can commonly be idiopathic. Less common causes are prescription drugs, Parkinson disease, connective tissue disease, amyloidosis, autonomic failure syndromes, and infections.

Diagnosis

Chronic nausea, vomiting, and early satiety should prompt suspicion for gastroparesis. Severe abdominal pain is not a typical feature of gastroparesis and should prompt a search for alternative diagnoses. It is important to establish whether the patient is actually vomiting or ruminating. Rumination is the act of effortless regurgitation of undigested and pleasant-tasting food within minutes of eating, usually followed by rechewing and reswallowing. If the patient is truly vomiting, the differential diagnosis is broad; however, the majority of alternative diagnoses can be ruled out based on history, physical examination, and laboratory and imaging tests, as shown in **Table 4**.

The cannabinoid hyperemesis syndrome has become increasingly recognized in the last decade. Its hallmarks include episodic abdominal pain, nausea, and vomiting in a

TABLE 4. Differential Diagnosis of Gastroparesis

Differential Diagnosis	Evaluation
Rumination syndrome	History of passive regurgitation of pleasant-tasting gastric contents, without preceding nausea
Cyclic vomiting syndrome	History of stereotypical bouts of vomiting with intervening periods without symptoms
Medication effect	Medication list: opioids, tricyclic antidepressants, calcium channel blockers, clonidine, dopamine agonists, lithium, nicotine, marijuana, progesterone
Pregnancy	Pregnancy test
Gastric outlet obstruction	Upper endoscopy or upper GI barium series
Complete small-bowel obstruction	Abdominal radiograph
Partial small-bowel obstruction	Small-bowel follow-through or CT enterography versus enteroclysis
Crohn disease with small-bowel stricture	Small-bowel follow-through
Intestinal pseudo-obstruction	Abdominal radiograph or CT with dilated small bowel in the absence of obstruction; ANA, anti-Scl 70, lactate, CPK, fat pad biopsy, ANNA-1
Cannabinoid hyperemesis syndrome	History of marijuana use; history of relief of nausea and vomiting with hot baths/showers
Hypothyroidism	TSH
Diabetes mellitus	Hemoglobin A_{1c}, plasma glucose
CNS disorders	Examination: cranial nerve palsies, cerebellar signs, CNS imaging
Functional dyspepsia	Symptoms are milder in severity; may have mildly delayed gastric transit

ANA = antinuclear antibody; ANNA-1 = type 1 antineuronal nuclear antibody; CNS = central nervous system; CPK = creatine phosphokinase; GI = gastrointestinal; TSH = thyroid-stimulating hormone.

patient using marijuana. Symptoms are associated with compulsive hot-water bathing. The syndrome is best treated by complete cessation of marijuana use.

Testing

Residual food in the stomach on upper endoscopy after an overnight fast can suggest gastroparesis but is not diagnostic. Consensus recommendations advise the use of a gastric emptying scan following a low-fat, egg-white meal labeled with technetium-99m sulfur colloid with images obtained at 0, 1, 2, and 4 hours after meal ingestion. Gastric retention greater than 60% at 2 hours and more than 10% at 4 hours is diagnostic for gastroparesis. Mathematical extrapolation using earlier images to estimate 4-hour results can lead to false-positive results. Use of opioid and anticholinergic medications also causes false-positive results. One third of patients with functional dyspepsia will have slow gastric emptying; it may be difficult to distinguish functional dyspepsia from mild gastroparesis.

Management

Small, frequent meals and avoidance of carbonated beverages and indigestible fiber (owing to increased risk of bezoar development) are beneficial. Because liquids empty from the stomach more rapidly, patients with gastroparesis should replace some calories from solid foods with calorically dense liquids. High-fat foods inhibit emptying and should be avoided.

Prokinetic medications are frequently the cornerstone of pharmacotherapy; their mechanism of action is summarized in **Table 5**. Metoclopramide is effective used at doses of 5 to 10 mg, 3 to 4 times daily (maximum: 40 mg/d) before meals, but the risk of irreversible tardive dyskinesia is 1% to 10% for patients taking this agent for more than 3 months. Erythromycin is a potent stimulant of gastric emptying. The usefulness of the oral formulation is limited owing to tachyphylaxis, but the intravenous formulation (3 mg/kg every 8 hours) is often utilized for an acute exacerbation in a hospitalized patient. Domperidone, cisapride, and tegaserod were removed from the market because of the excess risk of cardiac events and drug interactions. These drugs are now only available in the United States through "compassionate use" pathways, but patients sometimes seek out these agents from other countries or the "gray market" in their desperation for symptom relief. Antiemetics are frequently used to relieve nausea, but clinical trial data to support their use are limited. Opioid agents should be avoided. Additional management in patients with diabetic gastroparesis involves maintaining euglycemia. The choice of medication for patients with diabetes is important, as amylin analogues (pramlintide) and glucagon-like peptide 1 drugs (exenatide) reduce gastric emptying.

In severe, refractory cases, patients are at risk for malnutrition and dehydration. Gastroduodenal manometry can be used in patients with gastroparesis and small-bowel dysmotility to distinguish a myopathic from a neuropathic process, as it has been found to change management in up to 25% of refractory cases. Enteral nutrition support is indicated when there is unintentional weight loss greater than 10% of body weight over 3 to 6 months, repeated hospitalizations or nasogastric intubations to relieve symptoms, or inability to deliver proper nutrients or medications. Endoscopic placement of a percutaneous jejunostomy tube (with or without a venting gastrostomy tube) may be used under these circumstances and can improve nutrition, symptom control, and need for rehospitalization; however, it can be associated with a 10% rate of complications. Total parenteral nutrition is a last option for those who cannot tolerate jejunal feeding owing to an associated small-bowel dysmotility or the inability to place a percutaneous jejunostomy tube. Other options for refractory cases include endoscopic injection of botulinum toxin into the pylorus and electrical gastric stimulation (sometimes called the gastric pacemaker) to promote gastric emptying. Strong evidence to support these therapies is lacking. Surgical treatment such as gastrectomy is not recommended. **H**

TABLE 5. Prokinetic Agents for Gastroparesis		
Drug	**Mechanism**	**Adverse Effects**
Erythromycin	Motilin receptor agonist	Nausea, diarrhea, cramps, rash, *Clostridium difficile* susceptibility, cytochrome P450 drug interactions
Metoclopramide	Dopamine 2 receptor antagonist, 5-HT3 receptor antagonist, 5-HT4 receptor agonist	Extrapyramidal symptoms, dystonic reactions, tardive dyskinesia, drowsiness
Cisapride (removed from market)	5-HT4 receptor agonist	Cardiac arrhythmia (increased QTc), cramping, diarrhea
Domperidone (removed from market)	CNS dopamine receptor antagonist	Galactorrhea, breast tenderness, menstrual irregularities
Tegaserod (removed from market)	Partial 5-HT4 receptor agonist	Abdominal pain, diarrhea, cardiac arrhythmia

CNS = central nervous system; QTc = QT interval corrected for rate.

- Chronic nausea, vomiting, and early satiety should prompt suspicion for gastroparesis.
- Prokinetic medications are the cornerstone of pharmacotherapy for gastroparesis.

Gastric Polyps and Submucosal Lesions

Gastric Polyps

Gastric polyps are found in 2% to 4% of patients undergoing upper endoscopy and are generally asymptomatic, but bleeding or obstruction may occur rarely. Fundic gland polyps usually present as numerous, small lesions (<1 cm) located in the gastric fundus or body. Fundic gland polyps can develop sporadically with little or no malignant potential or in association with familial adenomatous polyposis syndrome, in which dysplasia may be observed in approximately 40% of cases. Management guidelines recommend that patients with numerous fundic gland polyps (with or without dysplasia) who are younger than 40 years of age should undergo colorectal evaluation for signs of possible familial adenomatous polyposis syndrome. Hyperplastic polyps present as single or multiple lesions in the gastric antrum or body that range in size from less than 1 cm to greater than 10 cm. Less than 3% of hyperplastic polyps exhibit dysplasia or cancer. Adenomatous polyps are often single, large lesions (>1 cm) in the gastric antrum that have features of chronic atrophic gastritis in the surrounding mucosa. Malignant transformation has been reported in as many as two thirds of gastric adenomatous polyps that are greater than 2 cm in diameter. Other less common gastric polyp subtypes are hamartomatous polyps and inflammatory fibroid polyps.

Gastric Subepithelial Masses

Gastric subepithelial masses are frequently observed during upper endoscopy, but accurate, population-based prevalence estimates have not been described. The differential diagnosis consists of both intramural and extramural lesions. Endoscopic ultrasound can be used to characterize the size, layer of origin, and general morphology of intramural lesions, as well as to obtain tissue samples for histologic evaluation. Cross-sectional imaging studies, such as CT and/or MRI, are preferred for determining the primary source and overall distribution of extramural lesions. Relevant examples of gastric subepithelial masses include:

- Intramural (benign): lipoma, leiomyoma, gastric varices, ectopic pancreatic tissue, and duplication cyst;
- Intramural (malignant or potentially malignant): gastrointestinal stromal tumor, carcinoid, lymphoma, glomus tumor, and metastatic disease;
- Extramural: normal abdominal structures (such as left hepatic lobe or gallbladder), intra-abdominal tumor or abscess, pancreatic pseudocyst, renal cyst, and aneurysm.

Gastrointestinal Stromal Tumors

Gastrointestinal stromal tumors are the most commonly reported mesenchymal tumors in the stomach, with an annual, age-adjusted incidence rate of approximately 6.8 per 1,000,000 population in the United States. Most patients are initially diagnosed between the ages of 50 and 69 years, often during evaluation of symptoms and signs such as anemia, early satiety, or abdominal discomfort. There may be single or multiple tumors with a median size of approximately 5 cm. Immunohistochemical testing for CD117 (also known as c-kit protein) and CD34 expression can help confirm the diagnosis. Surgical resection is the treatment of choice. Preoperative and/or postoperative chemotherapy with imatinib mesylate may be considered based on the staging evaluation.

Gastric Carcinoid Tumors

The estimated annual, age-adjusted incidence rate for gastric carcinoid tumors is 1.7 per 1,000,000 population in the United States, with an average age of 64 years at diagnosis. Gastric carcinoid tumors may present with nonspecific gastrointestinal symptoms such as abdominal pain, dyspepsia, or bleeding. They can be single or multiple. Type I and type II gastric carcinoids (associated with hypergastrinemia resulting from chronic atrophic gastritis or gastrinoma, respectively) account for approximately 70% to 80% of these tumors and have a relatively favorable prognosis. Endoscopic resection may be adequate for smaller lesions (≤2 cm), but surgical resection is recommended for larger tumors. Small lesions (≤2 cm) typically have an indolent natural history; metastases occur rarely and the 5-year survival rate exceeds 95%. For small lesions, endoscopic removal of the polyp followed by regular endoscopic surveillance (every 6 to 12 months for at least 3 years) is the preferred management strategy. Type III (sporadic) gastric carcinoids appear to be more aggressive and should be treated with radical gastrectomy and lymph node removal in the absence of distant metastases. Surgically unresectable disease should be treated with octreotide.

- Management guidelines recommend that patients with numerous gastric fundic gland polyps who are younger than 40 years should undergo colorectal evaluation for signs of possible familial adenomatous polyposis syndrome.
- Patients with small (≤2-cm) type I gastric carcinoid tumors should be followed with endoscopic surveillance every 6 to 12 months for at least 3 years after initial endoscopic removal.

Gastric Adenocarcinoma

Epidemiology and Risk Factors

Based on 2008 global registry data, gastric malignancies rank fourth (N = 989,000 cases per year) and second (N = 738,000 cases per year) in cancer incidence and mortality, respectively. More than 70% of newly diagnosed cases occur in Eastern Asia, particularly China. Overall, age-standardized incidence rates are approximately twofold higher for men than for women. Gastric cancer is considerably less common in developed regions such as the United States, where it ranks sixteenth with respect to both cancer incidence (N = 21,000 cases per year) and cancer mortality (N = 10,570 cases per year).

Adenocarcinomas are the most common histologic type of gastric malignancies (85% to 90%). Gastric adenocarcinomas are categorized as intestinal or diffuse. The intestinal subtype is predominant and tends to be diagnosed in older patients. Diffuse gastric cancers may affect younger patients and are often associated with a worse prognosis. Worldwide, *H. pylori* is the most common risk factor for gastric cancer. However, because 50% of the global population is estimated to be infected with *H. pylori* and only a fraction of these individuals develop stomach cancer, other genetic and environmental susceptibility factors must play a role and have not yet been fully defined. Other risk factors for gastric cancer are ionizing radiation, heavily salted foods, and a high-carbohydrate diet; fresh fruits and vegetables are thought to provide protective effects against gastric cancer. Predisposing conditions are pernicious anemia and gastric adenoma.

Although the majority of gastric malignancies are sporadic (arising unrelated to familial clustering), these tumors have also been associated with several hereditary cancer syndromes. Hereditary nonpolyposis colorectal cancer, familial adenomatous polyposis, Peutz-Jeghers syndrome, and juvenile polyposis syndrome can affect both the upper and lower gastrointestinal tract.

Screening and Surveillance

Population-based gastric cancer screening programs have been implemented in some high-risk geographic regions, but the methods used and benefits achieved are quite variable. Incidence rates in the United States do not warrant widespread screening of the general population. However, surveillance evaluations are appropriate for high-risk patients. Patients with a history of adenomatous gastric polyps should undergo upper endoscopy 1 year after polypectomy. If recurrent or residual adenomas are absent, future surveillance endoscopy should be repeated every 3 to 5 years. Insufficient data are available to recommend for or against routine gastric cancer screening among patients with pernicious anemia, intestinal metaplasia, or low-grade gastric dysplasia. However, if a diagnosis of high-grade gastric dysplasia is established, aggressive endoscopic resection or surgical gastrectomy should be considered.

Clinical Manifestations and Diagnosis

Early gastric cancers are often asymptomatic or may be associated with relatively nonspecific symptoms such as nausea, dyspepsia, or vague abdominal pain. Patients with advanced tumors often have more obvious symptoms such as emesis, early satiety, unintentional weight loss, abdominal mass, bowel obstruction, ascites, or lower-extremity edema. The diagnostic test of choice is an upper endoscopy. When the diagnosis has been established, CT of the chest, abdomen, and pelvis; PET; and endoscopic ultrasound may be performed for staging purposes. Only 10% to 20% of patients with gastric cancer present with localized disease. The 5-year relative survival rate for any gastric cancer is 26%. For management of gastric cancer, see MKSAP 16 Hematology and Oncology.

Complications of Gastric Surgical Procedures

Because of the significant increase in the prevalence of obesity, bariatric procedures have become the most common reason that patients undergo gastric surgery (see MKSAP 16 General Internal Medicine). Complications of bariatric surgery depend on the type of procedure performed (**Table 6**). Roux-en-Y gastric bypass (RYGB) is the most common bariatric procedure (**Figure 12**), followed by laparoscopic adjustable gastric banding.

Bariatric Surgery Complications

Postoperative Mortality

The most common causes of postoperative mortality in patients who undergo bariatric surgery are venous thromboembolism, anastomotic leaks, and exacerbation of preexisting medical comorbidities. The risk of venous thromboembolism extends beyond the hospital stay and is lower with laparoscopic approaches; however, preoperative inferior vena cava filter placement is not routinely recommended. Anastomotic leaks occur most commonly at the gastrojejunal anastomoses but can occur at any staple or suture line. Early detection is crucial to prevent peritonitis and death. The absence of fever, abdominal tenderness, and leukocytosis does not rule out a leak; tachycardia with

TABLE 6. Types of Bariatric Surgery

Category of Procedure	Types
Restrictive procedures	Laparoscopic adjustable gastric banding
	Vertical banded gastroplasty
	Sleeve gastrectomy
Combined restrictive-malabsorptive procedures	Roux-en-Y gastric bypass
	Biliopancreatic diversion with duodenal switch

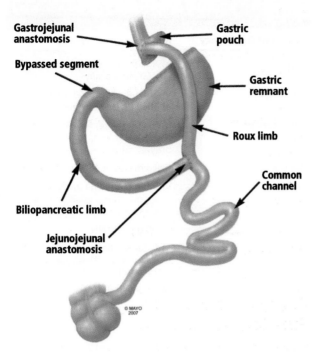

Gastrojejunal anastomosis
Gastric pouch
Bypassed segment
Gastric remnant
Roux limb
Common channel
Biliopancreatic limb
Jejunojejunal anastomosis

© MAYO 2007

FIGURE 12. Anatomy of a Roux-en-Y bypass

Adapted from: Mayo Clinic. Bariatric surgery: Types. Available at: www.mayoclinic.org/bariatric-surgery/types.html?mc_id=comlinkpilot&placement=bottom. By permission of Mayo Foundation.

CONT.

a heart rate greater than 120/min is the most reliable finding. Extravasated contrast on radiographic imaging is diagnostic, and surgical repair is necessary.

Restrictive Procedure Complications

Laparoscopic adjustable gastric banding is the most common restrictive procedure. Early complications consist of band infection, stomal obstruction, or rarely gastric perforation; local inspection and upper gastrointestinal radiographs can be used for evaluation. Late complications consist of erosion of the band into the gastric wall (which may lead to severe bleeding) and slipping of the gastric band proximally or distally (causing obstructive symptoms). Up to one third of all patients will require removal or revision of their laparoscopic adjustable gastric banding owing to complications.

Malabsorptive Procedure Complications

There are many potential complications after bariatric procedures in which there is a malabsorptive component, and the cause varies depending on the timing after surgery (**Table 7**). Internal hernias occur more commonly after laparoscopic bariatric surgeries because of fewer adhesions, which allows for increased bowel mobility and herniation through mesenteric defects. Herniated bowel may result in bowel ischemia; patients present with abdominal pain, nausea, and vomiting. Cross-sectional imaging should be performed but may not always be confirmatory; therefore, if clinical suspicion is high, surgical exploration is warranted.

Gastrointestinal bleeding can occur any time after bariatric surgery. Early postoperative bleeding may require intraoperative endoscopy for management, but later bleeding can be evaluated with routine upper endoscopy; in patients with RYGB, an extended or push endoscopy may be needed to reach the jejunojejunal anastomosis. If the biliopancreatic limb or remnant stomach needs to be evaluated, double-balloon endoscopy can be used. Marginal ulcers occur commonly on the jejunal side of the gastrojejunal anastomosis and can be seen in up to 20% of patients after RYGB.

Stomal stenosis can occur at the gastrojejunal anastomosis, which has a normal diameter of only 12 to 21 mm. Patients present with nausea and immediate postprandial emesis; endoscopic balloon dilation can be performed. Additional areas of potential bowel obstruction in patients after RYGB are at the jejunojejunal anastomosis, the mid

TABLE 7. Complications of Bariatric Surgery		
Complication	**Time of Occurrence**	**Cause**
Anastomotic leak	Early	Suture or staple disruption
Internal hernias	Early or late	Mesenteric defects, mobile bowel
Gastrointestinal bleeding	Early or late	Early: sites of sutures, staples, or anastomoses
		Late: PUD in gastric remnant and anastomotic margins; other nonsurgical-related causes (PUD, NSAIDs, diverticuli, etc.)
Marginal ulceration	Late	Acid, *Helicobacter pylori*, NSAIDs, bisphosphonates, smoking, sutures, ischemia
Stomal stenosis	Late > early	Early: ischemia, edema
		Late: adhesions, scarring from recurrent ulceration
Bowel obstruction	Late > early	Sites of anastomosis or compression, adhesions
Staple line dehiscence	Late > early	Early: ischemia, technique
		Late: dietary nonadherence
PUD = peptic ulcer disease.		

CONT.

portion of the Roux limb as it courses behind the transverse colon, and any area of adhesions. Small-bowel radiographs or CT can be used for diagnosis.

Dehiscence of the staple line separating the gastric pouch and gastric remnant can cause free communication of gastric contents into the excluded stomach; this is more common when the remnant stomach is simply stapled off rather than transected. Weight gain may occur because the restrictive component has been disrupted. Upper gastrointestinal radiograph can demonstrate a staple line dehiscence.

Biliary stone disease is common after bariatric surgery; more than one third of patients will develop new stones after surgery, with sludge in an additional 10% to 15%. For patients with symptomatic gallstones preoperatively, a cholecystectomy is performed in conjunction with the bariatric surgery; the role of prophylactic cholecystectomy for all patients has not been proved. Common bile duct stones (choledocholithiasis) can be difficult to manage after RYGB given that the working length of a typical endoscopic retrograde cholangiopancreatography scope is 124 cm, and the typical length of a Roux limb is 100 to 150 cm, so the ampullary region is rarely reached. Percutaneous transhepatic cholangiopancreatography or a surgical gastrostomy into the remnant stomach with intraoperative endoscopic retrograde cholangiopancreatography are ways to achieve biliary access in this setting.

Nutritional Complications

Up to one third of patients undergoing bariatric surgery will have micronutrient deficiencies preoperatively; it is therefore imperative to assess vitamin and mineral status before surgery. Deficiencies are common postoperatively and are related to inadequate oral intake, malabsorption, and nonadherence to the supplementation regimen (**Table 8**). Additionally, bioavailability of certain medications may be reduced after surgery.

Anemia is common after bariatric surgery, occurring in up to 40% of patients, and may be related to decreased iron, vitamin B_{12}, or folate. Iron absorption is affected by reduced gastric acid and bypass of the duodenum where iron absorption occurs. While a multivitamin containing iron may be adequate, many patients will require additional iron supplementation. Vitamin B_{12} levels are also altered after bariatric surgery owing to reduced gastric acid, decreased intrinsic factor, and/or small-intestinal bacterial overgrowth; all patients should receive supplementation. Calcium and vitamin D supplementation are also necessary. Thiamine deficiency leading to Wernicke-Korsakoff syndrome and death has been reported after bariatric surgery, given that thiamine stores can deplete very quickly with reduced oral intake. Wernicke-Korsakoff syndrome is characterized by nystagmus, ophthalmoplegia, ataxia, and confusion, and administration of intravenous thiamine should occur promptly.

TABLE 8. Nutritional Deficiencies and Replacement after Bariatric Surgery

Nutrient Deficiency	Replacement Therapy
Iron	MVI with iron, or elemental iron 80-100 mg/d orally
Vitamin B_{12}	Vitamin B_{12} 500-1000 µg/d orally, or 1000 µg IM monthly
Folic acid	MVI with folate; for women of childbearing age, folate 1 mg/d orally
Calcium	Calcium citrate 1500 mg/d orally
Vitamin D	Vitamin D 400-800 units/d orally or ergocalciferol 50,000 units orally weekly
Thiamine	25-50 mg/d orally
Vitamin A	MVI daily; if deficient, 2500 units/d orally with ongoing monitoring
Vitamin E	MVI daily; if deficient, 10 mg/d orally

IM = intramuscularly; MVI = multivitamin.

Other Gastric Resection Complications

Other complications can occur after gastric resection for any indication, the most common of which is dumping syndrome. This syndrome is seen in up to 25% of patients after gastric resection and up to 85% of patients after RYGB. Dumping syndrome occurs owing to the rapid emptying of refined sugars from the stomach, leading to an osmotic load in the small bowel and release of circulating digestive hormones. Early dumping, occurring 30 to 60 minutes postprandially, presents with gaseous distention, nausea, and diarrhea; late dumping occurs 1 to 3 hours after a meal and is associated with sweating, tremulousness, and confusion, all related to reactive hypoglycemia following an insulin surge. After bariatric surgery, patients should be counseled to eat small, frequent meals and to avoid foods rich in carbohydrates, which can lead to bloating and features of dumping syndrome. Other complications may include bile reflux gastropathy, afferent loop syndrome, postvagotomy diarrhea, and retained antrum syndrome.

KEY POINTS

- Because of the significant increase in the prevalence of obesity, bariatric procedures have become the most common reason that patients undergo gastric surgery.

- Sustained tachycardia with a heart rate greater than 120/min can be an indicator of an anastomotic leak after bariatric surgery in the absence of gastrointestinal bleeding.

- Nutritional deficiencies are common after bariatric surgery, and patients should receive appropriate supplementation.

- Patients who have recently undergone bariatric surgery may develop thiamine deficiency, which is characterized by confusion, ataxia, nystagmus, and ophthalmoplegia.

Disorders of the Pancreas

Acute Pancreatitis

Acute pancreatitis is the abrupt onset of pancreatic and peripancreatic inflammation. The rate of acute pancreatitis continues to rise, with an estimated 10 to 45 cases per 100,000 persons in Western countries. The mortality rate is approximately 5%.

Acute pancreatitis is classified as mild (interstitial) or severe. Eighty percent of patients with acute pancreatitis have interstitial pancreatitis, and these patients recover without sequelae. Severe pancreatitis is characterized by organ failure (hypoxemia, hypotension, kidney failure) or complications such as necrosis or fluid collections. Recent studies have demonstrated that necrosis is not as important as persistent organ failure in predicting the severity of the clinical course.

Pancreatitis is caused by premature activation of intracellular pancreatic trypsinogen to trypsin, triggering an inflammatory cascade that can cause capillary leak syndrome and sometimes the systemic inflammatory response syndrome. Causes of acute pancreatitis are shown in **Table 9**. In the United States, 80% of cases of acute pancreatitis are caused by gallstones or alcohol use. Multiple medications have been implicated as a cause of acute pancreatitis.

The pathophysiology of gallstone-induced pancreatitis is debated, but it is likely related to gallstone obstruction within the main pancreatic duct or reflux of bile into the pancreatic duct owing to impaction of the stone at the ampulla. The pathophysiology of alcoholic pancreatitis is unknown but is likely related to the direct toxic injury of alcohol on the pancreatic acinar cells.

Clinical Presentation and Diagnosis

Acute pancreatitis is diagnosed by the presence of at least two of the following: (1) typical clinical symptoms, (2) elevated serum amylase and/or lipase levels greater than three times the upper limit of normal, or (3) typical findings on cross-sectional imaging.

Acute pancreatitis is almost always associated with the sudden onset of pain. The pain is generally located in the epigastrium and radiates to the back; patients tend to be more comfortable in a seated position. Pain is often accompanied by fever, nausea, and vomiting. Patients are sometimes dyspneic secondary to pleural effusions that develop as a result of capillary leak syndrome.

The diagnosis is confirmed by an elevation in the serum amylase and lipase levels of at least three times the upper limit

TABLE 9.	Causes of Acute Pancreatitis
Common	
Biliary disease	
Gallstones	
Microlithiasis	
Alcohol use	
Occasional	
Medications	
Furosemide	
Didanosine	
Asparaginase	
Mesalamine	
Hydrochlorothiazide	
6-Mercaptopurine/azathioprine	
Simvastatin	
Hypertriglyceridemia	
Hypercalcemia	
Pancreas divisum	
Choledochocele	
Post-ERCP	
Rare	
Autoimmune	
Infectious	
Viral (cytomegalovirus, mumps)	
Parasitic (*Toxoplasma* species, *Ascaris lumbricoides*)	
Ischemia	
Genetic	

ERCP = endoscopic retrograde cholangiopancreatography.

of normal. Although both serum enzyme levels are usually elevated, either one alone is sufficient to corroborate the diagnosis after other causes of elevation have been excluded. Lipase has a longer half-life than amylase and tends to rise sooner. Although an elevated serum amylase level is usually from a pancreatic source, hyperamylasemia can be produced by abnormalities of other organs such as the salivary glands or fallopian tubes and can be seen in such conditions as a perforated ulcer, intestinal ischemia, acute cholecystitis, acute hepatitis, ruptured ectopic pregnancy, parotitis, or chronic kidney disease. Macroamylasemia, a benign condition in which large amylase multimers are poorly filtered from the blood, can be confused with acute pancreatitis, but it can be differentiated using serum protein electrophoresis. Benign pancreatic hyperenzymemia, or Gullo syndrome, is a rare cause of benign elevations in the amylase and/or lipase levels.

If the clinical picture is unclear, contrast-enhanced CT is the best imaging test to diagnose acute pancreatitis. Common findings include pancreatic or peripancreatic edema, inflammatory stranding, fluid collections, pancreatic necrosis, or splenic vein thrombosis (**Figure 13**). Obtaining a CT scan at the time of initial presentation will not worsen acute pancreatitis, but it should only be performed in cases of diagnostic uncertainty.

Prognostic Criteria

Multiple scoring systems have been devised to prognosticate outcomes in acute pancreatitis. The Ranson criteria rely on parameters that are measured at admission and at 48 hours; because of their complexity and the lag time for prognosis, these criteria are now rarely used. The Acute Physiology and Chronic Health Evaluation (APACHE) II score is more accurate than the Ranson criteria, but it is cumbersome to obtain.

Some studies have suggested hemoconcentration as a potential predictor of morbidity and mortality in acute pancreatitis because it serves as a marker of capillary leak. Patients with severe disease tend to have elevated levels of blood urea nitrogen, serum creatinine, and occasionally hematocrit (all markers of hemoconcentration). Of these factors, the blood urea nitrogen level appears to be the most accurate for predicting severity. Factors that predispose patients to a poor prognosis are multiple medical comorbidities, age greater than 70 years, and BMI greater than 30.

Management

All patients with acute pancreatitis should be admitted to the hospital. Most patients require narcotic pain medications and bowel rest. Aggressive fluid resuscitation should be started early because the inflamed pancreas can sequester significant fluid, leading to decreased effective circulating volume. Patients should be monitored closely and intensive care should be considered if there is hemodynamic instability.

Nasogastric tubes are not needed unless the patient has an ileus as a result of the pancreatitis. Antibiotics should not be given prophylactically and should be used only in the context of a documented source of infection; they do not confer any benefit on mortality and may predispose the patient to intra-abdominal fungal infections. In patients with documented necrotizing pancreatitis and clinical instability, endoscopic, percutaneous, or surgical sampling of the pancreatic bed should be performed to guide further therapy. In patients with documented infection, drainage, antibiotics, and supportive care are the cornerstone of management. Nasojejunal feedings should be started as soon as is feasible in patients who do not show signs of improvement within 72 to 96 hours. Parenteral nutrition should be avoided if possible because of significantly increased risk of bacteremia/fungemia.

Endoscopic retrograde cholangiopancreatography (ERCP) in acute pancreatitis should be used only in the following clinical scenarios: (1) in a patient with ascending cholangitis (fever, right upper quadrant pain, and jaundice) concomitant with acute pancreatitis, or (2) in a patient with gallstone pancreatitis who is not improving clinically and has worsening liver chemistry tests. Patients with gallstone pancreatitis and no complications should have a cholecystectomy prior to discharge.

Patients with interstitial pancreatitis generally recover within several days and are discharged without sequelae. Patients with severe disease may have a long, protracted course, remaining hospitalized for weeks to months. Approximately 20% of patients with severe acute pancreatitis die. Therefore, it is critically important to define and address the underlying cause if possible to avoid recurrence.

Complications

Pancreatic fluid collections arise secondary to disruption of the main pancreatic duct and/or its branches. These should be suspected in patients who continue to have abdominal pain or failure to thrive several weeks after their initial hospitalization. Pancreatic pseudocysts are encapsulated fluid collections without solid debris that do not contain an epithelial layer; they are the most common complication from acute pancreatitis. Walled-off pancreatic necrosis consists of fluid and solid debris that develops in the context of severe pancreatitis (**Figure 14**). Many collections will resolve spontaneously. However, if they persist and cause symptoms (such as pain or mass effect), surgical, percutaneous, or endoscopic decompression/debridement can be performed depending on local expertise.

Pancreatic duct leaks are relatively common (approximately 30%) following an episode of severe acute pancreatitis. If untreated, patients can develop pancreatic fistulas, especially to cutaneous tissues. Duct leaks are generally treated with endoscopic stenting, octreotide, pancreatic enzymes, and bowel rest. Splenic vein thrombosis (leading occasionally to gastric varices) can also occur, but anticoagulation is generally not recommended in this setting. Patients can develop diabetes mellitus if they have extensive necrosis. ◨

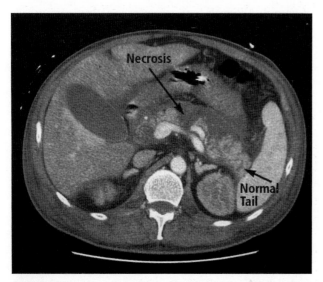

FIGURE 13. CT scan demonstrating acute pancreatitis, with hypoperfusion of the pancreatic body indicating necrosis. Note that the distal tail is perfusing normally.

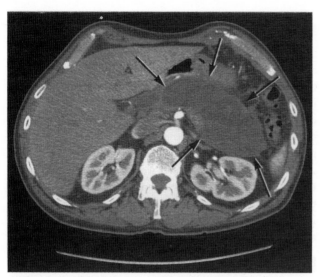

FIGURE 14. CT scan demonstrating walled-off pancreatic necrosis (*arrows*) virtually replacing the entire pancreatic body and tail

---

KEY POINTS

- Most cases of acute pancreatitis are mild; however, 20% of patients develop severe disease and approximately 5% of patients die.

- Eighty percent of cases of acute pancreatitis in the United States are caused by alcohol use or gallstones.

- Serial blood urea nitrogen measurements may be the most reliable routine laboratory test to predict severity of acute pancreatitis.

- Early aggressive fluid resuscitation should be undertaken as soon as the diagnosis of acute pancreatitis is made or suspected.

- Endoscopic retrograde cholangiopancreatography should be avoided in patients with acute pancreatitis unless there is cholangitis or worsening clinical symptoms in the context of rising liver chemistry tests.

- Asymptomatic pancreatic pseudocysts following acute pancreatitis typically resolve spontaneously and do not require treatment.

Chronic Pancreatitis

Chronic pancreatitis is defined as the irreversible destruction of the pancreatic parenchyma, which causes varying degrees of endocrine and exocrine dysfunction. Chronic pancreatitis is a heterogeneous disorder with wide phenotypic variation; however, the vast majority of patients have abdominal pain. It is estimated to affect approximately 5 in 100,000 persons in the United States and has a male predominance.

The most common cause of chronic pancreatitis is habitual alcohol use. The majority of patients with alcohol-related chronic pancreatitis are heavy users (more than 10 years and

50 g/d), but the amount and duration of consumption can be variable. Tobacco use confers a risk for chronic pancreatitis independent of alcohol use. Causes of chronic pancreatitis are listed in **Table 10**.

Clinical Presentation and Diagnosis

Approximately 90% of patients with chronic pancreatitis have abdominal pain as their main clinical symptom. The pain can be variable, but in most patients it is constant, severe, and radiates to the back. Patients can develop symptoms of exocrine dysfunction, including weight loss and diarrhea. Fat-soluble vitamin deficiency is common. Endocrine dysfunction can also occur, and many patients eventually become insulin dependent as their disease progresses.

Chronic pancreatitis is classified as either large-duct or small-duct (also known as minimal change) disease. Small-duct disease can be difficult to diagnose because changes are often subtle and are not seen on standard cross-sectional imaging.

The diagnosis of chronic pancreatitis can be challenging because no gold standard exists. Agreement has not been reached regarding the extent of fibrosis needed in resected pathology specimens to make the diagnosis. Diagnosis is often based on clinical symptoms and cross-sectional imaging that demonstrates pancreatic calcifications, ductal dilatation, parenchymal atrophy, and/or focal inflammatory masses (**Figure 15**).

Direct tests of pancreatic function, using either cholecystokinin or secretin stimulation, can be used to evaluate for minimal change disease by measuring early changes in exocrine function. However, these tests are technically difficult to perform and are not universally available, limiting practical clinical application.

For imaging of the pancreatic duct, magnetic resonance cholangiopancreatography (MRCP) should be performed rather than ERCP for diagnosis of chronic pancreatitis because of the high risk of post-ERCP pancreatitis. Endoscopic ultrasound (EUS) is a newer tool being used to diagnose chronic pancreatitis, but more experience is needed before recommendations for its use can be made.

TABLE 10.	Causes of Chronic Pancreatitis
Type	**Cause**
Toxic	Alcohol
	Tobacco
Genetic	Pancreatic secretory trypsin inhibitor
	Cystic fibrosis transmembrane conductance regulator
	Serine protease inhibitor, Kazal type I
Obstructive	Pancreatic solid tumor
	Intraductal papillary mucinous neoplasm
	Pancreas divisum
	Trauma
Other	Recurrent acute pancreatitis
	Autoimmune pancreatitis

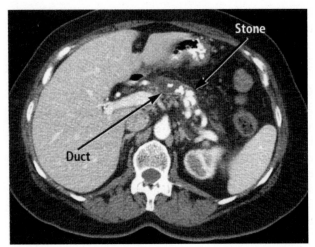

FIGURE 15. CT scan demonstrating chronic pancreatitis including pancreatic ductal dilatation and parenchymal stones

Management

Management of chronic pancreatitis is primarily targeted at preventing further parenchymal damage and treating clinical symptoms. Patients should be counseled to avoid toxic exposures, most commonly alcohol and tobacco. If an obstruction such as a pancreatic duct stricture or stone is present, it should be stented or removed.

Exocrine insufficiency is treated using enteric-coated pancreatic enzymes. Enzymes should be taken with meals and, depending on the severity of insufficiency, patients should receive at least 30,000 units of lipase daily. Fat-soluble vitamin replacement is also important. Endocrine insufficiency can be difficult to manage, because patients with chronic pancreatitis often lose counterregulatory hormones such as glucagon when their islet cells are destroyed, rendering their plasma glucose levels more labile. If diabetes mellitus occurs, it should be treated with insulin.

Pain can be difficult to treat in patients with chronic pancreatitis. Opiates should be avoided for as long as possible, because opioid dependence is a major problem in this patient population. Non–enteric-coated pancreatic enzymes, which theoretically limit stimulation of the pancreas by inhibiting the cholecystokinin feedback loop, should be used for pain control. All non–enteric-coated enzymes should be used with acid-suppressing medications, because these enzymes can be denatured by gastric acid secretion. Antioxidant combinations (vitamin A, vitamin E, selenium) have shown some efficacy for improving pain in chronic pancreatitis. Transcranial magnetic stimulation has been shown in preliminary studies to improve the pain of chronic pancreatitis through neuron depolarization, but this modality is not widely available. Celiac plexus blockade (using corticosteroids) or neurolysis (using ethanol) can be performed percutaneously or via EUS, but any relief from this procedure tends to be short lived. It is generally recommended that this therapy be tried once in patients with severe pain from chronic pancreatitis.

Surgical management of chronic pancreatitis is reserved for patients in whom conventional medical management is unsuccessful. Surgical management is categorized into operative resection (pancreaticoduodenectomy or distal pancreatectomy) and drainage procedures (lateral pancreaticojejunostomy), and the choice of surgery is dependent on the clinical situation. Patients with obstruction of the pancreatic duct are more likely to be considered candidates for drainage procedures. Total pancreatectomy is rarely performed for chronic pancreatitis because it renders patients insulin dependent and does not always control pain. Total pancreatectomy with autologous islet cell transplantation is increasingly being used, but its long-term benefit for pain control and insulin independence is unknown.

KEY POINTS

- The hallmark symptom of chronic pancreatitis is abdominal pain, which is accompanied by varying degrees of exocrine and endocrine insufficiency.

- There is no gold standard diagnostic test for chronic pancreatitis, but typical findings on cross-sectional imaging include pancreatic calcifications, ductal dilatation, parenchymal atrophy, and/or focal inflammatory masses.

- Management of chronic pancreatitis includes counseling to avoid alcohol and tobacco, pain control, pancreatic enzyme supplementation to treat malabsorption, and insulin treatment of diabetes mellitus if and when it occurs.

- Surgical therapies for chronic pancreatitis should be reserved for patients in whom all medical management strategies have been exhausted.

Pancreatic Adenocarcinoma

Pancreatic adenocarcinoma is one of the deadliest malignancies; about 32,000 cases are identified each year. The 5-year survival rate of 5% has not improved in decades, owing to the advanced degree of disease at the time of diagnosis and the lack of effective treatments other than complete surgical resection. No current effective screening modality exists. Approximately 80% of newly diagnosed patients have unresectable disease at presentation.

Age greater than 50 years is the most important risk factor. Cigarette smoking and chronic pancreatitis increase the risk of disease 20-fold. Hereditary pancreatitis, caused by a mutation in the cationic trypsinogen gene, causes cancer in up to 40% of affected patients. The number of persons in the United States with hereditary pancreatitis is estimated at 1000. Intraductal papillary mucinous neoplasms, most commonly affecting the main duct, are an important risk factor.

Clinical Presentation

Most patients present with painless jaundice if the tumor is in the pancreatic head; pancreatic or biliary malignancy should be the leading differential diagnosis in patients older than 50 years who present with this symptom. Patients often present with anorexia and weight loss. Up to 60% of patients will have new or worsening glucose intolerance at the time of diagnosis secondary to the tumor affecting the insulin-producing islet cells. Pain, usually in the back, is present only if the tumor arises in the body and tail of the pancreas and affects the celiac ganglia. Acute pancreatitis is a less common presenting symptom of malignancy; however, any patient older than 50 years with idiopathic acute pancreatitis should undergo cross-sectional imaging to evaluate for a tumor.

Physical examination most commonly discloses weight loss and jaundice. Rarely, Trousseau syndrome (migratory thrombophlebitis) or Courvoisier sign (palpable gallbladder due to compression of the distal bile duct) is observed.

Diagnosis and Staging

Contrast-enhanced multiplanar CT is 90% sensitive in detecting pancreatic malignancy, but lesions less than 2 cm in diameter often cannot be visualized (**Figure 16**). EUS permits more sensitive analysis of tumors less than 2 cm and can facilitate tissue sampling by fine-needle aspiration if the diagnosis is in question. CT also permits evaluation of local and regional spread. Common locations for vascular metastases include the portal and splenic veins, superior mesenteric artery, and celiac axis. Adenocarcinoma will most commonly metastasize to the liver through the portal vein, but lung and peritoneal involvement is also common.

Diagnosis of adenocarcinoma is definitively made by tissue sampling. The modality depends on local expertise, and options include operative, percutaneous, or EUS-guided techniques. In patients who have imaging that is characteristic of resectable pancreatic cancer, tissue sampling prior to potential curative resection is not required. CA 19-9 is a serum test that can support the diagnosis, but it is neither sensitive nor specific enough to reliably make the diagnosis.

Staging is best accomplished with multiplanar CT (to evaluate vascular invasion and metastases) and EUS (if no obvious metastases are noted on CT). **Table 11** describes the staging, treatment, and prognosis of pancreatic adenocarcinoma. For further information on treatment of pancreatic cancer, see MKSAP 16 Hematology and Oncology.

> **KEY POINTS**
>
> - The 5-year survival rate of 5% for pancreatic adenocarcinoma has not improved in decades, owing to the advanced stage of disease at the time of diagnosis and the lack of effective treatments other than complete surgical resection.
> - Staging of pancreatic adenocarcinoma is best accomplished with multiplanar CT (to evaluate vascular invasion and metastases) and endoscopic ultrasound (to further stage if there are no metastases on CT).

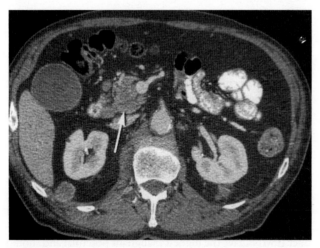

FIGURE 16. CT scan of pancreatic adenocarcinoma, with a large mass in the head of the pancreas (*arrow*)

Autoimmune Pancreatitis and IgG4 Disease

Autoimmune pancreatitis (AIP) is the pancreatic manifestation of a systemic fibroinflammatory disease that affects the pancreas, bile duct, salivary glands, retroperitoneum, and lymph nodes. Organs affected by AIP have a lymphoplasmacytic

TABLE 11. Staging, Treatment, and Prognosis of Pancreatic Adenocarcinoma

Stage	Findings	Treatment	Prognosis
Localized disease	No vascular involvement of the celiac axis or SMA; no extrapancreatic metastases	Surgical resection combined with neoadjuvant or adjuvant chemoradiotherapy	20% survival at 5 years
Locally advanced disease	Vascular invasion of the celiac axis or SMA; occlusion of the portal/SMV; no extrapancreatic metastases	Neoadjuvant chemoradiotherapy, with restaging thereafter	10 months
Metastatic disease	Extrapancreatic metastases	Palliative chemotherapy	6 months

SMA = superior mesenteric artery; SMV = superior mesenteric vein.

infiltrate rich in immunoglobulin IgG subclass 4 (IgG4)–positive cells, and the inflammatory process responds to corticosteroid therapy. The systemic disease of which AIP is a manifestation has been called IgG4-associated systemic disease.

AIP is rare; in Japan, where most cases of AIP have been described, the prevalence is estimated to be 0.82 per 100,000 persons. Men are nearly twice as likely as women to develop AIP, and the average age of onset is in the fifth decade of life. The pathogenesis of AIP is unknown, but it almost certainly reflects an immune-mediated process. AIP has been linked to other autoimmune conditions such as Sjögren syndrome, retroperitoneal fibrosis, and primary sclerosing cholangitis. The biliary involvement in IgG4-associated systemic disease has recently been called IgG4-associated cholangitis and may resemble cholangiocarcinoma or primary sclerosing cholangitis.

Idiopathic duct-centric chronic pancreatitis, or type II autoimmune pancreatitis, is a newly described entity not related to IgG4 cell deposition. Affected patients tend to be younger and male, and they often have inflammatory bowel disease.

Clinical Presentation and Diagnosis

Patients with AIP most commonly present with painless obstructive jaundice. Very rarely, patients may present with typical acute pancreatitis. Patients can also present with a pancreatic mass found incidentally on cross-sectional imaging. It is essential that pancreatic adenocarcinoma be excluded prior to diagnosing AIP. The most commonly involved extrapancreatic organ is the biliary tree, where distal biliary involvement mimics a pancreatic-cancer–related stricture.

Characteristic cross-sectional imaging demonstrates diffusely enlarged pancreatic parenchyma, forming a "sausage-shaped" gland with featureless borders (**Figure 17**). Increased

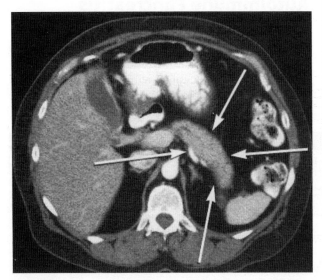

FIGURE 17. CT scan demonstrating autoimmune pancreatitis with the classic "sausage-shaped" pancreas (*arrows*)

numbers of circulating immunoglobulins, specifically IgG4, are a hallmark of the disease. Making the diagnosis generally requires diagnostic pancreatic histology or the finding of greater than or equal to ten IgG4-positive cells per high-power field on immunostain of lymphoplasmacytic infiltrate with storiform fibrosis. Definitive diagnosis often requires a combination of imaging, histopathology, and serology.

Treatment

Corticosteroids are the cornerstone of treatment for AIP. Between 30% and 40% of patients will have clinical or radiographic relapse following prolonged treatment with corticosteroids, and retreatment with a second prolonged course is required. Patients with relapse after a second prolonged course of corticosteroids may require chronic prednisone therapy or another agent such as azathioprine or 6-mercaptopurine.

KEY POINTS

- Autoimmune pancreatitis is a chronic inflammatory disease characterized by an IgG4 lymphoplasmacytic infiltrate that may affect other organs such as the biliary tree, salivary glands, retroperitoneum, and lymph nodes.
- Corticosteroids are the cornerstone of treatment for autoimmune pancreatitis.

Cystic Neoplasms of the Pancreas

The incidence of pancreatic cystic neoplasms is increasing owing to incidental detection by cross-sectional imaging. The prevalence of pancreatic cysts may be as high as 20% in the population; however, malignant cystic neoplasms represent only 1% of all pancreatic adenocarcinoma. Pancreatic cystic neoplasms are associated with von Hippel-Lindau disease.

Intraductal papillary mucinous neoplasms (IPMN) are the most common cystic neoplasms of the pancreas. These lesions involve the main duct, the ductal side braches, or a combination of the two (**Figure 18**). Main- and combined-duct IPMNs have the highest malignant potential and should be resected. Side-branch IPMNs do not require resection as long as they are less than 3 cm in diameter, do not connect

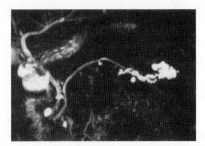

FIGURE 18. Magnetic resonance cholangiopancreatography demonstrating main-duct intraductal papillary mucinous neoplasm in the pancreatic tail

with the main duct, do not cause symptoms such as pancreatitis, and do not have worrisome features on imaging such as nodularity or a thickened cyst wall.

Mucinous cystadenoma and cystadenocarcinoma are less common than IPMN. They are typically located in the body and tail of the pancreas and are defined histologically by the presence of ovarian stroma. The rate of transformation to malignancy is likely low, but operative resection is recommended for these lesions. These are usually diagnosed via sampling performed during EUS. Serous cystadenomas are benign neoplasms of the pancreas that can grow large enough to cause localized obstruction. The morphologic features of microcysts and a central scar are pathognomonic for a serous cystadenoma. Pancreatic pseudocysts result from direct ductal injury to the pancreas and should be resected or drained only if they cause localized symptoms or become infected.

Differentiation of these cystic lesions is usually made with sampling of the cystic contents using EUS. Cysts high in carcinoembryonic antigen are typically IPMN or mucinous lesions (**Table 12**).

KEY POINTS

- The prevalence of pancreatic cysts may be as high as 20% in the population; however, malignant cystic neoplasms represent only 1% of all pancreatic adenocarcinoma.
- Differentiation of cystic lesions of the pancreas is usually made with sampling of the cystic contents using endoscopic ultrasound.

Pancreatic Neuroendocrine Tumors

Pancreatic neuroendocrine tumors (islet cell tumors) arise from pancreatic endocrine tissue and can cause hormonal hypersecretion. Neuroendocrine tumors, however, can arise from other regions of the gastrointestinal system, and many of these tumors do not cause hormonal hypersecretion (known as nonfunctioning tumors). These tumors are associated with multiple endocrine neoplasia type 1 and von Hippel-Lindau disease.

Table 13 describes the types and clinical features of pancreatic neuroendocrine tumors. The most common pancreatic neuroendocrine tumor is a gastrinoma, which causes excessive gastrin production leading to increased number and activity of parietal cells with subsequent marked oversecretion of acid. All localized gastrinomas should be resected. Metastatic gastrinomas should be treated with acid suppression and octreotide to suppress diarrhea.

Other pancreatic neuroendocrine tumors include insulinomas (**Figure 19**), glucagonomas, and vasoactive intestinal polypeptide–secreting tumors (known as VIPomas). All should be removed operatively. Insulinomas are the least likely to metastasize, but associated hypoglycemia often necessitates their removal. Neuroendocrine tumors are often best localized using EUS or pentetreotide scintigraphy (octreotide scanning); however, insulinomas will generally not be seen with scintigraphy because they do not produce adequate numbers of somatostatin receptors. EUS has an approximately 90% detection rate for insulinomas.

TABLE 12. Cyst Fluid Analysis of Pancreatic Cystic Lesions

Lesion	Carcinoembryonic Antigen	Amylase	CA 19-9
Pseudocyst	Low	High	Low
IPMN	High	Low	Low
Mucinous cystadenoma	High	Variable	Variable
Serous cystadenoma	Low	Low	Variable

IPMN = intraductal papillary mucinous neoplasm.

TABLE 13. Clinical Characteristics of Pancreatic Neuroendocrine Tumors

Tumor Type	Hormone	Symptoms	Criteria for Diagnosis
Gastrinoma	Gastrin	Peptic ulcers, diarrhea, esophagitis (Zollinger-Ellison syndrome)	Elevated serum gastrin >1000 pg/mL (1000 ng/L), secretin stimulation test
Insulinoma	Insulin	Hypoglycemia; associated with MEN-1	Inappropriately high insulin level during hypoglycemia
VIPoma	Vasoactive intestinal peptide	Watery diarrhea, hypokalemia, hypochlorhydria (Verner-Morrison syndrome)	Elevated serum VIP level >75 pg/mL (75 ng/L)
Glucagonoma	Glucagon	Dermatitis (necrolytic migratory erythema), diabetes mellitus	Elevated serum glucagon >1000 pg/mL (1000 ng/L)

MEN-1 = multiple endocrine neoplasia type 1; VIP = vasoactive intestinal peptide.

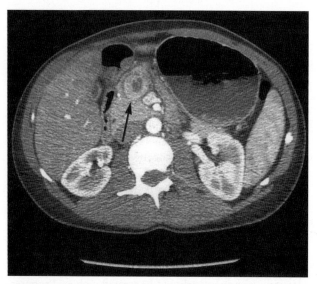

FIGURE 19. Contrast-enhanced CT scan demonstrating insulinoma in the pancreatic head (*arrow*)

In patients with metastatic disease, limited treatment options are available. Treatment options are chemotherapy, hepatic artery embolization, or radiolabeled somatostatin analogues such as octreotide or lanreotide.

KEY POINTS

- Pancreatic neuroendocrine tumors (islet cell tumors) arise from pancreatic endocrine tissue and can cause hormonal hypersecretion.
- Endoscopic ultrasound has an approximately 90% detection rate for insulinomas.

Disorders of the Small and Large Bowel

Diarrhea

Characterization

Diarrhea is defined as an increase in frequency or liquidity of stool or as stool weight greater than 200 g/d. Diarrhea may be classified by duration (acute, <14 days; subacute, 14 days-4 weeks; chronic, >4 weeks) or by specific features (osmotic, secretory, inflammatory, or malabsorptive).

Osmotic and secretory diarrhea can often be distinguished by clinical history. Patients with osmotic diarrhea often have stool volumes of less than 1 L/d and have cessation of stooling when they are fasting; those with secretory diarrhea may pass liters of stool daily, causing severe dehydration and electrolyte disturbances, with persistent stooling despite fasting. If it is not evident by the clinical presentation, a stool osmotic gap can be used to distinguish between secretory and osmotic diarrhea.

The stool osmotic gap calculation is:

$$290 - 2 \times [\text{stool sodium} + \text{stool potassium}]$$

A gap less than 50 mOsm/kg (50 mmol/kg) indicates secretory diarrhea; a gap greater than 100 mOsm/kg (100 mmol/kg) suggests osmotic diarrhea.

Inflammatory diarrhea is often but not always characterized by blood or mucus in the stool. Malabsorptive diarrhea is the loss of fat, carbohydrates, or protein in the stool secondary to an underlying disease (see Malabsorption). Some diseases, such as Crohn disease or celiac disease, may cause a combination of these categories of diarrhea.

Evaluation and Management

Acute diarrhea is most commonly caused by infectious pathogens and is often self-limited. See MKSAP 16 Infectious Disease for a discussion of infectious diarrhea. Evaluation is necessary only in patients with the clinical and demographic characteristics described in **Table 14**. Adequate oral fluid resuscitation is necessary to avoid dehydration in patients with acute diarrhea.

The causes and evaluation of chronic diarrhea are broad (**Table 15**). Diagnosis relies on a careful assessment of the patient history. Key clinical features include travel, medications, surgical history, family history, types of foods regularly ingested, stool timing and characterization, and the presence of associated features such as weight loss, joint pains, skin lesions, or fevers. The evaluation for chronic diarrhea is stepwise and often involves a combination of stool studies (cultures, fecal fat quantification), endoscopic evaluation (upper endoscopy with small-bowel biopsies and cultures, colonoscopy with terminal ileal examination and random biopsies), and radiographic images of the pancreas and small bowel. Any time a patient is referred for an endoscopic evaluation for diarrhea, biopsies should be obtained from the duodenum and colon, even if they appear endoscopically normal, to evaluate for conditions such as celiac disease and microscopic colitis, respectively. Other tests, such as breath testing (for lactose, fructose, or sucrose) or

TABLE 14. Clinical and Demographic Indications for the Evaluation of Acute Diarrhea
Bloody stools
Fever ≥38.5 °C (101.3 °F)
Significant abdominal pain
Severe diarrhea leading to volume depletion
Inflammatory bowel disease
Recent antibiotic use
Elderly patients
Hospitalized patients
Pregnant women
Immunocompromised patients
Food handlers

evaluation of secretagogues (serum levels of gastrin, calcitonin, vasoactive intestinal peptide, tryptase, and urine 5-hydroxyindoleacetic acid), are indicated only in the setting of suggestive clinical features.

The evaluation and management of acute and chronic diarrhea are described in **Figure 20**.

KEY POINTS

- Acute diarrhea typically lasts less than 2 weeks; chronic diarrhea lasts longer than 4 weeks.

- Diarrhea can be categorized as osmotic, secretory, inflammatory, or malabsorptive.
- Adequate oral fluid resuscitation is necessary to avoid dehydration in patients with acute diarrhea.

Malabsorption

Types
Malabsorption is the generalized loss of nutrients, fat, carbohydrate, or protein in the digestive tract.

TABLE 15. Causes and Evaluation of Chronic Diarrhea

Disorder	Diagnosis	Clues or Risk Factors
Inflammatory bowel disease		
Ulcerative colitis	Colonoscopy with biopsies	Bloody diarrhea, tenesmus
Crohn disease	Ileocolonoscopy with biopsies, small-bowel imaging (SBFT, CTE, MRE)	Weight loss, abdominal pain, perianal disease
Microscopic colitis	Colonoscopy with biopsies	Secretory diarrhea
Celiac disease	Serologies (tTG IgA), upper endoscopy with small-bowel biopsies	Extraintestinal features, family history
Small intestinal bacterial overgrowth	Upper endoscopy with small-bowel cultures, hydrogen breath testing	Bloating, excess flatus, malabsorption
Carbohydrate malabsorption	Detailed history, hydrogen breath testing, stool osmotic gap, avoidance trial	Bloating, excess flatus
Pancreatic insufficiency	Features of chronic pancreatitis on imaging (CT, EUS, MRCP), 48- to 72-hour fecal fat quantitation, pancreatic function tests	Known pancreatic disease/resection, weight loss
Bile acid malabsorption	Compatible history, clinical response to cholestyramine	Terminal ileal resection (<100 cm)
Bile acid deficiency	Compatible history, steatorrhea, response to medium-chain triglyceride diet	Terminal ileal resection (>100 cm)
Ischemia	Colonoscopy with biopsies (for colonic ischemia), duplex ultrasound or MRA (for chronic mesenteric ischemia)	Low-flow states, cardiovascular risk factors
Radiation enteropathy/proctopathy	Compatible history, small-bowel imaging, colonoscopy with biopsies	Any previous radiation to abdomen or pelvis
Irritable bowel syndrome	Compatible history, fulfills Rome criteria, exclude other diseases	Symptoms relieved after a bowel movement
Eosinophilic enteritis	Eosinophilia on small-bowel biopsies (for mucosal-based disease) or full-thickness bowel biopsy (for submucosal- or serosal-based disease)	Atopic history, peripheral eosinophilia (not required)
Whipple disease	Small-bowel biopsies showing PAS+ macrophages that are acid-fast negative, polymerase chain reaction on any biopsied affected tissue	Arthralgia, lymphadenopathy, neurologic symptoms
Iatrogenic	Detailed history and review of chart	New medications, initiation of enteral nutrition
Factitious diarrhea	Diagnosis of exclusion	Often high volume and frequency, bulimia, anorexia, weight loss, stool osmolality and osmolar gaps may be helpful (>50 mOsm/kg [50 mmol/kg]),stool magnesium >90 meq/L may be diagnostic

CTE = computed tomography enterography; EUS = endoscopic ultrasound; MRA = magnetic resonance angiography; MRCP = magnetic resonance cholangiopancreatography; MRE = magnetic resonance enterography; PAS = periodic acid–Schiff; SBFT = small-bowel follow-through; tTG = tissue transglutaminase antibody.

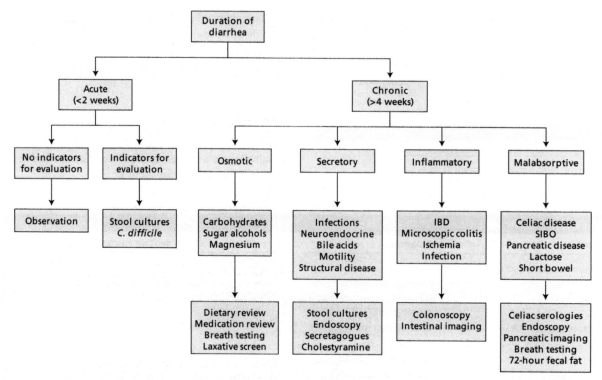

FIGURE 20. Evaluation of diarrhea. *C. difficile* = *Clostridium difficile*; IBD = inflammatory bowel disease; SIBO = small intestinal bacterial overgrowth.

Patients with fat malabsorption (steatorrhea) present with diarrhea and weight loss as the predominant features. To document steatorrhea, patients should undergo quantitative fecal fat collection for 48 to 72 hours, with fat intake of 100 g/d for several days before and during the stool collection. After steatorrhea has been documented, the cause must be determined. Fat malabsorption is most often caused by pancreatic insufficiency or small-bowel diseases such as celiac disease, autoimmune enteropathy, or small intestinal bacterial overgrowth. Abdominal imaging of the pancreas and upper endoscopy with small-bowel biopsies and cultures are usually performed.

Patients with carbohydrate malabsorption present with diarrhea, bloating, and excess flatus but no weight loss. Lactose is the most commonly malabsorbed carbohydrate, but malabsorption of fructose and sucrose also occurs. Hydrogen breath testing can confirm malabsorption, which should be correlated with clinical symptoms during the test. This is because some patients may have detectable carbohydrate malabsorption without clinical intolerance, in which case further evaluation into the cause of clinical symptoms would be required.

Protein malabsorption presents with diarrhea, edema, ascites, and anasarca. Protein malabsorption usually occurs along with malabsorption of other nutrients; it is unusual for it to occur in isolation. To document protein malabsorption, a stool α_1-antitrypsin clearance test should be performed.

When protein malabsorption is verified, the underlying cause should be evaluated and managed. Causes of protein malabsorption include but are not limited to *Clostridium difficile* infection, inflammatory bowel disease, celiac disease, Whipple disease, amyloidosis, constrictive pericarditis, lymphangiectasia, and lymphatic obstruction.

Malabsorption Syndromes

Celiac Disease
Celiac disease is an immunologic response to dietary gliadins in patients who are genetically at risk as deemed by the presence of *HLA-DQ2* or *HLA-DQ8*. Celiac disease is thought to affect nearly 1% of individuals in the United States. The typical features of celiac disease are diarrhea, bloating, and weight loss, but extraintestinal manifestations of celiac disease are increasingly being seen (**Table 16**).

The best serologic test to screen for celiac disease is the tissue transglutaminase (tTG) IgA antibody, but the sensitivity (69%-93%) and specificity (96%-100%) vary significantly among laboratories. IgA-based tTG testing may result in false negatives in the small proportion (<5%) of patients who have selective IgA deficiency; however, it is more useful for screening than an IgG-based tTG, which has poor sensitivity in non–IgA-deficient patients. Any patient with a positive serologic test or clinical features of celiac disease despite negative serologic tests should undergo small-bowel biopsies.

TABLE 16. Extraintestinal Manifestations of Celiac Disease

Category	Examples
Hematologic	Anemia (low iron, vitamin B$_{12}$, folate), functional asplenia (Howell-Jolly bodies)
Musculoskeletal	Osteopenia/osteoporosis, osteomalacia, arthropathy
Neurologic	Seizures, peripheral neuropathy, ataxia
Reproductive	Infertility, recurrent miscarriages
Skin	Dermatitis herpetiformis
Renal	Glomerular IgA deposition
Other	Enamel defects, abnormal liver chemistry tests, vitamin-deficient states

TABLE 17. Risk Factors for Small Intestinal Bacterial Overgrowth

Category	Examples
Dysmotility	Scleroderma, intestinal pseudo-obstruction, autonomic neuropathy, amyloidosis, systemic myopathies
Altered gastric acid	Achlorhydria, gastric resection, pharmacologic acid suppression
Structural	Small-bowel strictures (NSAIDs, Crohn disease, anastomotic), small-bowel diverticula, enterocolonic fistula, radiation enteropathy
Altered anatomy	Resected ileocecal valve, blind loops, afferent limbs, any intestinal bypass, short-bowel syndrome
Others	Advancing age, immunodeficiency, celiac disease, pancreatic insufficiency, cirrhosis

Reprinted with permission from Dukowicz AC, Lacy BE, Levine GM. Small intestinal bacterial overgrowth: a comprehensive review. Gastroenterol Hepatol. 2007;3(2):112-122. Copyright 2007, Millennium Medical Publishing, Inc.

Testing of *HLA* status is not routinely recommended because 30% to 40% of the general population has *HLA-DQ2* or *HLA-DQ8* positivity. However, *HLA* testing could be considered in patients with nondiagnostic histology or negative serologic markers. It may also be considered in patients who are following a gluten-free diet before diagnosis and who refuse to reintroduce gluten to undergo testing.

All patients with celiac disease should adhere to a gluten-free diet by avoiding wheat, barley, and rye. Because of cross-contamination with other cereal grains, oats should be avoided for the first year and should only be introduced if the patient is doing well clinically. In patients whose symptoms are recurrent or do not respond to a gluten-free diet, gluten ingestion (either surreptitious or inadvertent) is the most likely explanation. Associated conditions that may account for recurrent diarrhea are microscopic colitis (70-fold increased risk), lactose malabsorption, small intestinal bacterial overgrowth, pancreatic insufficiency, inflammatory bowel disease, refractory celiac disease, or enteropathy-associated T-cell lymphoma. Disorders associated with celiac disease include Down syndrome, type 1 diabetes mellitus, juvenile rheumatoid arthritis, thyroid disease, and autoimmune liver conditions.

Patients with celiac disease should undergo baseline bone densitometry, evaluation of vitamin and mineral levels, and vaccination against encapsulated organisms.

Small Intestinal Bacterial Overgrowth

Small intestinal bacterial overgrowth (SIBO) is an excess number (>10^5 organisms/mL) and alteration in type (resembling colonic flora) of bacteria cultured from the small intestine. Digestive enzymes and intestinal motility normally limit the growth of excessive bacteria, but SIBO can occur in conditions in which these functions are disrupted (**Table 17**). Clinical features of SIBO are diarrhea, bloating, and weight loss. Patients may have a combination of fat, protein, or carbohydrate malabsorption. In addition to nutritional deficiencies that may be noted on laboratory testing, patients may have macrocytosis secondary to vitamin B$_{12}$ deficiency (due to

bacterial consumption of the vitamin as well as the premature cleavage from intrinsic factor). Folate levels may be elevated owing to production from intestinal bacteria. The diagnosis of SIBO can be established with hydrogen breath testing (often with lactulose as a substrate) showing an early peak of hydrogen production due to fermentation of the carbohydrate by small intestinal bacteria. Results of hydrogen breath testing can be affected by rapid intestinal transit (false positives) and recent antibiotic use (false negatives). The diagnosis can also be established by upper endoscopy with small-bowel cultures that disclose greater than 10^5 organisms/mL of aerobes and anaerobes. Although patients may have clinical improvement with a single course of antibiotic therapy, many patients will require rotating antibiotics that may include amoxicillin-clavulanate, fluoroquinolones, tetracycline derivatives, metronidazole, or rifaximin. Lactose avoidance can be used as adjunctive therapy.

Short-Bowel Syndrome

Short-bowel syndrome is defined as the presence of less than 200 cm of remaining small bowel (normal is 600 cm) and usually follows massive resection of intestine. The most common causes of short-bowel syndrome in adults are Crohn disease, ischemia, volvulus, trauma, and certain tumors (desmoids). Other causes of intestinal failure in adults include intestinal motility disorders and radiation enteritis.

Critical to the ability to adapt after significant small-bowel resection is whether the colon remains in continuity with the small bowel. Over time, the colon can compensate by absorbing increasing amounts of water and electrolytes, and calories from carbohydrate malabsorption can be reclaimed when colonic bacteria ferment these maldigested products. Gastric acid suppression and electrolyte monitoring are critical; in the early postoperative period, there is a surge of gastric acid secretion that can worsen diarrhea, because of the inactivation of pancreatic digestive enzymes from the high-acid state. Although oral rehydration and antidiarrheal agents are used in these patients, many will require parenteral nutrition. Enteral nutrition is encouraged to stimulate bowel adaptation, even if parenteral nutrition is required. Long-term complications include catheter-related infections, liver disease, SIBO, and micronutrient deficiencies. Intestinal transplantation is performed at selective centers, mostly in children. The role of growth factors to promote bowel adaptation is being studied.

Lactose Malabsorption

Although lactose intolerance is commonly reported, the true prevalence of lactose malabsorption and intolerance is not known. Certain ethnic groups (black, American Indian, Hispanic, and Asian) are at increased risk for primary lactase deficiency. There are insufficient data to support the belief that lactose malabsorption increases with advancing age; population-based studies are needed to answer this question more definitively. Lactose malabsorption may also occur after any process that affects the small-bowel mucosa (because lactase resides on the brush border), such as celiac disease, Crohn disease, radiation enteritis, and small-bowel resection. Gastroenteritis may cause self-limited lactose malabsorption.

Most patients with lactose malabsorption report osmotic diarrhea, bloating, and excess flatus. Weight loss and gastrointestinal bleeding are not expected; if present, they may point to an underlying diagnosis causing secondary lactase deficiency. The diagnosis can be supported by hydrogen breath testing with lactose as the substrate. An increase in breath hydrogen greater than 20 parts per million (which results from colonic bacteria breaking down the unabsorbed carbohydrate) indicates lactose malabsorption; if symptoms are also reproduced during the test, a diagnosis of lactose malabsorption with intolerance is supported.

Traditional management has consisted of lactose avoidance, but this can lead to inadequate intake of calcium and vitamin D. Evidence suggests that patients with documented lactose malabsorption can ingest 12 g of lactose (equivalent to 1 cup of milk) with few, if any, symptoms. Also, ingesting lactose throughout the day rather than in large boluses helps with tolerance, as does ingesting lactose with other food products. Certain dairy products such as yogurt may be better tolerated by patients with lactose malabsorption, because yogurt is emptied from the stomach at a slower rate than milk, which allows for more controlled digestion and absorption. Yogurt may also contain lactase as a result of the bacterial cultures that are present. Although patients may report benefit from the use of lactase enzyme supplementation, the amount and dosing pattern of such supplements are not well described.

KEY POINTS

- Malabsorption is the generalized loss of nutrients, fat, carbohydrate, or protein in the digestive tract.

- The typical features of celiac disease are diarrhea, bloating, and weight loss, but extraintestinal manifestations of celiac disease are increasingly being seen.

- Treatment for celiac disease consists of a gluten-free diet; baseline bone densitometry and evaluation of vitamin and mineral levels are recommended.

- Patients with lactose malabsorption tend to have osmotic diarrhea, bloating, and excess flatus, but weight loss and gastrointestinal bleeding are not present.

Inflammatory Bowel Disease

Inflammatory bowel disease consists primarily of Crohn disease and ulcerative colitis. However, as better diagnostic and genetic approaches evolve, evidence suggests that additional subtypes of inflammatory bowel disease may exist. Most patients have distinct features of either Crohn disease or ulcerative colitis, but approximately 5% to 10% have features of both diseases (known as indeterminate colitis).

Crohn disease and ulcerative colitis are most commonly diagnosed in the second or third decade of life but may occur at any age. There may be a second peak in incidence in the seventh and eighth decades of life. There is no gender predominance, and approximately 1.5 million Americans have these diseases.

Risk Factors

Both Crohn disease and ulcerative colitis are believed to be caused by a combination of genetic alterations, immune system dysregulation, and environmental triggers. Ashkenazi (Eastern European) Jewish descendants have a higher prevalence of inflammatory bowel disease than other ethnic or religious groups, likely based on genetic similarities within this relatively small group. Genetic determinants predisposing to inflammatory bowel disease are much more common than the occurrence of the disease, implicating environmental triggers as probable important factors for disease expression.

The second part of the triad leading to inflammatory bowel disease is dysregulation of the immune system. A simplified paradigm has attributed Crohn disease to an abnormal CD4+ T-cell T-helper 1 (Th1) response, whereas ulcerative colitis is believed to be predominantly a CD4+ T-cell Th2 response. The importance of the T-helper cell Th17 has recently been identified to be associated with Crohn disease. There is significant crossover between multiple immunologic pathways, with production of inflammatory cytokines leading to mucosal and/or structural damage being the common endpoint.

It is likely that multiple environmental exposures contribute to Crohn disease or ulcerative colitis. Putative agents include infections, antibiotics, NSAIDs, and other medications. Smoking is a risk factor for Crohn disease, whereas the cessation of smoking appears to be a risk factor for new diagnoses of ulcerative colitis in some older patients. An interesting north-south gradient of higher to lower prevalence of inflammatory bowel disease has been reported both in the United States and France and in a similar pattern to other immune-mediated disease (such as multiple sclerosis). Inflammatory bowel disease is more prevalent in westernized societies than in third-world countries and is overrepresented in higher socioeconomic groups. This geographic variation supports the hypothesis that environmental or lifestyle factors may be important in the pathogenesis of Crohn disease and ulcerative colitis.

Clinical Manifestations

Although ulcerative colitis and Crohn disease both are characterized by bowel inflammation, the clinical manifestations of these diseases can be very different. Ulcerative colitis causes mucosal inflammation isolated to the colon, and Crohn disease causes transmural bowel wall inflammation that may affect the entire gastroenterologic tract from the mouth to the anus. Symptoms vary widely in severity and are directly related to the extent of bowel involvement and the complications that can develop. Inflammatory bowel disease may be mild, causing only occasional symptoms, or severe, causing significant impact on quality of life.

Ulcerative Colitis

Patients with ulcerative colitis almost always have a sense of bowel urgency due to rectal inflammation. Frequent watery bowel movements are typical, and bleeding occurs with more severe inflammation. The onset of ulcerative colitis is typically acute, and patients often remember when symptoms first started.

Ulcerative colitis almost always starts at the rectum and involves a varying length of colon. It may be limited to the rectum (proctitis), extend from the rectum to the sigmoid or descending colon (left-sided colitis), or continue proximal to the splenic flexure to include the entire colon (extensive colitis or pancolitis). Typical endoscopic findings of ulcerative colitis are a continuous pattern of inflammation with varying severity of mucosal granularity, edema, loss of the normal vascular pattern, friability, and ulceration. A diffuse pattern of microulcerations is commonly seen, and frank ulcers are atypical. The transition from abnormal to normal tissue is usually abrupt, with a very clear line of demarcation. Pseudopolyps (inflammatory polyps) may be seen in patients with long-standing disease, sometimes with hundreds throughout the colon. If a stricture develops in a patient with ulcerative colitis, this suggests either the wrong diagnosis or malignancy.

Abdominal pain is an unusual manifestation of ulcerative colitis and suggests a complication such as toxic megacolon or perforation. Toxic megacolon is the most severe complication associated with ulcerative colitis; it is associated with a 40% mortality rate in patients undergoing emergency colectomy after a perforation has occurred (compared with 2% without a perforation). Most patients with toxic megacolon related to ulcerative colitis have at least 1 week of bloody diarrhea symptoms that are unresponsive to medical therapy. On examination, patients have tachycardia, fever, hypotension, decreased or absent bowel sounds, and lower abdominal distention and tenderness, often with peritoneal signs. On plain film radiography, the transverse colon is most affected, with dilatation exceeding 6 cm. About 50% of patients with toxic megacolon may improve with medical therapy (bowel rest, intravenous corticosteroids, antibiotics, and fluids); however, progressive abdominal distention and tenderness with hemodynamic instability are indications for immediate surgery.

Crohn Disease

Crohn disease has variable manifestations and is typically more indolent in onset. Most patients recall gradually feeling worse over time, sometimes with nonspecific symptoms. One third to one half of patients have disease that involves both the small bowel and colon. About one third have disease confined to the small bowel (most often the terminal ileum), and approximately 20% have isolated colonic disease. Upper gastrointestinal tract involvement is less common (<10%) and is rarely present without lower gastrointestinal tract findings. Perianal disease (fissures, fistulas, abscesses) occurs in roughly one quarter of patients with Crohn disease.

Symptoms depend on the location of the disease and presence of complications such as strictures or fistulas. If the colon is predominantly affected, diarrhea and bleeding similar to ulcerative colitis may be the main symptoms. When the small bowel is involved or any stricturing is present, postprandial pain and obstructive-type symptoms (pain, nausea, vomiting, bloating) may occur. Transmural disease may cause perforations, leading to acute symptoms of peritonitis or long-standing pain and/or fevers due to abscess or phlegmon formation. Fistulizing disease can lead to some of the most troublesome symptoms. Fistulas may occur around the anus (perianal fistulas), from bowel to bowel (entero-entero fistulas), from the bowel to other organs (enterovesicular or enterovaginal fistulas), or from the bowel to the skin (enterocutaneous fistulas). Symptoms from fistulas can range from occasional painless drainage to painful cycles of abscess formation followed by drainage.

Typical endoscopic findings of Crohn disease are a patchy pattern of inflammation with spared regions of normal-appearing mucosa interspersed between abnormal regions ("skip lesions"). It is common for the rectum to be completely spared. Aphthoid ulcerations can range from a few millimeters to a few centimeters in diameter, and stricturing of the bowel is not unusual. As with ulcerative colitis, pseudopolyps may be seen in the colon; however, if a cluster of polyps is noted, this may represent an internal orifice of a fistula.

Extraintestinal Manifestations

Crohn disease and ulcerative colitis can lead to manifestations outside of the bowel. Approximately 15% of patients experience some form of extraintestinal symptoms over the course of their disease. Ocular manifestations include episcleritis, iritis, or uveitis. Oral aphthous ulcers are more common in Crohn disease than ulcerative colitis but may occur in the latter. Rheumatologic diseases such as enteropathic arthritis are fairly common; they are typically symmetric and can involve both large and small joints. Sacroiliitis and ankylosing spondylitis are associated with inflammatory bowel disease; patients with ankylosing spondylitis are often *HLA-B27* positive. The most common dermatologic manifestations of inflammatory bowel disease are erythema nodosum (painful subcutaneous nodules most often seen on the extensor surface of the leg) and pyoderma gangrenosum (ulcers on the skin that can mimic cellulitis). Erythema nodosum and pyoderma gangrenosum associated with ulcerative colitis typically resolve with treatment of the underlying inflammatory bowel disease. Primary sclerosing cholangitis is more common in patients with ulcerative colitis; these patients may represent a distinct phenotype of disease with a particularly high rate of colorectal cancer. Some extraintestinal symptoms track with the luminal disease activity (episcleritis, iritis, skin manifestations, and peripheral arthritis) and others are independent of disease activity (uveitis, axial arthritis, primary sclerosing cholangitis).

Diagnosis

Endoscopy with histopathology is the gold standard for the diagnosis of inflammatory bowel disease. Although other diseases such as acute infectious colitis, ischemia, or drug toxicity may have a similar endoscopic appearance, inflammatory bowel disease will invariably show chronic inflammatory changes and/or granuloma formation on biopsy. It can occasionally be very difficult to distinguish Crohn disease or ulcerative colitis from chronic infections (tuberculosis, *Yersinia* species), NSAID-induced colitis, or small-bowel lymphoma. Cultures, NSAID avoidance, or serial studies with repeat biopsies may be necessary. If ulcerative colitis is suspected, a complete colonoscopy should be performed with inspection of the terminal ileum. If Crohn disease is suspected, both colonoscopy and upper endoscopy should be performed to determine the full extent of disease. Backwash ileitis refers to distal ileal involvement with severe extensive ulcerative colitis and may be confused with ileocolonic Crohn disease.

Radiographic imaging plays a key role in evaluating the small bowel in Crohn disease and in identifying complications of Crohn disease and ulcerative colitis. A small-bowel follow-through can reveal small-bowel Crohn disease that is out of the reach of upper endoscopy or colonoscopy and may demonstrate fistulas or strictures. CT enterography has recently gained a prominent role in evaluating Crohn disease because it allows better visualization of the extent and severity of disease. CT enterography offers luminal images similar to those of small-bowel follow-through but can also reveal extraluminal findings such as lymphadenopathy, mesenteric fat inflammation, or abscess/phlegmon. Patients with Crohn disease typically have many imaging studies over the course of their disease; owing to concerns about excessive radiation exposure leading to a possible increased risk for malignancy, magnetic resonance enterography has developed increasing popularity. As radiologists gain experience with magnetic resonance enterography, the accuracy can be as good as that of CT enterography. Ultrasound is used more frequently in Europe and more often in children than in adults. Gastroenterologists in the United States are not trained in the use of transabdominal ultrasound as they are in European countries, and as patients with Crohn disease develop more complications over time, leading to distorted anatomy, ultrasound becomes more difficult to interpret. Small-bowel capsule endoscopy has allowed for a better understanding of proximal small-bowel Crohn disease, but it should only be performed after ruling out strictures by one of the above radiographic images because of concern about capsule retention.

Serologic markers have been recently identified that are seen more often in patients with Crohn disease or ulcerative colitis compared with patients without inflammatory bowel disease. These markers are related to antibodies against microbial antigens or specific carbohydrates. A high percentage of patients with known Crohn disease or ulcerative colitis have these markers, but the accuracy is not high enough to be relied on without confirmatory endoscopy. Because these blood tests alone cannot establish or rule out a diagnosis of inflammatory bowel disease or clearly differentiate Crohn disease from ulcerative colitis in patients with indeterminate colitis, their value for diagnosis is limited. However, the number and magnitude of identified serologic markers correlate with the risk of Crohn disease complications. Genetic markers are not currently clinically useful. Caution should be used when ordering tests for serologic and genetic markers for diagnosis, because a false-positive result can lead to unnecessary testing and higher insurance premiums, and false negatives can lead to neglect of a proper evaluation.

For disease flares, stool studies (routine enteric pathogens, ova and parasites, and *C. difficile*) should be performed, because superimposed infections are not uncommon. *C. difficile* is now well recognized as a cause of significant morbidity and mortality in patients with inflammatory bowel disease and is being reported more often in ambulatory patients without recent antibiotic use. Patients with colitis (ulcerative colitis or Crohn colitis) whose disease becomes refractory to corticosteroid therapy should undergo colonoscopy with biopsies to evaluate for cytomegalovirus infection, which is found in up to 30% of patients undergoing colectomy. For obstructive symptoms, severe pain, or fever, three-dimensional imaging (CT or MRI) should be performed to rule out complications. If there is no evidence of infection or complications requiring surgery, medical therapy should be initiated. **H**

Treatment

The treatment of Crohn disease and ulcerative colitis are similar but have slightly different approaches within the same classes of medications. The available medical therapies and their indications and side effects are described in **Table 18**.

Crohn Disease

The standard treatment approach for Crohn disease has been to (1) initiate therapy with 5-aminosalicylate drugs at diagnosis; (2) begin thiopurine therapy with azathioprine or 6-mercaptopurine if a patient requires repeated courses of corticosteroids; and (3) begin therapy with anti–tumor necrosis factor (anti-TNF) agents if these other therapies are unsuccessful (**Figure 21**). This paradigm has been challenged by newer studies showing that 5-aminosalicylates have only minimal efficacy in Crohn disease, and the success of treatment is significantly higher when anti-TNF therapy is begun alone or in combination with thiopurines earlier in the disease course. Many experts have abandoned the use of 5-aminosalicylates entirely for Crohn disease except for those with mild Crohn

colitis. The decision to use thiopurine or anti-TNF monotherapy versus combination therapy is based on an individual patient's severity of symptoms and risk factors for

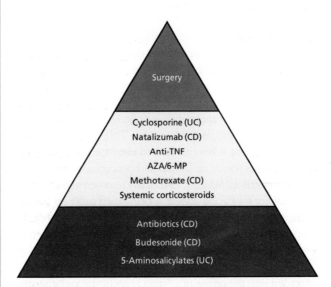

FIGURE 21. Standard treatment approach for Crohn disease and ulcerative colitis. Typically, treatment for inflammatory bowel disease begins with agents at the base of the pyramid and progresses sequentially toward the tip of the pyramid if patients do not have an adequate response to treatment. Although this algorithm still applies for ulcerative colitis, newer data for Crohn disease suggest that the earlier use of thiopurines and anti-TNF agents prior to the use of medications at the base of the pyramid or systemic corticosteroids leads to a more favorable treatment response. AZA = azathioprine; CD = used for Crohn disease only; MP = mercaptopurine; TNF= tumor necrosis factor; UC = used for ulcerative colitis only.

TABLE 18. Medical Therapy for Inflammatory Bowel Disease		
Medication	**Indication**	**Side Effects/Adverse Events**
5-ASA (sulfasalazine, olsalazine, balsalazide, mesalamine: oral, rectal)	UC: induction/maintenance CD (mild) involving the colon: induction/maintenance	Interstitial nephritis (rare) Diarrhea (olsalazine)
Antibiotics (metronidazole, ciprofloxacin)	CD: perianal and colonic disease	Metronidazole: peripheral neuropathy, metallic taste, antabuse effect Ciprofloxacin: arthropathy, tendon injury, sun sensitivity
Corticosteroids (oral, intravenous, rectal)	UC/CD: induction, not maintenance	Acne, moon facies, truncal obesity, osteoporosis, osteonecrosis, diabetes mellitus, hypertension, cataracts, infection
Budesonide	CD (ileal/right colon): induction	Minimal corticosteroid effects
Methotrexate	CD: induction/maintenance	Nausea, fatigue, hepatotoxicity, pneumonitis
6-MP, azathioprine	UC/CD: corticosteroid withdrawal, maintenance	Pancreatitis, fever, infection, leukopenia, hepatotoxicity, lymphoma
Anti–TNF-α (adalimumab, certolizumab pegol, infliximab)	UC/CD: induction/maintenance	Infusion/injection-site reaction, tuberculosis reactivation, demyelination, infection, heart failure, lymphoma
Cyclosporine	UC: corticosteroid refractory	Hypertension, nephro- and neurotoxicity
Natalizumab	CD: induction/maintenance for disease refractory to anti-TNF agents	Progressive multifocal leukoencephalopathy

ASA = aminosalicylate; CD = Crohn disease; MP = mercaptopurine; TNF = tumor necrosis factor; UC = ulcerative colitis.

developing complications of their disease balanced against the potential side effects of these treatments. As treatment algorithms evolve, early referral soon after diagnosis to an expert in inflammatory bowel disease can be very helpful to establish an initial treatment plan.

Antibiotics can be useful as adjunctive therapy in patients with Crohn disease involving the colon and in perianal disease, because they seem to have both an anti-inflammatory and antimicrobial effect. Methotrexate administered with 1 mg of folic acid can be used instead of thiopurines when azathioprine or 6-mercaptopurine is not tolerated. Natalizumab is effective for patients in whom anti-TNF therapy has been unsuccessful, but it has had limited use based on an association with progressive multifocal leukoencephalopathy due to JC virus infection. Surgery, historically reserved as the last line of treatment for Crohn disease, is being used more commonly if there is a limited segment of diseased bowel that can be managed with a minimally invasive procedure. Patients with perianal disease may need surgical therapy for drainage of abscesses or placement of a seton (a rubber band that is threaded into the orifice of a fistula and out through the anus to develop a loop through the fistula tract to prevent recurrent abscess formation) to aid in fistula healing. When there are no signs of active perianal infection, anti-TNF agents are very effective in healing perianal and other enterocutaneous fistulas. Approximately 40% of patients with Crohn disease require some type of bowel surgery within the first 5 years of their disease; 80% require surgery by 20 years of disease.

Ulcerative Colitis

The therapeutic approach to ulcerative colitis should follow the sequence of medical therapy described in Figure 21. Unlike Crohn disease, patients with ulcerative colitis respond well to 5-aminosalicylate agents. Patients with proctitis or left-sided colitis should receive topical therapy with 5-aminosalicylate suppositories and enemas or hydrocortisone enemas. If patients require repeated courses of corticosteroids or become corticosteroid dependent, thiopurines should be initiated (methotrexate has not been shown to be effective in ulcerative colitis). Anti-TNF agents should be used in patients who do not maintain remission with thiopurines. In hospitalized patients whose disease is refractory to corticosteroids, infliximab or cyclosporine can be very effective. If a patient responds and is able to discontinue corticosteroids, infliximab can then be continued as a maintenance drug or cyclosporine can be used as a short-term bridge to a thiopurine for maintenance. Colectomy with end-ileostomy or ileal pouch-anal anastomosis (also referred to as a J-pouch) is usually considered the last resort of treatment; however, some patients may prefer surgery over the potential long-term toxicity from treatment with immunosuppressive medications. Approximately 20% of patients with ulcerative colitis ultimately require colectomy over the course of their lifetime.

Health Care Maintenance for the Patient with Inflammatory Bowel Disease

Because treatment of inflammatory bowel disease frequently requires suppression of the immune system (owing to corticosteroid and other immunosuppressive therapies), patients require more frequent and intensive monitoring for long-term complications of therapy and aggressive disease-prevention strategies. Osteopenia and osteoporosis are common in patients with inflammatory bowel disease as a result of a chronic inflammatory state, corticosteroid use, and malabsorption (especially in patients with Crohn disease of the small bowel). Patients should receive calcium and vitamin D supplementation as well as a baseline dual-energy X-ray absorptiometry (DEXA) scan. Immunosuppressed patients should receive influenza vaccination every year and pneumococcal vaccination every 5 years. Live vaccinations (varicella, intranasal influenza vaccines, measles, mumps, rubella) should be avoided in immunosuppressed patients. Patients with ulcerative colitis (except those with only proctitis) and Crohn colitis (with at least one third of the colon involved) are at increased risk of colorectal cancer after approximately 8 years of disease. These patients should undergo surveillance colonoscopy with biopsies every 1 to 2 years. If flat dysplasia is present, the benefits and risks of prophylactic colectomy should be discussed with the patient. Because smoking (for Crohn disease) and NSAID use (for Crohn disease and ulcerative colitis) are known to exacerbate disease activity, patients should be routinely reminded to stop smoking and avoid or limit NSAID use. Hospitalized patients with inflammatory bowel disease are at an increased risk for deep venous thrombosis and should receive anticoagulation as a routine prophylactic measure.

Microscopic Colitis

Microscopic colitis is a distinct entity from Crohn disease and ulcerative colitis. It is characterized by histologic inflammation in endoscopically normal-appearing colonic mucosa. Patients typically lack signs of systemic inflammation and present with painless watery diarrhea without bleeding. Diagnosis can only be made when biopsies of the colon show a predominance of intraepithelial lymphocytes in the colonic mucosa (lymphocytic colitis) or the addition of a thickened subepithelial collagen band (collagenous colitis).

Microscopic colitis may be idiopathic or may be a side effect of medications (Table 19) or systemic disease. A diagnosis of microscopic colitis should prompt a careful review of prescription and over-the-counter medications; celiac disease should also be considered, as it can be associated with microscopic colitis. Treatment may be as simple as drug withdrawal or treatment of celiac disease. Medical therapy, if needed, begins with antidiarrheal agents or high-dose bismuth. Other therapies shown to be effective include delayed-release budesonide, cholestyramine, and 5-aminosalicylate agents. If these medications are ineffective, systemic corticosteroids may be used. There is limited evidence that thiopurines may be helpful for corticosteroid-refractory or corticosteroid-dependent disease. Rarely, colectomy is required for medically refractory disease.

KEY POINTS

- Ulcerative colitis causes mucosal inflammation isolated to the colon, and Crohn disease causes transmural bowel wall inflammation that may affect the entire gastroenterologic tract from the mouth to the anus.

- Ulcerative colitis is characterized by the acute onset of bowel urgency, frequent watery bowel movements, and often bleeding; patients often remember when symptoms first started.

- Crohn disease is characterized by indolent onset and variable clinical manifestations that depend on the location of disease and the presence of complications; most patients recall gradually feeling worse over time.

- Microscopic colitis presents with painless watery diarrhea without bleeding and is diagnosed with biopsy showing histologic inflammation in endoscopically normal-appearing colonic mucosa.

TABLE 19. Drugs That May Cause Microscopic Colitis

High Likelihood

Acarbose

Aspirin

Lansoprazole (possibly other PPIs)

NSAIDs

Ranitidine

Sertraline

Ticlopidine

Intermediate Likelihood

Carbamazepine

Flutamide

Lisinopril

Levodopa with benserazide

Paroxetine

Simvastatin

Low Likelihood

Cimetidine

Gold salts

PPI = proton pump inhibitor.

Data from: Beaugerie L, Pardi DS. Review article: drug-induced microscopic colitis - proposal for a scoring system and review of the literature. Aliment Pharmacol Ther. 2005;22(4):277-284. [PMID: 16097993]

Constipation

Constipation is often defined based on infrequent stool production, but increasing importance is being placed on stool consistency and effort required for defecation. The Bristol Stool Form Scale may be useful to objectively assess bowel habits (**Figure 22**). Functional constipation can affect up to 8% of the population and is assessed using the Rome III criteria, which evaluate straining, stool form and frequency, ease of evacuation, and manual maneuvers to defecate. Causes of constipation are described in **Table 20**.

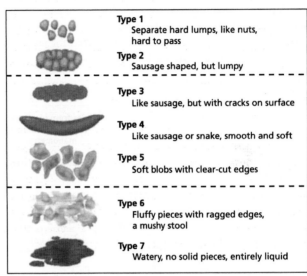

FIGURE 22. Bristol Stool Form Scale

Reprinted with permission from Macmillan Publishers Ltd: American Journal of Gastroenterology. Spiller RC, Thompson WG. Bowel disorders. 105:775-785. Copyright 2010.

TABLE 20. Causes of Constipation

Category	Examples
Metabolic	Hypothyroidism, hypercalcemia, diabetes mellitus, pregnancy
Structural	Colorectal cancer, strictures (ischemia, Crohn disease), hernias, mass lesions, endometriosis, rectocele, dyssynergic defecation
Medication-induced	Opiates, tricyclic antidepressants, iron, calcium channel blockers, aluminum- and calcium-containing antacids, antipsychotics
Neuromuscular	Intestinal pseudo-obstruction, spinal cord lesions, multiple sclerosis, autonomic neuropathy, Hirschsprung disease, colonic inertia
Inflammatory	Radiation, inflammatory bowel disease
Functional	Constipation-predominant irritable bowel syndrome
Toxicities	Bismuth, lead, herbal supplements

Evaluation and management of chronic constipation are described in **Figure 23**. History alone may often provide helpful clues in establishing the diagnosis. Patients with constipation should be asked about time of onset, stool frequency and form, alarm features (weight loss, rectal bleeding, sudden change in bowel habits, family history of colorectal cancer, or onset at greater than 50 years), new medications, dietary changes (decreased fluid intake, reduced fiber), altered activity level, other gastrointestinal symptoms (nausea, vomiting, abdominal pain), and effort with defecation (excessive straining, digitation for stool evacuation, repositioning on the toilet, and incomplete evacuation).

A physical examination that includes careful assessment of the abdomen, perineum, and rectum may uncover systemic diseases. The perianal area should be inspected for fissures, hemorrhoids, or other external lesions, and sensation of the perineum should be assessed. Rectal examination is useful to evaluate perineal descent, resting and squeeze tone, and the ability to relax the puborectalis and external anal sphincter when instructed. Masses or hard stool within the rectal vault should be noted.

Baseline laboratory studies should include a complete blood count, thyroid-stimulating hormone, serum calcium, and fasting glucose levels. Patients older than 50 years or those with alarm features should undergo colonoscopy. For patients with clinical features (digitation with defecation and sense of blockage in the anorectal region) or examination features (paradoxical contraction of the puborectalis or external anal sphincter) suggestive of dyssynergic defecation, anorectal manometry should be performed.

The initial management for constipation consists of treating reversible causes (medications, metabolic causes, or diet). Adequate fluid and fiber (25 to 30 g/d) intake is

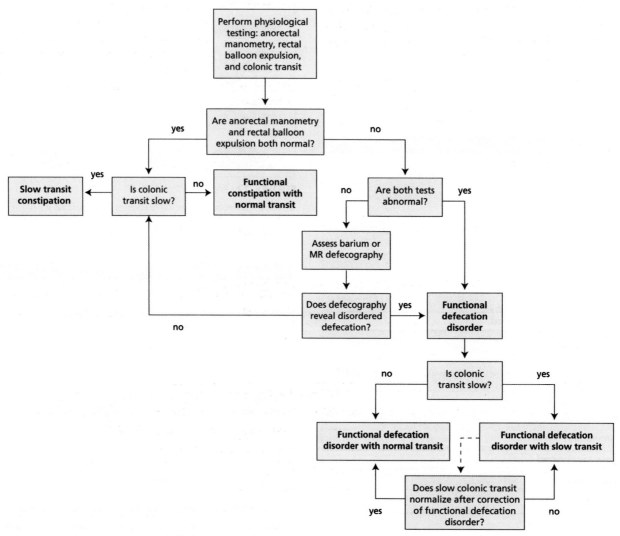

FIGURE 23. Evaluation and management of patients with functional constipation. MR = magnetic resonance.

essential. Fiber should be gradually escalated to prevent gaseous distention. Polyethylene glycol is well tolerated and is superior to other osmotic agents such as lactulose in improving stool frequency and form. Magnesium-containing antacids can be used but should be avoided in patients with chronic kidney disease or hypermagnesemia. A stool softener such as docusate sodium can be used as adjunctive therapy to ease evacuation in patients with hemorrhoids or hard stools. Stimulant laxatives, such as bisacodyl or senna, may be considered in patients with slow-transit constipation. Lubiprostone, a chloride channel activator that increases intestinal fluid secretion, can be used in patients with constipation-predominant irritable bowel syndrome or chronic idiopathic constipation. Methylnaltrexone can help with opioid-induced constipation without negating the benefits of the analgesia. Bowel obstruction should be excluded before initiating lubiprostone or methylnaltrexone. Patients with dyssynergic defecation should be referred for biofeedback. A subtotal colectomy with ileorectal anastomosis should be reserved for patients with refractory constipation after dyssynergic defecation has been ruled out and motility consultation has been completed. **H**

KEY POINTS

- Functional constipation can affect up to 8% of the population and is assessed using the Rome III criteria, which evaluate straining, stool form and frequency, ease of evacuation, and manual maneuvers to defecate.

- Patients with constipation who are older than 50 years or have alarm features (weight loss, rectal bleeding, sudden change in bowel habits, family history of colorectal cancer) should undergo colonoscopy.

Irritable Bowel Syndrome

Irritable bowel syndrome (IBS) is an intestinal syndrome defined by abdominal discomfort and altered bowel habits without an organic cause. It is common, with an estimated prevalence of 7% (range 1% to 20%), and is more common in women (1.5:1 female to male ratio), patients less than 50 years of age, and patients of lower socioeconomic status. Prevalence estimates are similar across all countries that have been studied. Risk factors for IBS are a family history of IBS, physical or sexual abuse, food intolerance, estrogen use, somatization traits, psychological distress, and low birth weight. The most widely studied and accepted risk factor is a history of infectious gastroenteritis; 7% to 30% of affected patients develop IBS.

The pathophysiology of IBS is poorly understood. Some evidence suggests altered motility, low-grade inflammation, dysfunctional serotonin signaling, altered intestinal bacterial flora, intestinal gas retention, and visceral hypersensitivity, all of which may interact with a genetic predisposition and environmental factors. Motility disorders such as gastroparesis, slow-transit constipation, and chronic intestinal pseudo-obstruction are not synonymous with IBS. The low-grade inflammation and abnormal cytokine milieu suspected to play a role in IBS are different from the overt intestinal inflammation that is seen on endoscopic evaluation of inflammatory bowel disease.

Evaluation

The history and physical examination are crucial to diagnosing IBS. Individual symptoms are not useful for distinguishing IBS from alternative diagnoses, and therefore clinical criteria have been proposed for the diagnosis of IBS. The Rome III criteria are used frequently in clinical practice to diagnose IBS but are not yet validated (**Table 21**). The

---

TABLE 21. Rome III Diagnostic Criteria and Subtyping for Irritable Bowel Syndrome

Recurrent abdominal pain or discomfort (abnormal sensation not described as pain) at least 3 days a month in past 3 months (with onset >6 months prior) associated with two or more of the following:

Improvement with defecation

Onset associated with change in frequency of stool

Onset associated with change in form (appearance) of stool

1. IBS with constipation (IBS-C)—hard or lumpy stools[a] ≥25% and loose (mushy) or watery stools[b] <25% of bowel movements[c]
2. IBS with diarrhea (IBS-D)—loose (mushy) or watery stools[b] ≥25% and hard or lumpy stools[a] <25% of bowel movements[c]
3. Mixed IBS (IBS-M)—hard or lumpy stools[a] ≥25% and loose (mushy) or watery stools[b] ≥25% of bowel movements[c]
4. Unsubtyped IBS (IBS-U)—insufficient abnormality of stool consistency to meet criteria IBS-C, D, or M[c]

[a]Bristol Stool Form Scale type 1-2 (separate hard lumps like nuts [difficult to pass] or sausage-shaped but lumpy).

[b]Bristol Stool Form Scale type 6-7 (fluffy pieces with ragged edges, mushy stool, or watery, no solid pieces, entirely liquid).

[c]In the absence of use of antidiarrheals or laxatives.

IBS = irritable bowel syndrome.

Reprinted from Alimentary Pharmacology & Therapeutics. 26(6). Ersryd A, Posserud I, Abrahamsson H, Simrén MM. Subtyping the irritable bowel syndrome by predominant bowel habit: Rome II versus Rome III; 953-961. Copyright 2007, with permission from John Wiley and Sons. AND Reprinted from The Lancet. Vol. 369. Spiller R. Clinical update: irritable bowel syndrome; 1586-1588. Copyright 2007, with permission from Elsevier.

American College of Gastroenterology recommends a simple definition: abdominal pain or discomfort that occurs in association with altered bowel habits over a period of at least 3 months. The diagnosis of IBS is further subtyped into diarrhea predominant (IBS-D), constipation predominant (IBS-C), or mixed (IBS-M), which alternates between diarrhea and constipation.

In the absence of alarm symptoms, a diagnosis of IBS can be made without many additional tests. Routine use of thyroid function tests, erythrocyte sedimentation rate, C-reactive protein level, stool study for ova and parasites, abdominal imaging, and colonoscopy are not recommended in the absence of alarm features, because they are unlikely to change the diagnosis. Serologic tests for celiac disease are recommended for IBS-M and IBS-D because the prevalence of celiac disease in patients with IBS symptoms is as high as 4%. A food diary is reasonable for patients with IBS-M or IBS-D because lactose malabsorption may be more prevalent in patients with IBS. Testing for small-bowel bacterial overgrowth is not recommended. The diagnosis of IBS may be established through the use of validated clinical symptom criteria and without extensive testing in the majority of cases, although in situations with an atypical presentation or with other factors leading to diagnostic uncertainty, the judicious use of specific, appropriate studies may be indicated.

The presence of alarm symptoms should prompt further diagnostic testing tailored to the clinical scenario. Alarm symptoms include age of onset greater than 50 years; nocturnal symptoms; anemia; weight loss; rectal bleeding; family history of colon cancer, inflammatory bowel disease, or celiac disease; or abnormal physical examination findings. Anemia and weight loss provide the best specificity for making an alternative diagnosis of colorectal cancer at 89% and 90%, respectively.

Management

Management of IBS begins by educating the patient on the disease and providing reassurance, both of which improve the patient-physician relationship. Patients commonly are concerned with the interaction of diet with IBS; however, current evidence does not suggest a role for food allergy testing or restrictive diets. Consideration of lactose malabsorption is reasonable, however. Modest evidence suggests that the probiotic *Bifidobacterium infantis* improves IBS symptoms.

Loperamide can be used to improve stool consistency and frequency in IBS-D, but it is not efficacious for IBS symptoms overall. Low-dose tricyclic antidepressants provide improvement of global symptoms of IBS and abdominal pain (number needed to treat = 4); they may be more efficacious in IBS-D owing to the anticholinergic effect on accelerated intestinal transit. Rifaximin, a nonabsorbed oral antibiotic, is not FDA approved for treatment of IBS but has been shown to improve global IBS symptoms. Alosetron, a 5-HT3 antagonist, is effective for IBS-D; however, it is monitored by the

FDA through a prescribing program because of an increased risk of severe constipation and colonic ischemia.

A high-fiber diet or fiber supplementation has been the cornerstone of treatment of IBS. Insoluble fiber (psyllium, ispaghula, calcium polycarbophil) appears to be modestly effective; however, soluble fiber (corn, wheat bran) is no better than placebo. Limited data on osmotic laxatives have shown improvement in bowel frequency but not abdominal pain. Lubiprostone is FDA approved for use in women with IBS-C; however, it is pregnancy category C, and a negative pregnancy test is required before starting therapy in women of childbearing age. Contraception should be used while taking lubiprostone. Lubiprostone is not a first-line agent in IBS-C, but it is appropriate for patients whose symptoms persist despite the use of fiber and standard laxatives.

For treatment of abdominal pain or discomfort, smooth-muscle relaxants such as hyoscine and peppermint oil show some short-term benefit; however, safety is not well documented. Selective serotonin reuptake inhibitors (SSRIs) are more effective than placebo at relieving global IBS symptoms and abdominal pain (number needed to treat = 3.5). SSRIs may be theoretically better for patients with IBS-C than those with IBS-D, because SSRIs may accelerate transit. Low-dose tricyclic antidepressants are effective for treatment of abdominal discomfort. Narcotic pain medications should not be given to patients with abdominal pain from IBS because they may lead to narcotic bowel syndrome and paradoxical worsening of pain.

The prognosis for patients with IBS is generally excellent. However, patients with IBS can develop serious conditions, and changes in symptoms should prompt reassessment. Patients with IBS are three times more likely to undergo cholecystectomy and twice as likely to receive an appendectomy or hysterectomy; continued assessment may help the patient avoid potentially unnecessary surgeries.

KEY POINTS

- Irritable bowel syndrome is a clinical diagnosis based on the Rome III criteria; in the absence of alarm features, extensive diagnostic evaluation is unnecessary.

- The three irritable bowel syndrome subtypes are diarrhea predominant (IBS-D), constipation predominant (IBS-C), or mixed (IBS-M), which alternates between diarrhea and constipation.

- The American College of Gastroenterology recommends routine serologic testing for celiac disease in patients with symptoms of diarrhea-predominant or mixed irritable bowel syndrome.

Diverticular Disease

Colonic diverticulosis is extremely common in Western populations, with prevalence estimates of 40% by age 60 years and 60% by age 80 years. The distal (sigmoid and descending) colon is most often affected. Among Asian populations, diverticula tend to be more densely clustered in the proximal (cecum, ascending, and transverse) colon. Affected patients may present with one to hundreds of diverticula, which usually measure 5 to 10 mm in diameter. Although definitive data are lacking, colonic diverticula appear to result from a combination of anatomic factors (intrinsic weakness where vasa recta penetrate the colon wall), motility factors (simultaneous or excessive haustral contractions), and dietary causes (decreased fiber intake). Genetic associations are inconclusive.

Approximately one in five patients with diverticulosis will experience at least one episode of diverticulitis, which presents with left lower quadrant pain, fever, and leukocytosis. Other features are anorexia, nausea, vomiting, dysuria, abdominal mass, guarding, and rebound tenderness. Conditions to consider in the differential diagnosis are appendicitis; Crohn disease; colorectal neoplasia (benign or malignant); ischemic or pseudomembranous colitis; ovarian cyst, abscess, or torsion; and ectopic pregnancy. Abdominopelvic CT is the test of choice if the diagnosis is not obvious from the history and examination. Colonoscopy and flexible sigmoidoscopy are relatively contraindicated owing to the potential for procedure-induced perforation.

The natural history of diverticulitis and general management recommendations are shown in **Table 22**. Following resolution of acute diverticulitis, the entire colorectum should be evaluated with colonoscopy to rule out other diagnoses that may mimic diverticulitis, such as adenocarcinoma or Crohn disease. Immunocompromised patients are at increased risk for secondary complications from acute diverticulitis and should be offered elective surgery following a single episode of disease. Data from large cohort studies do not support an association between nut, corn, or popcorn consumption and risk of diverticular disease.

For a discussion of diverticular bleeding, see Gastrointestinal Bleeding.

Ischemic Bowel Disease

Intestinal ischemic disease can be caused by a variety of factors and may be acute or chronic. Both the small bowel and colon can be affected by ischemia, but these typically have different clinical manifestations. The clinical presentation is broad, ranging from mild abdominal cramping and bleeding to severe, life-threatening surgical emergencies. Colonic ischemia is the most common form of intestinal ischemia; acute mesenteric ischemia is less common but is potentially more serious.

Acute Mesenteric Ischemia

Clinical Features and Diagnosis

Acute mesenteric ischemia is inadequate blood flow to all or part of the small bowel. Causes include superior mesenteric artery (SMA) embolus, SMA thrombosis, nonocclusive mesenteric ischemia (usually due to splanchnic vasoconstriction), mesenteric venous thrombosis, and focal segmental ischemia. SMA embolus from the left atrium or ventricular mural thrombi is the most common cause. The next most common cause is nonocclusive mesenteric ischemia after a cardiovascular event. These two causes account for approximately 75% of all cases of acute mesenteric ischemia.

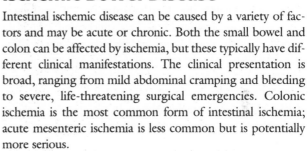

TABLE 22. Natural History of Diverticulitis

Subgroup	Features	Management
Isolated, uncomplicated	Solitary episode of acute diverticulitis	Antibiotics[a], bowel rest, analgesia
Recurrent, uncomplicated	Multiple discrete episodes of acute diverticulitis	Surgical resection on a case-by-case basis
Complicated	Acute diverticulitis with abscess, fistula, obstruction, perforation, or stricture	Antibiotics[a], percutaneous drainage[b], endoscopic stent[b], surgical resection
Smoldering	Acute diverticulitis with ongoing, chronic symptoms	Antibiotics[a], surgical resection

[a]Antibiotics should cover gram-negative rods and anaerobic bacteria; outpatient oral therapy may be adequate for patients with mild symptoms; inpatient intravenous therapy should be used for patients with severe symptoms and/or features of complicated disease.

[b]May be used as a temporizing measure as needed to convert from emergency to elective surgery

Reprinted from Gastroenterol Clin North Am. 38(3). Touzios JG, Dozois EJ. Diverticulosis and acute diverticulitis; 513-525. Copyright 2009, with permission from Elsevier.

Patients with acute mesenteric ischemia are typically older than 50 years and have underlying cardiac disease. The classic presentation is acute onset of severe abdominal pain; the abdomen is typically soft and less tender than expected based on the patient's symptoms (pain out of proportion to the examination). It is rare for a young person to develop acute mesenteric ischemia, but when it occurs it is usually caused by vasoactive medications such as cocaine and triptans.

Diagnosis of acute mesenteric ischemia requires a high level of suspicion. An elevated leukocyte count, metabolic acidosis, and elevated serum lactate level are common, but their absence should not exclude the diagnosis. Plain abdominal films may be normal early in the course of disease, but later they may show dilated loops of bowel and thumbprinting of the small bowel and right colon (the SMA also supplies the right colon). Ultrasound has a limited role because it may not adequately visualize the distal vasculature. CT may show intestinal pneumatosis and bowel wall thickening. Like plain films, CT may be normal early, and findings may not be obvious until necrotic bowel is present. CT and MR angiography are able to better diagnose acute intestinal ischemia earlier and define the vascular distribution of the insult. The gold standard is classic angiography. Although it is invasive, it allows the highest diagnostic accuracy and the potential for therapeutic intervention.

Treatment

The treatment of acute mesenteric ischemia is based on the underlying cause. For all patients, initial treatment should consist of cardiovascular resuscitation and initiation of antibiotics (to address the high frequency of sepsis secondary to bacterial translocation). Papaverine, a phosphodiesterase inhibitor, can be used at the time of angiography to relieve mesenteric vasoconstriction in patients with embolic and nonembolic arterial occlusion as well as nonocclusive mesenteric ischemia. For persistent signs of peritonitis, laparotomy is typically required. The use of anticoagulants is controversial because intestinal and intraperitoneal hemorrhage can occur. **H**

Chronic Mesenteric Ischemia

Clinical Features and Diagnosis

Chronic mesenteric ischemia, also called intestinal angina, is a manifestation of mesenteric atherosclerosis. The typical symptom is abdominal pain beginning approximately 30 minutes after eating, which is believed to be due to diversion of small-bowel blood flow to the stomach as digestion begins. The blood flow to the small bowel, which is already compromised, then has even more limited oxygen supply, leading to ischemia and subsequent abdominal pain. This typical symptom leads to a fear of eating (sitophobia), which causes the weight loss that is seen in most patients with chronic mesenteric ischemia. The natural history is progression of mild pain with eating to food avoidance, weight loss, and eventually

pain without eating. If progressive and left untreated, chronic mesenteric ischemia can rarely lead to intestinal infarction.

Diagnosis is made by clinical history and imaging. Doppler ultrasound is a screening test, but it cannot confirm the diagnosis and is often of limited use if patients are obese. MR or CT angiography may be more sensitive and specific, but an abnormal study still warrants confirmatory splanchnic angiography. Angiography should show occlusion of at least two of the major splanchnic arteries to make the diagnosis.

Treatment

Surgical revascularization is the definitive treatment for chronic mesenteric ischemia. Percutaneous angioplasty with or without stenting can be attempted in patients who are poor surgical candidates for bypass surgery. Short-term success rates are high with this percutaneous procedure, but long-term recurrence rates are significantly higher compared with surgical bypass.

Colonic Ischemia

Clinical Features and Diagnosis

Colonic ischemia comprises 75% of all cases of intestinal ischemia. The range of severity is broad, from a mild, reversible, transient colitis to gangrene and fulminant colitis with a high mortality rate. There are many causes of ischemic colitis; the most common are summarized in **Table 23**. Typical symptoms are the acute onset of mild, crampy abdominal pain with tenderness on examination over the affected region of colon. Bleeding may not occur early but often occurs within a few days of pain onset. Although plain abdominal films or CT may show thumbprinting, diagnosis is made by colonoscopy or flexible sigmoidoscopy. The most

TABLE 23. Causes of Ischemic Colitis
Arterial
Hypoperfusion: decreased cardiac output, cardiac arrhythmias, sepsis with shock
Thrombotic: thrombosis of the inferior mesenteric artery
Embolic: arterial emboli, cholesterol emboli
Drug-induced
Cocaine
Digoxin
Estrogens
Pseudoephedrine
Postoperative
Coronary artery bypass graft surgery
Abdominal aortic surgery
Vasculitis
Systemic lupus erythematosus
Hypercoagulable state
Protein C and S and antithrombin III deficiency; factor V Leiden mutation

commonly affected sites are the sigmoid and descending colon, as well as the "watershed" regions at the splenic flexure and rectosigmoid junction. The rectum is typically spared owing to its dual blood supply.

Treatment

Treatment is largely supportive. Most patients improve with intravenous fluids, broad-spectrum antibiotics, and reversal of any obvious causative agents. Even patients with severely ischemic colonic mucosa can have a remarkable and rapid reversal of signs and symptoms. Rarely, patients may develop peritoneal signs and shock and require urgent laparoscopy and colectomy. **H**

KEY POINTS

- Patients with acute mesenteric ischemia are typically older than 50 years and have underlying cardiac disease.
- The classic presentation of acute mesenteric ischemia is acute onset of severe abdominal pain; the abdomen is typically soft and less tender than expected based on the patient's symptoms (pain out of proportion to the examination).
- The natural history of chronic mesenteric ischemia is progression of mild abdominal pain with eating to food avoidance, weight loss, and eventually pain without eating.
- Typical symptoms of colonic ischemia are the acute onset of mild, crampy abdominal pain with tenderness on examination over the affected region of colon.

Colorectal Neoplasia

Epidemiology

Worldwide, colorectal malignancies rank third (N = 1,230,000 cases per year) in cancer incidence and fourth (N = 608,000 cases per year) in cancer mortality. Age-standardized incidence rates are higher for men than for women (gender ratio = 1.4:1). Incidence rates demonstrate considerable geographic variation; the majority of cases (approximately 60%) are reported from developed regions. In the United States, colorectal cancer ranks third in cancer incidence and mortality for both men and women. Colorectal cancer mortality rates have recently declined in the United States (for men, by 32% from 1990 to 2005; for women, by 28% from 1991 to 2005), presumably owing to improved early detection and treatment strategies. For reasons that remain incompletely defined, black patients have higher colorectal cancer incidence and mortality rates than other racial and ethnic groups in the United States.

KEY POINTS

- In the United States, colorectal cancer ranks third in cancer incidence and cancer mortality in both men and women.
- Colorectal cancer mortality rates have recently declined in the United States, presumably owing to improved early detection and treatment strategies.

Pathophysiology

Colorectal carcinogenesis is a complex process with heterogeneous outcomes. The full spectrum of genetic and epigenetic alterations is currently unknown, but most tumors are thought to proceed through the sequence of normal epithelium to premalignant adenoma to invasive adenocarcinoma. There are three major colorectal cancer subtypes based on molecular patterns of chromosomal instability (CIN), microsatellite instability (MSI), and CpG island methylator phenotype (CIMP).

Approximately two thirds of all colorectal cancers develop through the CIN pathway. CIN-positive tumors exhibit aberrant chromosomal content that varies between cells, with loss of heterozygosity as a characteristic feature.

MSI is observed in 15% to 20% of sporadic colorectal cancer cases. Microsatellites, which are small regions of repetitive nucleotide sequences, are prone to slippage-induced frameshift mutations during DNA replication. In the presence of genetically altered or epigenetically silenced DNA mismatch repair genes, these replication errors go uncorrected and can be detected as bandshifts on gel electrophoresis. MSI is categorized as MSI-high if greater than or equal to 30% of ten standard microsatellite markers display abnormal bandshifts. Clinicopathologic characteristics of MSI-high tumors are female preponderance, proximal colonic location, lower stage, higher grade, increased peritumoral lymphocyte infiltration, and diploid chromosome number.

CIMP is defined by the extent of promoter hypermethylation detected in select growth-regulating genes. Overall, 20% to 40% of colorectal cancers demonstrate a CIMP-positive phenotype. Emerging data suggest that some CIMP-positive tumors may evolve from serrated polyps rather than through the classic adenoma-carcinoma sequence. Inactivation of the *BRAF* gene appears to be an important early event in the proposed serrated pathway.

Risk Factors

Environmental Exposures

Diets higher in fruits, vegetables, and fiber have been associated with decreased colorectal cancer risk, but convincing prevention benefits have not yet been demonstrated. Calcium supplementation seems to have a favorable, albeit relatively modest, effect on colorectal cancer risk, but the putative benefit must be balanced against possible toxicities in other organ systems. Calcium binds to potentially harmful substances in the colorectal lumen and may also directly reduce mucosal proliferation. Although folate plays a role in DNA synthesis and gene expression, risks and benefits of supplementation remain unclear. Limited data suggest potential benefit of folate supplementation in lowering the risk for development of disease but also possible acceleration of tumor growth if unrecognized disease is already present. Excess red meat consumption, particularly when cooked at high temperatures or with a heavily charred surface, has also been linked to increased risk for colorectal cancer.

Cigarette smoking exposes the colorectal epithelium to a variety of potential carcinogens through both topical and systemic routes. Alcohol intake of 30 g/d or more increases colorectal cancer risk by approximately 25%; alcohol may disrupt normal DNA processing. Excess body weight (BMI >30), which can lead to higher circulating concentrations of growth hormones, cytokines, or energy substrates, has been associated with a 40% greater colorectal cancer risk. A high level of physical activity may reduce colorectal cancer risk by approximately 20%, which appears to be independent of BMI status.

Predisposing Conditions

Chronic inflammatory bowel disease (ulcerative colitis and Crohn disease) has been associated with increased risk for colorectal cancer; however, the magnitude of this risk increase is unclear. Duration of inflammatory bowel disease is an important factor; colorectal cancer incidence is low in patients with less than 8 years of disease, but incidence progressively increases after 10 years (2%), 20 years (8%), and 30 years (18%) of disease. The extent and location of colorectal involvement are also relevant. Pancolitis and distal colitis confer high and intermediate colorectal cancer risks, respectively, but proctitis appears to confer minimal (if any) increased risk compared with the general population. Age of onset of disease has not been clearly shown to increase malignant potential. Other risk factors include a concomitant diagnosis of primary sclerosing cholangitis and family history of colorectal cancer (especially when diagnosed at age <50 years).

Type 2 diabetes mellitus may increase colorectal cancer risk, perhaps owing to higher concentrations of circulating insulin and/or insulin-like growth factors related to obesity. Based on a meta-analysis of more than 2.5 million participants, diabetes was associated with a 30% higher risk for colorectal cancer than no diabetes. Although some studies have shown a higher risk for women than for men, and for proximal versus distal colorectal cancers, existing data are not conclusive.

Ureterosigmoidostomy is associated with a markedly elevated colorectal cancer risk (100 to 500 times higher than the general population), with a prolonged latency period that can exceed 50 years. Cholecystectomy has been associated with modestly increased colorectal cancer risk, perhaps as a consequence of altered fecal bile acid composition.

Nonsyndromic Family History

The strength of the association between family history of colorectal neoplasia and colorectal cancer risk is influenced by the degree of relationship, number of relatives affected, and age at diagnosis. In the setting of one first-degree relative or two second-degree relatives with colorectal cancer diagnosed at any age, the lifetime risk of developing colorectal cancer is elevated two- to threefold compared with the general population. When two first-degree relatives are affected, the cumulative risk is increased by three- to fourfold. Diagnosis of colorectal cancer in a first-degree relative at age 50 years or younger is also associated with a three- to fourfold risk increase.

A family history of colorectal adenoma appears to confer similarly increased colorectal cancer risks.

Hereditary Colorectal Cancer Syndromes

Hereditary Nonpolyposis Colorectal Cancer

Although the population prevalence of hereditary nonpolyposis colorectal cancer (HNPCC) is incompletely defined, this syndrome is thought to be the most common type of hereditary colorectal cancer (2% to 3% of all cases). The inheritance pattern is autosomal dominant. Colorectal adenomas develop at a relatively young age (by age 20 to 30 years) and are thought to progress to colorectal cancer more quickly than sporadic adenomas. The lifetime risk of colorectal cancer is approximately 80%, with a mean age at diagnosis of 44 years. Clinicopathologic features of HNPCC-associated colorectal cancers include proximal colon location (up to two thirds of all cases), poorly differentiated histology, and MSI-high phenotype. Endometrial adenocarcinoma is the second most common cancer in HNPCC, with a lifetime risk of approximately 30% to 60%. Additional HNPCC-related malignancies are gastric, biliary tract, urinary tract, ovarian, and small-bowel cancer. Pedigree analysis, with or without molecular testing, can be used to help identify possible HNPCC kindreds using the Amsterdam criteria II or the revised Bethesda guidelines, as shown in **Table 24.**

More recently, different cancer profiles have been described for Amsterdam criteria–positive families with a demonstrable DNA mismatch repair gene defect. The terms Lynch syndrome (mutation identified) and familial colorectal cancer type X (mutation not identified) have been proposed to distinguish these kindreds. Emerging data suggest that familial colorectal cancer type X may be associated with a more modest increase in colorectal cancer risk, along with a slightly later age at onset (50 to 60 years) compared with Lynch syndrome. In addition, endometrial and other extracolonic cancer risks appear to be lower in familial colorectal cancer type X than Lynch syndrome.

Familial Adenomatous Polyposis

The estimated incidence of familial adenomatous polyposis (FAP) is 1 in 6000 to 13,000 live births. This syndrome accounts for less than 1% of all cases of colorectal cancer.

TABLE 24. Criteria for Hereditary Nonpolyposis Colorectal Cancer Screening

Amsterdam Criteria II[a]
≥3 relatives with an HNPCC-associated cancer
≥2 successive generations affected
≥1 first-degree relative of at least 2 other cancer cases
≥1 cancer diagnosed before age 50 years

Revised Bethesda Guidelines[b]
Colorectal cancer diagnosed in a patient less than 50 years of age
Presence of synchronous, metachronous colorectal or other HNPCC-associated tumors, regardless of age
Colorectal cancer with the MSI-H histology diagnosed in a patient less than 60 years of age
Colorectal cancer diagnosed in one or more first-degree relatives with an HNPCC-related tumor, with one of the cancers diagnosed under age 50 years
Colorectal cancer diagnosed in two or more first- or second-degree relatives with HNPCC-related tumors, regardless of age

[a]Suspect HNPCC if all criteria are met. Used to identify families likely to represent HNPCC. Reprinted from Gastroenterology. 116(6). Vasen HF, Watson P, Mecklin JP, Lynch HT. New clinical criteria for hereditary nonpolyposis colorectal cancer (HNPCC, Lynch syndrome) proposed by the International Collaborative group on HNPCC; 1453-1456. Copyright 1999, with permission from Elsevier.

[b]Proceed with microsatellite instability testing if any criterion is met. Used to select colorectal cancer cases for molecular analyses of the DNA mismatch repair system. Reprinted from Umar A, Boland CR, Terdiman JP, et al. Revised Bethesda Guidelines for hereditary nonpolyposis colorectal cancer (Lynch syndrome) and microsatellite instability. J Natl Cancer Inst. 2004;96(4):261-268, by permission of Oxford University Press.

HNPCC = hereditary nonpolyposis colorectal cancer; MSI-H = microsatellite instability–high.

Germline mutations in the *APC* gene are inherited in an autosomal dominant pattern. Classically, FAP is characterized by hundreds to thousands of adenomatous polyps distributed throughout the colorectum, with a mean age at polyp diagnosis of 16 years. Without intervention, nearly all patients with FAP will develop colorectal cancer, with a mean age at cancer diagnosis of 39 years. Duodenal adenomas, particularly in the periampullary region, can be found in 50% to 90% of patients with FAP and portend a lifetime risk for duodenal cancer of 4% to 12% in affected patients. Other associated malignancies are papillary thyroid cancer, childhood hepatoblastoma, and gastric adenocarcinoma. Benign conditions linked to FAP include gastric fundic gland polyps, small-bowel adenomas, osteomas, desmoid tumors, supernumerary teeth, and congenital hypertrophy of the retinal pigment epithelium. Medulloblastoma, glioma, or ependymoma may occur in a subset of families with the Turcot variant, which can also be associated with HNPCC. Classic FAP should be suspected when more than 100 colorectal adenomas are identified. *APC* mutational analysis can be used to confirm the diagnosis.

Attenuated Familial Adenomatous Polyposis
Attenuated familial adenomatous polyposis (AFAP) is a subset of FAP in which affected individuals develop fewer (<100), often more proximally distributed, colorectal adenomas. Clinical presentation may be delayed until the fourth or fifth decade of life. The cumulative colorectal cancer risk appears to be slightly lower for AFAP (approximately 70%) than for classic FAP (approximately 100%). Extracolonic features include upper gastrointestinal tract polyps but are otherwise less prominent than in classic FAP. Germline mutations are typically found in the extreme distal or proximal ends of the *APC* gene.

MYH-Associated Polyposis
MYH-associated polyposis (MAP) is characterized by heterozygous and homozygous mutations in the *MYH* gene (involved in DNA base-excision repair). These mutations may be found in approximately 1% (heterozygous) and 0.5% to 1% (homozygous) of the general population. The inheritance pattern is autosomal recessive, with biallelic *MYH* mutations predisposing to somatic alterations in *APC* and/or other key growth-regulating genes. The clinical spectrum of MAP often resembles AFAP, but emerging data suggest that the full spectrum of extracolonic neoplasia may be much broader, depending on which genes are secondarily affected. Genetic testing for *MYH* germline mutations is not yet routinely performed in clinical practice.

Peutz-Jeghers Syndrome
The estimated incidence of Peutz-Jeghers syndrome (PJS) is 1 in 8300 to 280,000 live births. Germline mutations in the *STK11/LKB1* gene are inherited with an autosomal dominant pattern. Clinical manifestations consist of mucocutaneous melanocytic macules (particularly in the perioral region and over the buccal mucosa) and gastrointestinal hamartomatous polyps, which may present during adolescence or early adulthood with symptoms of abdominal pain, bleeding, obstruction, or intussusception. PJS-associated hamartomatous polyps are most commonly located in the small intestine (60% to 90%) but can also be found in the colorectum, biliary tract, respiratory tract, or genitourinary tract. Colorectal adenomas can also be observed in patients with PJS. Cancer risk

is markedly increased, with 50% to 90% of affected individuals developing at least one malignancy over the course of a lifetime. By site, cumulative cancer risks are: colorectal cancer, 40%; gastric, 30% to 60%; pancreas, 35%; small intestine, 15% to 30%; esophagus, 0.5% to 33%; breast, 54%; ovary, 21%; lung, 15%; cervix, 10%; uterus, 9%; and testes, 9%. Proposed diagnostic criteria vary slightly but generally require a combination of histologically confirmed hamartomatous polyp(s) with distinctive PJS features (arborizing smooth muscle fibers), mucocutaneous melanocytic macules, and/or a known family history of PJS. *STK11/LKB1* mutational analysis can also be performed to confirm a suspected PJS diagnosis.

Juvenile Polyposis Syndrome

The estimated incidence of juvenile polyposis syndrome (JPS) is 1 in 16,000 to 100,000 live births. Germline mutations in the *BMPR1A*, *SMAD4*, or *PTEN* genes can be detected in JPS families. Benign juvenile hamartomatous polyps are relatively common, occurring as solitary, sporadic lesions in up to 2% of children younger than 10 years and characterized pathologically with dilated, mucus-filled crypts with an inflammatory infiltrate in the lamina propria. In contrast, patients with JPS have multiple polyps that are distributed throughout the gastrointestinal tract. Abdominal pain, diarrhea, bleeding, obstruction, or intussusception may occur during childhood or adolescence, with an average age at JPS diagnosis of 18.5 years. Approximately two thirds of untreated patients with JPS develop colorectal cancer by age 60 years. Other associated malignancies are gastric, duodenal, and pancreatic cancer. Some patients with JPS may also have hereditary hemorrhagic telangiectasia, which can present with digital clubbing. A clinical diagnosis of JPS can be made based on any of the following: (1) three or more juvenile polyps in the colorectum, (2) multiple juvenile polyps throughout the gastrointestinal tract, or (3) any number of juvenile polyps coupled with a family history of JPS. Genetic testing is not yet routinely performed in clinical practice.

Hyperplastic Polyposis

Hyperplastic polyposis (HPP), a familial predisposition to multiple and/or large hyperplastic polyps in the colorectum, has been recognized; however, the population-based prevalence, underlying genetic alteration, and usual inheritance pattern remain incompletely defined. Colorectal cancer risk is increased to an unknown degree. According to the World Health Organization, the diagnosis of HPP can be made if any of the following criteria are met: (1) five or more histologically confirmed hyperplastic polyps located proximal to the sigmoid colon, of which two or more are larger than 1 cm in diameter; (2) any number of hyperplastic polyps located proximal to the sigmoid colon in a person who has one or more first-degree relatives with documented HPP; or (3) more than 30 hyperplastic polyps distributed throughout the colorectum.

KEY POINTS

- Smoking, alcohol consumption, excess body weight, and diet high in red meat have been linked to an increased risk for colorectal cancer.
- Patients with inflammatory bowel disease or type 2 diabetes mellitus are at higher risk for developing colorectal cancer.
- The most common hereditary colon cancer syndrome is hereditary nonpolyposis colorectal cancer, which confers a lifetime risk of colorectal cancer of approximately 80%.

Screening

Average Risk

Approximately three quarters of all colorectal cancers are diagnosed in average-risk persons (that is, persons without previously identified colorectal cancer risk factors). Approximately 90% occur during the sixth decade of life or later. The American College of Physicians issued a guidance statement in 2012 on screening for colorectal cancer based on a rigorous and comprehensive review of existing guidelines. They recommend that clinicians perform an individualized assessment of risk for colorectal cancer in all adults. Those with average risk should begin screening at age 50 years (age 40 years for black patients) and continue at intervals based on the method of screening chosen and the results of screening until age 75 years or until there is a life expectancy of less than 10 years. Multiple test options have been endorsed by national organizations, and their recommendations for screening for colorectal cancer in average-risk individuals with different modalities are shown in **Table 25**. The American Cancer Society, the U.S. Multi-Society Task Force on Colorectal Cancer, and the American College of Radiology divide colorectal cancer screening options into two categories: (1) tests that detect premalignant adenomas and colorectal cancer (flexible sigmoidoscopy, colonoscopy, double-contrast barium enema, and CT colonography) and (2) tests that primarily detect colorectal cancer (stool assays). Conversely, based on strict rules of evidence and computer simulation models, the U.S. Preventive Services Task Force interpreted existing data as insufficient to support CT colonography or stool DNA testing for average-risk colorectal cancer screening. The ACP guidance statement recommends using a stool-based test, flexible sigmoidoscopy, or optical colonoscopy for screening in patients at average risk. Further description of the endorsed screening tests (except barium enema) is provided in the following sections.

Guaiac Fecal Occult Blood Test

Guaiac fecal occult blood testing (gFOBT) uses a reagent that changes color in the presence of peroxidase, which is found in human blood, animal blood, and other dietary sources. Proper test performance typically requires the collection of two samples

TABLE 25. Colorectal Cancer Screening Guidelines for Average-Risk Persons

Screening Option	ACP	ACS-USMSTF-ACR	USPSTF	Screening Interval[a]
Guaiac fecal occult blood testing	Recommended	Recommended if >50% sensitivity for CRC	Recommended	1 year
Fecal immunochemical test	Recommended	Recommended if >50% sensitivity for CRC	Recommended	1 year
Stool DNA test	Recommended	Recommended if >50% sensitivity for CRC	Not recommended owing to insufficient evidence	Uncertain
Flexible sigmoidoscopy	Recommended	Recommended if sigmoidoscope is inserted to 40 cm of the colon or to the splenic flexure	Recommended, with fecal occult blood test every 3 years	5 years
CT colonography	Uncertain	Recommended, with referral for colonoscopy if polyps ≥6 mm in diameter are detected	Not recommended owing to insufficient evidence	5 years
Colonoscopy	Recommended	Recommended	Recommended	10 years
Barium enema	Not recommended	Recommended, but only if other endorsed options are not available	Not recommended	5 years

[a]Assuming a negative/normal test result

ACP = American College of Physicians; ACS-USMSTF-ACR = American Cancer Society, U.S. Multi-Society Task Force on Colorectal Cancer, and American College of Radiology; CRC = colorectal cancer; USPSTF = U.S. Preventive Services Task Force.

Reprinted from Gastroenterology. 138(6). Lieberman D. Progress and challenges in colorectal cancer screening and surveillance; 2115-2126. Copyright 2010, with permission from Elsevier.

from three consecutive stools (six samples total). Samples can be obtained at home and mailed in to a clinical laboratory for processing and analysis. Randomized, controlled trials have shown statistically significant reductions in colorectal cancer incidence (17% to 20%) and mortality (15% to 33%) with regular gFOBT screening. Limitations of gFOBT screening are low sensitivity for advanced adenomas (11% to 41%), diet and medication interactions that may produce false-positive or false-negative results, the need for annual testing if negative, and the need for appropriate diagnostic follow-up (ideally by colonoscopy) if testing is positive to achieve maximum benefit. For any positive screening gFOBT result, colonoscopy is the indicated diagnostic test. Current recommendations from the U.S. Multi-Society Task Force on Colorectal Cancer specify that a high-sensitivity gFOBT be used if this colorectal cancer screening option is pursued.

Fecal Immunochemical Test

Fecal immunochemical test (FIT) assays incorporate antibodies directed against the human globin protein, improving its specificity over gFOBT assay methodology. In cross-sectional studies, single-episode screening estimates of FIT sensitivity have ranged from 60% to 85% for colorectal cancer and 25% to 50% for advanced adenomas. Sample collection can be completed at home, and pretest dietary restrictions are not necessary. As with gFOBT screening, FIT screening requires annual testing for negative results and appropriate diagnostic follow-up for a positive result.

Stool DNA Test

Unlike fecal occult blood tests, stool DNA (sDNA) assays target molecular alterations that originate directly from the lesion of interest. Currently, an entire stool specimen (30 g minimum) must be submitted for evaluation. In two prospective screening studies reported to date, multi-marker sDNA assays demonstrated moderate sensitivity for colorectal cancer (25% to 58%) and lower sensitivity for adenomas 1 cm or larger (8% to 45%). Evolving DNA extraction and analysis protocols, as well as iterative marker selection, may lead to improved performance characteristics. At present, sDNA testing is not routinely available for colorectal cancer screening.

Flexible Sigmoidoscopy

Flexible sigmoidoscopy is endoscopic evaluation of the lower colorectum (up to 60 cm). It is typically performed after limited bowel preparation (two enemas) and without conscious sedation during the procedure. Patients with adenomas of any size or polyps larger than 5 mm (if biopsies are not obtained) should undergo full colonoscopy. Screening benefits appear to be most pronounced in the examined bowel segment, with mortality reduced by approximately 60%. Because proximal neoplasia is reportedly more common among black patients and older women, proceeding directly to colonoscopy for screening may be more prudent in these patients. A potential complication of flexible sigmoidoscopy is bowel perforation, which occurs in less than 1 in 20,000 examinations.

CT Colonography

CT colonography provides radiologic evaluation of the entire colorectum, as well as limited evaluation of extracolonic structures in the abdomen and pelvis. Dietary restrictions, full cathartic preparation, and oral contrast ingestion are required prior to CT colonography. During the examination, a small rectal catheter is placed to insufflate the colon with room air or carbon dioxide. Conscious sedation is not required. Compared with colonoscopy as the structural reference standard, CT colonography has estimated sensitivities of greater than 90% for colorectal cancer and 85% to 93% for polyps 1 cm or larger. Diagnostic and/or therapeutic colonoscopy is recommended for one or more polyps 1 cm or larger, or three or more polyps 6 mm or larger. Bowel perforation can occur from CT colonography, but the rate appears to be extremely low (<1 in 10,000 examinations).

Colonoscopy

Colonoscopy permits endoscopic evaluation of the entire colorectum. Dietary restrictions and full cathartic preparation are required prior to the procedure, and conscious sedation is administered during the procedure. In contrast to other endorsed screening options, therapeutic polypectomy can be completed during the baseline procedure.

Although colonoscopy screening has not been rigorously investigated in randomized, controlled trials, observational data suggest that substantial reductions in colorectal cancer incidence (53% to 72%) and mortality (31%) may be obtained from this strategy. If no polyps are detected during a high-quality baseline colonoscopy evaluation (cecal intubation accomplished, mucosa well visualized with minimal fecal debris, and withdrawal time ≥6 minutes), the next colonoscopy can be performed in 10 years. As defined by the American Society for Gastrointestinal Endoscopy/American College of Gastroenterology task force on quality in endoscopy, an adequate bowel preparation allows confidence that mass lesions other than small (<5 mm) polyps were generally not obscured by residual debris. If the bowel preparation is not adequate, the screening evaluation should be repeated before planning a long-term surveillance program. It is important to recognize colonoscopy "miss rates" when determining an appropriate surveillance interval; miss rates are 5% for colorectal cancer, 2% to 12% for polyps

TABLE 26. Colorectal Cancer Surveillance for Patients at Increased Risk

Patient Group	Preferred Test	Onset	Surveillance Interval[a]	Other Considerations[a]
Inflammatory Bowel Disease				
UC, pancolitis	Colonoscopy	IBD duration >8 years	1-2 years	
UC, distal colitis	Colonoscopy	IBD duration >8 years	1-2 years	
UC, proctitis	Colonoscopy	IBD duration >8 years	10 years	
Crohn disease, ≥1/3 of colon involved	Colonoscopy	IBD duration >8 years	1-2 years	
With PSC	Colonoscopy	At PSC diagnosis	1 year	
Nonsyndromic Family History				
1 first-degree relative with CRC[b]	Colonoscopy	Age 40 years or age 10 years before youngest age at CRC diagnosis in the family, whichever is younger	5 years	
Hereditary Cancer Syndromes				
Lynch syndrome	Colonoscopy	Age 20-25 years[b]	1-2 years	Transvaginal ultrasound or endometrial aspirate at age 25-30 years, repeat every 1 year (women) Urine cytology at onset of CRC screening, repeat every 1 year Upper endoscopy screening may be offered in families with gastric cancer
Familial CRC type X	Colonoscopy	Age 5-10 years before youngest age at CRC diagnosis in the family	3-5 years	

(continued on next page)

TABLE 26. Colorectal Cancer Surveillance for Patients at Increased Risk *(continued)*

Patient Group	Preferred Test	Onset	Surveillance Interval[a]	Other Considerations[a]
Hereditary Cancer Syndromes *(continued)*				
Familial adenomatous polyposis, classic	Flexible sigmoidoscopy	Age 10-12 years	1 year	Abdominal ultrasound and serum α-fetoprotein, age 0-6 years, repeat every 1 year Upper endoscopy (with side-viewing examination of the duodenal papilla) when CRN detected or by age 25 years, repeat every 1-3 years Palpation of thyroid gland, repeat every 1 year
Familial adenomatous polyposis, attenuated	Colonoscopy	Age 5-10 years before youngest age at CRC diagnosis in the family	1 year	
MYH-associated polyposis	Colonoscopy	Age 25-30 years	3-5 years	Upper endoscopy (with side-viewing examination of the duodenal papilla) at age 30-35 years, repeat every 3-5 years
Peutz-Jeghers syndrome	Colonoscopy	Age 25 years	2-3 years	Upper endoscopy and small-bowel radiography at age 10 years, repeat every 2 years Testicular exam at age 10 years, repeat every 1 year (men) Pelvic exam with cervical smear at age 20 years, repeat every 1 year (women) Mammography at age 25-35 years, repeat every 1 year (women)
Juvenile polyposis	Colonoscopy	Age 12 years	3 years	Upper endoscopy by age 15 years, then repeat every 1-3 years
Hyperplastic polyposis	Colonoscopy	Age 40 years[b]	5 years	

[a]Assuming negative/normal test result

[b]The U.S. Multi-Society Task Force on Colorectal Cancer recommends colonoscopic screening for patients with a first-degree relative with CRN at age <60 years or ≥2 first-degree relatives with CRC diagnosed at any age beginning at age 40 years or age 10 years before youngest age at CRN or CRC diagnosis in the family, whichever is younger, and any modality screening beginning at age 40 years for 1 first-degree relative with CRN diagnosed at age >60 years or ≥2 second-degree relatives with CRC diagnosed at any age.

CRC = colorectal cancer; CRN = colorectal neoplasia (adenoma or adenocarcinoma); IBD = inflammatory bowel disease; PSC = primary sclerosing cholangitis; UC = ulcerative colitis.

1 cm or larger, and more than 20% for polyps 6 mm or larger. Other potential risks associated with colonoscopy screening are clinically significant bleeding (2 to 6 per 1000 examinations) and bowel perforation (approximately 1 per 1000 examinations).

Increased Risk

Colorectal cancer screening guidelines for patients at increased risk owing to chronic inflammatory bowel disease, nonsyndromic family history, or a hereditary cancer syndrome are provided in **Table 26.** Specific early detection algorithms for potentially higher-risk patients with type 2 diabetes, ureterosigmoidostomy, or cholecystectomy have not been established, so colorectal cancer screening strategies for these patients should be formulated on an individual basis.

KEY POINTS

- Approximately three quarters of all colorectal cancers are diagnosed in average-risk persons (persons without previously identified colorectal cancer risk factors).
- Age 50 years is the accepted threshold for initiating screening in average-risk persons; screening should be continued until age 75 years or until there is a life expectancy of less than 10 years.

Surveillance

Postpolypectomy

Patients with one or more adenomas detected during a colorectal cancer screening evaluation are at increased risk for developing subsequent advanced colorectal neoplasia.

Adenoma multiplicity, size, morphology, and histology are thought to be the strongest predictors of future risk. If a high-quality baseline colonoscopy evaluation was performed, the postpolypectomy surveillance interval can be stratified based on these characteristics. For low-risk patients (1 to 2 adenomas, <1 cm, tubular morphology, and low-grade dysplasia), surveillance colonoscopy can be repeated in 5 to 10 years. For high-risk patients (≥3 adenomas, ≥1 cm, villous morphology, or high-grade dysplasia), surveillance colonoscopy should be repeated in 3 years, assuming complete removal of the index lesion(s). If more than 10 adenomas are detected during a single evaluation, the next colonoscopy should be repeated in less than 3 years and the possibility of an underlying hereditary cancer syndrome should be considered. Patients with large, sessile adenomas that are removed piecemeal should undergo repeat colonoscopy at a relatively short interval (2 to 6 months) to ensure complete resection. Patients with small, hyperplastic, rectal polyps only (without meeting criteria for hyperplastic polyposis syndrome) should undergo surveillance according to average-risk screening guidelines.

Post–Colorectal Cancer Treatment

Patients with colorectal cancer who receive potentially curative treatment (such as surgery, chemotherapy, radiation therapy, or a combination of these) should be monitored aggressively to detect early recurrence and perform surveillance for metachronous colorectal neoplasia in the remaining colorectal segment. Preoperative clearing colonoscopy (or CT colonography for obstructing tumors) is recommended to identify synchronous malignancies, which occur in approximately 2% to 7% of all patients with colorectal cancer. Following treatment, surveillance colonoscopy should be repeated 1 year after the clearing examination. If normal findings are observed, subsequent surveillance colonoscopies can be performed at 3 years and 5 years after the clearing examination, respectively. If adenomas are detected, surveillance intervals can be tailored according to postpolypectomy guidelines.

> **KEY POINTS**
>
> - Patients with one or more adenomas detected during a colorectal cancer screening evaluation are at increased risk for developing subsequent advanced colorectal neoplasia; these patients should receive surveillance colonoscopy.
> - Patients with colorectal cancer who receive potentially curative treatment should be monitored aggressively to detect early recurrence and/or to prevent metachronous colorectal neoplasia in the remaining colorectal segment.

Clinical Presentation

Symptoms of colorectal cancer are often related to anatomic location and size of the tumor. For tumors originating in the proximal colon (cecum to splenic flexure), common symptoms include nonspecific abdominal pain, unintentional weight loss, and occult gastrointestinal bleeding. Tumors arising from the distal colon (descending and sigmoid) or rectum can present with increased stool frequency (small caliber), incomplete evacuation, constipation, or hematochezia. Clinical signs that may be related to colorectal cancer are anemia, fistula, mass lesion, or unexplained abscess. At presentation, approximately 40% of patients have localized disease, 36% have regional metastases, 19% have distant metastases, and 5% are unstaged. Relatively frequent sites for distant metastases are the liver, peritoneal cavity, and lungs; the adrenal glands, ovaries, and skeletal system are less commonly involved. Metastases to the brain or central nervous system are rare.

Diagnosis and Staging

Colonoscopy is the initial test of choice for evaluating symptoms suggestive of colorectal cancer because biopsy samples can be obtained during the diagnostic procedure. Staging is determined by depth of tumor invasion, extent of nodal involvement, and presence or absence of distant metastases. For colon cancers, the clinical (or preoperative) stage is generally based on the physical examination, abdominopelvic CT, and chest radiography findings. The rectal cancer staging evaluation usually includes endoscopic ultrasonography or pelvic MRI in addition to the tests for colon cancers. The final pathologic stage is determined following surgery. Based on Surveillance Epidemiology and End Results (SEER) program data from 1999 to 2006, the 5-year relative survival rate for patients with any colorectal cancer is 65%, with estimates of 90%, 70%, and 12% for localized, regional, and distant stages of disease, respectively. For management of colorectal cancer, see MKSAP 16 Hematology and Oncology.

Chemoprevention

The goal of colorectal cancer chemoprevention is to apply pharmaceutical and/or nutritional compounds to prevent, inhibit, or reverse the carcinogenic process prior to the malignant transformation of premalignant dysplasia. Leading candidate agents include NSAIDs, difluoromethylornithine (DFMO), exogenous estrogen, calcium carbonate, and vitamin D. However, existing data do not support routine clinical application of any candidate agent strictly for colorectal cancer chemoprevention outside of high-risk patient populations.

> **KEY POINT**
>
> - Outside of hereditary cancer syndromes, the risks outweigh the benefits of using NSAIDs or estrogen replacement therapy strictly for colorectal cancer chemoprevention.

Disorders of the Liver

Approach to the Patient with Abnormal Liver Chemistry Studies

Abnormal liver chemistries are found in as many as 13% of patients undergoing medical evaluations for any cause. Serum aspartate aminotransferase (AST) and alanine aminotransferase (ALT) elevations indicate hepatocyte inflammation or injury. In addition to the liver, AST is produced in the heart, skeletal muscles, and kidneys. However, ALT is produced minimally in nonhepatic tissues, so ALT elevations are more specific for diagnosing liver disease.

Serum alkaline phosphatase and bilirubin elevations imply biliary injury or abnormalities in the flow of bile. However, alkaline phosphatase elevations can also reflect bone injury or pregnancy. Laboratory fractionation of alkaline phosphatase can clarify the tissue of origin. Bilirubin is measured in conjugated (direct) and unconjugated (indirect) forms. Predominance of conjugated bilirubin indicates disease of the liver; predominance of unconjugated bilirubin indicates non–liver-disease states such as hemolysis or Gilbert syndrome, which is characterized by benign defects in bilirubin conjugation.

Measurements of serum albumin and prothrombin time reflect the synthetic function of the liver. However, albumin level can be affected by nutritional state and renal or gastrointestinal protein losses. Prothrombin time can also be adversely affected by nutritional state, specifically vitamin K deficiency.

It is common for elevations of hepatocellular (AST, ALT) and cholestatic (alkaline phosphatase, bilirubin) injury markers to coexist. The relative pattern and severity of these injury markers give important clues to the cause of liver inflammation, as described in **Table 27**. The duration of liver test elevation can also aid in diagnosis. Acute hepatitis exists when abnormalities have been present for less than 6 months; chronic hepatitis occurs when abnormalities have been present for more than 6 months. **H**

TABLE 27. Liver Chemistry Studies as Clues to the Diagnosis of Liver Inflammation

Disease	AST	ALT	Alkaline Phosphatase	Bilirubin	Other Features
Acute viral hepatitis	↑↑↑	↑↑↑	↑↑	Normal to ↑↑↑	Exposure history; constitutional symptoms
Chronic viral hepatitis	↑	↑↑	Normal to ↑	Normal	History of percutaneous, sexual, or perinatal exposure
Nonalcoholic steatohepatitis	↑	↑↑	Normal to ↑	Normal	Metabolic syndrome
Alcoholic hepatitis	↑↑	↑	Normal to ↑	Normal to ↑↑↑	History of alcohol abuse
Acute autoimmune hepatitis	↑↑↑	↑↑↑	Normal to ↑	Normal to ↑↑↑	Positive autoantibodies
Chronic autoimmune hepatitis	↑	↑↑	Normal to ↑	Normal	Positive autoantibodies
Wilson disease (acute or chronic)	↑↑	↑↑	↓	↑ (unconjugated)	Hemolysis, neuropsychiatric abnormalities, renal tubular acidosis
α₁-Antitrypsin deficiency (chronic)	↑	↑	Normal to ↑	Normal	Lung disease
Hemochromatosis (chronic)	↑	↑	Normal to ↑	Normal	Elevated ferritin
Primary biliary cirrhosis (chronic)	↑	↑	↑↑↑	Normal to ↑↑	Antimitochondrial antibodies
Primary sclerosing cholangitis (chronic)	↑	↑	↑↑↑	Normal to ↑↑	Presence of inflammatory bowel disease
Large bile duct obstruction (acute)	↑↑	↑↑	↑↑	↑↑	Abdominal pain
Infiltrative liver disease (such as lymphoma)	↑	↑	↑↑↑	Normal	Malaise, hepatomegaly
Ischemic hepatitis ("shock liver")	↑↑↑	↑↑↑	Normal to ↑	Normal	History of hypotension, rapid resolution of liver tests

ALT = alanine aminotransferase; AST = aspartate aminotransferase.

Viral Hepatitis

Hepatitis A

Hepatitis A virus (HAV) is a common cause of acute hepatitis in the United States. Clinical symptoms such as malaise, fatigue, nausea, and right upper quadrant discomfort develop 2 to 6 weeks after exposure. Jaundice and cholestasis can develop 1 to 2 weeks after the onset of symptoms. Symptoms are typically more severe in adults than children, in whom acute HAV infection can be clinically silent. Acute HAV is diagnosed by detecting serum anti-HAV IgM antibodies. Jaundice peaks in severity 2 weeks after onset, and clinical recovery is typically complete by 3 months. Occasionally, a relapsing or prolonged cholestasis syndrome develops. Overt liver failure is very rare. HAV is a self-limited infection and does not cause chronic hepatitis.

Persons at risk for HAV infection are travelers to endemic areas and men who have sex with men; vaccination of high-risk populations can prevent infection. Infected patients are contagious during the incubation period and for approximately 1 week after the onset of jaundice. Because infection is transmitted enterically, hand-washing and proper cooking of foods are crucial in preventing the spread of HAV.

Prompt vaccination of patients exposed to HAV can prevent the development of acute infection. For patients in whom vaccination may be unreliable (such as immunocompromised patients), immune globulin should be administered as postexposure prophylaxis.

Hepatitis B

Approximately 350 million persons worldwide and 1.25 million in the United States have hepatitis B virus (HBV) infection. HBV can cause both acute and chronic hepatitis. HBV is highly transmissible by blood (including needlestick), mucocutaneous (such as sexual contact), or perinatal exposures.

Diagnosis

HBV is diagnosed by serologic tests for HBV antigens and antibodies as well as direct HBV DNA assays, as described in Table 28. Acute HBV is characterized by symptoms similar to those of acute HAV. The incubation period of HBV is 4 to 16 weeks. HBV acquired in adulthood commonly results in an acute infection followed by resolution. In contrast, patients infected during childhood will typically develop chronic HBV infection. Adult patients who acquired HBV perinatally often are in an immune-tolerant state, which is characterized by high levels of HBV DNA but no active hepatic inflammation; these patients are at risk for conversion to active HBV. Inactive carriers of HBV have low levels of HBV DNA and are believed to be at low risk of progression of liver disease; therefore, initiation of medications to treat HBV in these patients is not justified. These patients maintain risk for reactivation of HBV, which may cause subsequent progression of liver disease. Monitoring for the development of chronic active HBV is therefore warranted for HBV immune-tolerant patients or HBV inactive carriers.

Management

The goal of HBV treatment is to reduce progression to significant chronic liver disease and complications of chronic HBV such as hepatocellular cancer.

Management of HBV is dependent on the interpretation of the serologic studies as described in Table 28. Acute HBV infection is managed with supportive care. Acute HBV in the adult patient is typically self limited. The role of oral antiviral medications in the management of acute HBV is restricted to patients who are developing liver failure from severe acute HBV. Fulminant liver failure caused by HBV may require liver transplantation.

Patients with chronic active HBV infection, defined by elevated hepatic aminotransferases or active inflammation on liver biopsy, should receive antiviral therapy. Clinical outcomes are improved in patients with chronic active HBV with effective viral suppression. The available antiviral medications for HBV are shown in **Table 29**. The goal of antiviral treatment is ideally to convert hepatitis B surface antigen (HBsAg)–positive status to HBsAg-negative status, although a more common goal is to induce suppression of viral replication without necessarily obtaining clearance of virus.

TABLE 28. Interpretation of Hepatitis B Virus Serologic Studies

Condition	HBsAg	HBsAb	HBc IgM	HBc IgG	HBeAg	HBeAb	HBV DNA	AST, ALT
Acute HBV	+	−	+	−	+	−	+	↑↑
Chronic active HBV	+	−	−	+	+ or −	+ or −	High	↑
Inactive HBV carrier	+	−	−	+	−	+ or −	Low	Normal
Immune-tolerant HBV	+	−	−	+	+ or −	+ or −	High	Normal
Resolved HBV	−	+	−	+	−	+	−	Normal
Previously immunized	−	+	−	−	−	−	−	Normal

ALT = alanine aminotransferase; AST = aspartate aminotransferase; HBc IgG = IgG antibody to hepatitis B core antigen; HBc IgM = IgM antibody to hepatitis B core antigen; HBeAb = antibody to hepatitis B e antigen; HBeAg = hepatitis B e antigen; HBsAb = antibody to hepatitis B surface antigen; HBsAg = hepatitis B surface antigen; HBV = hepatitis B virus.

TABLE 29. Medical Therapy for Hepatitis B Virus Infection

Medication	Duration of Therapy	Expense	Potency	Resistance
Peginterferon	1 year	↑↑↑		None
Lamivudine	6 months after HBeAg seroconversion, or loss of HBsAg if HBeAg negative to start	↑	High	High
Telbivudine	6 months after HBeAg seroconversion, or loss of HBsAg if HBeAg negative to start	↑↑	High	High
Adefovir	6 months after HBeAg seroconversion, or loss of HBsAg if HBeAg negative to start	↑↑	Moderate	Moderate
Tenofovir	6 months after HBeAg seroconversion, or loss of HBsAg if HBeAg negative to start	↑↑	High	Low
Entecavir	6 months after HBeAg seroconversion, or loss of HBsAg if HBeAg negative to start	↑↑	High	Low

HBeAg = hepatitis B e antigen; HBsAg = hepatitis B surface antigen.

Peginterferon can be considered in patients with elevated hepatic aminotransferases (greater than two times the upper limit of normal) and low HBV DNA levels. Patients without increased liver inflammation markers or who have high HBV DNA levels are unlikely to respond to peginterferon therapy. The oral nucleoside/nucleotide analogues (lamivudine, adefovir, telbivudine, entecavir, and tenofovir) effectively suppress HBV replication and can improve markers of liver inflammation. Entecavir and tenofovir are the favored agents, because viral resistance to lamivudine, telbivudine, and adefovir has been increasingly recognized.

Inactive carriers of HBV and immune-tolerant patients do not benefit from antiviral therapy.

Extrahepatic Manifestations

The two primary extrahepatic manifestations of HBV are polyarteritis nodosa and kidney disease, most commonly membranous glomerulonephritis (both mediated by circulating immune complexes). Extrahepatic manifestations indicate the need for viral suppression, typically with oral antiviral therapy. Hepatocellular cancer risk is increased in patients with HBV-related cirrhosis and in adults who acquired HBV infection perinatally.

Prevention

HBV prevention consists of vaccination of newborns and those at risk of infection, such as health care workers. Infected patients should be counseled on lifestyle factors that can prevent spread of infection. Vertical transmission of HBV can be minimized by prompt vaccination and administration of HBV immune globulin to newborns immediately after delivery if the mother has HBV infection.

Hepatitis C

As many as 4 to 5 million persons in the United States are estimated to be infected with hepatitis C virus (HCV). Infection occurs through percutaneous exposure, primarily by injection drug use or blood transfusion prior to 1992. Most acute HCV infections are asymptomatic. Chronic infection develops in up to 85% of patients with anti-HCV antibodies. HCV results in cirrhosis within 30 years of infection in 25% of chronically infected patients. Risk factors for progression to cirrhosis are male sex, obesity, alcohol use, and daily marijuana use. Patients with chronically elevated hepatic aminotransferases or a history of injection drug use, percutaneous exposure, or blood transfusion prior to 1992 should be screened for HCV infection.

Diagnosis

Patients with chronic HCV often have fatigue, mild right upper quadrant abdominal discomfort, and arthralgia. Extrahepatic manifestations of HCV are mixed cryoglobulinemia, membranoproliferative glomerulonephritis, porphyria cutanea tarda, and non-Hodgkin lymphoma. Testing for HCV consists of detecting anti-HCV antibodies and has a very high positive predictive value in patients with elevated liver tests and risk factors for HCV infection. The recombinant immunoblot assay (RIBA) or HCV RNA by polymerase chain reaction confirms HCV infection.

Treatment

Treatment of HCV consists of a regimen of peginterferon and ribavirin. NS3/4A protease inhibitors have recently been developed and have activity against HCV genotype 1. These are now combined with peginterferon and ribavirin in the treatment of this genotype. The available NS3/4A protease inhibitors, boceprevir and telaprevir, increase the likelihood of successful therapy when either is combined with peginterferon and ribavirin for the treatment of genotype 1. Liver biopsy is not necessary for HCV diagnosis but can be helpful in determining which patients may benefit from antiviral therapy. Clinical observation is an option for patients with minimal fibrosis on liver biopsy. When significant fibrosis is found, however, the benefits of antiviral therapy may outweigh the side effects of treatment (**Table 30**). Hepatitis C treatment has significant side effects, and the benefits of therapy should be weighed against the risks. Contraindications to antiviral therapy with peginterferon and ribavirin include decompensated liver disease, pregnancy, severe psychiatric disease, and severe preexisting cytopenias.

The goal of antiviral therapy is to obtain a sustained virologic response (SVR), defined as undetectable HCV viral levels by polymerase chain reaction 6 months after completion of antiviral therapy. Although all genotypes of HCV cause similar disease, responses to peginterferon and ribavirin differ by genotype. Treatment of genotype 1 with peginterferon, ribavirin, and an NS3/4A protease inhibitor has an up to 80% likelihood of SVR after a course of antiviral therapy. Genotypes 2 and 3 have a likelihood of SVR greater than 80% after a course of antiviral therapy with peginterferon and ribavirin. Viral levels are measured during treatment to determine the effectiveness of therapy. In addition, viral levels monitored during therapy help to determine the optimal duration of antiviral therapy to be administered. Undetectable viral levels after 4 weeks (rapid virologic response) or 12 weeks (early virologic response) of antiviral therapy indicate an improved chance of obtaining SVR. A viral level that has not decreased by 2-log at 12 weeks compared with the starting viral level is predictive of a lack of SVR, and treatment is typically terminated.

Prevention

There is no vaccination for HCV; therefore, prevention of HCV infection consists of minimizing risks of percutaneous exposure and effective screening of blood donors for the presence of HCV.

TABLE 30. Common Side Effects of Antiviral Therapy for Hepatitis C Virus
Peginterferon
Influenza-like symptoms (fatigue, headache, fevers)
Psychiatric side effects (depression, insomnia, irritability)
Cytopenias (neutropenia, anemia, thrombocytopenia)
Autoimmune thyroiditis
Ribavirin
Hemolytic anemia
Hyperuricemia
Rash
Teratogenicity
NS3/4A Protease Inhibitors
Rash
Anemia

Coinfection of Hepatitis C Virus and HIV

Risk factors for acquisition of HCV are similar to risk factors for acquisition of HIV, and therefore many patients are found to be infected with both viruses. As treatment for HIV has become significantly more effective over the last several years, chronic liver disease due to HCV is emerging as a major cause of morbidity and mortality in this patient population.

Patients with HIV should be assessed for HCV and should be offered antiviral therapy unless otherwise contraindicated. Patients with HIV/HCV coinfection progress to cirrhosis faster than patients with HCV alone, and therefore treatment can be offered to them at earlier stages of fibrosis than patients with HCV infection alone. The rates of success of therapy (obtaining an SVR) are typically lower in patients with HIV/HCV coinfection than in patients with HCV alone. Patients with AIDS or a CD4 cell count of less than 500/microliter should be started on antiretroviral therapy prior to consideration of HCV therapy, as a restored immune system may result in better treatment outcomes for HCV.

Hepatitis D

Hepatitis D virus (HDV) is an incomplete virus that requires the presence of HBV for replication. It is seen as a coinfection with HBV or a superinfection in a patient already infected with HBV; the latter manifests as severe acute hepatitis. HDV is diagnosed by identifying anti-HDV antibodies in the serum. HDV is transmitted via similar routes as HBV. Coinfection of HDV and HBV does not have significant clinical differences from infection with HBV alone. Resolution of HBV infection will result in resolution of HDV infection. Prevention of HDV infection is identical to that of HBV infection.

Hepatitis E

Hepatitis E virus (HEV) is similar to HAV in that it is transmitted via an enteric route, causes acute hepatitis, and does not cause chronic liver disease. HEV has a high incidence in Asia, Africa, and Central America. Fulminant HEV is rare. The incubation period for HEV is between 2 weeks and 2 months, and cholestasis can be prolonged. Overall mortality due to HEV is low; however, pregnant women infected during the third trimester can have a mortality rate as high as 25%. Acute HEV is diagnosed by detecting IgM antibodies to HEV. These tests are not commercially available and clinical samples must be sent to reference laboratories. There is no defined prophylaxis such as vaccination or postexposure immune globulin. Prevention consists of good hygiene and avoiding potentially contaminated substances such as drinking water and poorly cooked foods in endemic areas.

- Hepatitis A infection is self limited and only rarely causes liver failure.
- Hepatitis B infection is an important cause of chronic liver disease, and antiviral therapy should be considered for patients at risk of progression to significant liver disease.
- Hepatitis C treatment has significant side effects, and the benefits of therapy should be weighed against the risks.

Alcohol- and Drug-Induced Liver Disease

Alcohol-Induced Liver Disease

Approximately 4% of U.S. adults have been diagnosed with alcohol abuse or dependence. Alcohol-induced liver disease (ALD) can range from simple steatosis (fatty liver) to cirrhosis. The dose, duration, drinking pattern, and type of alcohol consumed influence the risk for developing ALD. Other risk factors include female sex, Hispanic and American Indian ethnicity, obesity, iron overload, chronic viral hepatitis, and genetic factors. Fatty liver is usually asymptomatic and resolves after 4 to 6 weeks with alcohol abstinence. However, continued alcohol use (>40 g/d) increases the risk of progression to cirrhosis by 30%. Severe alcoholic hepatitis occurs acutely in some patients with chronic liver injury and has a poor short-term prognosis.

ALD is diagnosed by a history of significant alcohol intake and clinical evidence of liver disease. Serum AST is typically elevated two to six times the upper limit of normal in severe alcoholic hepatitis. AST levels above 500 units/L and ALT levels above 200 units/L are uncommon. An AST/ALT ratio above 2 to 3 is typical for ALD. Liver biopsy can confirm ALD and exclude a superimposed condition like viral hepatitis.

The prognosis for ALD has traditionally been estimated using the Maddrey discriminant function (MDF) score, which is calculated as follows:

$$MDF = 4.6 \text{ (prothrombin time [s] − control prothrombin time [s]) + total bilirubin (mg/dL)}$$

Patients with MDF scores of 32 or greater (indicating severe alcoholic hepatitis) have short-term mortality risks as high as 50%.

The Model for End-Stage Liver Disease (MELD) score, which is a prognostic index based on serum values of total bilirubin, creatinine, and INR, has also been used to assess mortality in patients with ALD. A MELD score of 18 or greater was recently observed to have similar prognostic implications as the MDF score.

Treatment for ALD consists of promoting alcohol abstinence and relapse prevention strategies. Abstinence may improve histologic features of hepatic injury, decrease the risk of cirrhosis, and improve survival. In addition to abstinence and efforts to improve nutrition, patients with severe alcoholic hepatitis (MDF score ≥32 with or without hepatic encephalopathy) may benefit from short-term prednisolone or pentoxifylline if corticosteroid therapy is contraindicated by infection or kidney failure.

Drug- and Toxin-Induced Liver Disease

Worldwide, the annual incidence of drug- or toxin-induced liver disease is estimated between 13.9 and 24 cases per 100,000 persons. Drug-induced liver injury is the most common cause of acute liver failure requiring liver transplantation in the United States. Risk factors are age and female sex. An estimated 70% of cases are caused by prescription medications, and 9% are attributed to herbal and dietary supplements. Dose-dependent drug-induced liver injury is most commonly observed in association with acetaminophen use. For a discussion of acetaminophen toxicity, see Fulminant Hepatic Failure. For idiosyncratic drug-induced liver injury, the major classes of implicated agents are antibiotics, central nervous system agents (phenytoin, valproic acid), immunomodulatory agents, and lipid-lowering agents. Among the antibiotics, the most commonly implicated drug is amoxicillin-clavulanate, yet serious adverse clinical outcomes, including death or the need for liver transplantation, are exceedingly rare.

Patients may present with AST, ALT, and/or alkaline phosphatase elevations without jaundice and may be asymptomatic or have nonspecific symptoms such as fatigue and nausea. These patients tend to have a benign course if the offending agent is identified and discontinued. Abdominal pain, jaundice, and pruritus usually accompany severe drug-induced liver injury. Fever, rash, and eosinophilia occur with hypersensitivity-type reactions. Coagulopathy, kidney dysfunction, and mental status changes are seen in fulminant liver disease. The diagnosis is made after the exclusion of viral hepatitis (A, B, and C), alcoholic liver disease, autoimmune liver disease, and metabolic liver disease. Cross-sectional imaging to rule out biliary tract disease is also recommended. If the diagnosis of drug-induced liver injury remains uncertain, a liver biopsy is recommended. Histology may demonstrate prominent eosinophilia, granulomas, zonal or massive necrosis, or cholestasis with hepatitis. The diagnosis is further supported when symptoms and elevated liver enzymes resolve after drug or toxin withdrawal ("dechallenge").

A benign prognosis is typical. However, jaundice due to idiosyncratic drug-induced liver injury has a 10% mortality rate without transplantation, even when the causative drug is discontinued promptly. A recent study suggested that mortality could be improved with *N*-acetylcysteine for idiosyncratic drug-induced liver injury. *N*-acetylcysteine should also be given for acetaminophen toxicity. H

Autoimmune Hepatitis

Autoimmune hepatitis is characterized by serum autoantibodies, hypergammaglobulinemia, and histologic features of interface hepatitis. The mean incidence and prevalence rates are 1.9 and 16.9 per 100,000 persons among white Northern Europeans, but many ethnic groups can develop autoimmune hepatitis. Women are nearly four times more susceptible than men.

The clinical presentation of autoimmune hepatitis ranges from asymptomatic mild disease to fulminant hepatic failure. Common features are fatigue, jaundice, and pruritus. Nausea, vomiting, skin rash, and joint pain are less common. Serum AST and ALT levels are often 2 to 10 times above the upper limit of normal; elevated serum alkaline phosphatase levels occur in 20% of cases without significant biliary injury on histology. Total bilirubin and albumin levels are usually normal unless advanced cirrhosis or severe inflammation is present. Serum antinuclear and smooth muscle antibodies are observed together in 60% of cases. Serum titers greater than 1:40 suggest autoimmune hepatitis. Elevated serum γ-globulin levels (>2.0 g/dL [20 g/L]) are helpful for diagnostic verification. Serum p-ANCA levels may be helpful for the 10% to 15% of patients with negative antinuclear antibody, smooth muscle antibody, and γ-globulin levels less than 2.0 g/dL (20 g/L). Liver biopsy is typically required for diagnosis. The most specific histologic criteria are interface hepatitis with lymphocytes and plasma cells in portal, periportal, or lobular areas.

The absolute indications for treatment are: (1) AST levels greater than 10 times normal, (2) AST levels greater than five times normal with γ-globulin levels greater than two times normal, (3) bridging or confluent necrosis on liver biopsy, or (4) symptomatic disease (fever, nausea, vomiting, jaundice). Induction therapy consists of corticosteroids or combined treatment with azathioprine and corticosteroids. Both treatment regimens induce remission in more than 80% of patients; however, the combined regimen often has fewer side effects. Maintenance therapy with the same regimen should be provided for 12 to 18 months to increase the likelihood of histologic remission. Cessation of therapy before 12 months is associated with high rates of relapse even though liver biochemistries may have normalized quickly. Only 20% of patients remain in remission after the complete withdrawal

of medical therapy; therefore, medication doses should be tapered to monotherapy with azathioprine at the minimum dose needed to maintain remission.

A minority of patients with autoimmune hepatitis will have adverse drug effects or treatment failure that requires salvage therapies (mycophenolate mofetil, cyclosporine, or tacrolimus). Liver transplantation is effective in patients who develop end-stage liver disease. The overall 10-year survival after transplantation is estimated at 75%. Disease recurs in 20% to 30% of patients after transplantation and is usually managed by conventional immunosuppressive regimens.

Metabolic Liver Disease

Nonalcoholic Fatty Liver Disease

Nonalcoholic fatty liver disease (NAFLD) can range from asymptomatic hepatic steatosis to cirrhosis. NAFLD usually results from insulin resistance and the metabolic syndrome (obesity, diabetes mellitus, dyslipidemia, and hypertension). Inflammation and fibrosis associated with NAFLD is referred to as nonalcoholic steatohepatitis (NASH). NAFLD affects as much as 30% of the adult population in the United States, and as many as 20% of these patients have NASH. NASH progresses to cirrhosis in 10% of affected patients and is increasingly recognized as a cause of what would otherwise be labeled cryptogenic cirrhosis.

NAFLD and NASH are diagnosed after exclusion of other causes of liver disease by serologic evaluation. Abdominal imaging with ultrasound, CT, or MRI can demonstrate significant hepatic steatosis but cannot reliably identify hepatic inflammation or fibrosis. NASH may be inferred in patients who have the metabolic syndrome and elevated hepatic aminotransferases in the absence of other causes of liver disease. Liver biopsy confirms NASH and identifies the degree of hepatic inflammation and fibrosis. There are no reliable noninvasive indicators of hepatic fibrosis. Risk factors for progressive hepatic fibrosis are age greater than 50 years, BMI greater than 28, serum triglyceride levels greater than 150 mg/dL (1.7 mmol/L), and ALT level greater than twice the upper limit of normal.

The mainstay of treatment of NAFLD and NASH is weight loss and management of comorbidities. Monitoring of hepatic aminotransferases and markers of liver function is typically performed at intervals of every 3 to 6 months. Medical therapies for NASH remain investigational. The use of statins as indicated for the management of dyslipidemia is not contraindicated in the setting of elevated liver tests due to NASH. Antioxidants and oral hypoglycemic medications (metformin, thiazolidinediones) have been assessed in clinical trials but have not demonstrated improved clinical outcomes.

Hereditary Hemochromatosis

Hereditary hemochromatosis is the most common genetic disorder in white patients and is characterized by excessive iron deposition in the liver, heart, pancreas, and other glands. Hepatic iron overload can lead to cirrhosis and hepatocellular cancer.

Patients with persistently elevated liver tests should be screened for iron overload with measurement of serum ferritin and transferrin saturation (iron/total iron-binding capacity). Chronic inflammatory conditions such as alcoholic liver disease and chronic viral hepatitis can also lead to elevated iron indices. Elevated iron indices in the setting of chronic liver disease should prompt genetic testing for hemochromatosis. Patients with hereditary hemochromatosis who are older than 40 years or have a serum ferritin level greater than 1000 ng/mL (1000 micrograms/L) are at risk for cirrhosis. Liver biopsy is warranted, because confirmation of cirrhosis prompts surveillance for hepatocellular cancer and other complications of cirrhosis (such as esophageal varices). Extrahepatic manifestations of hemochromatosis are diabetes mellitus, cardiomyopathy, arthropathy, and skin color changes.

Treatment of hereditary hemochromatosis consists of therapeutic phlebotomy to normalize iron stores. In patients who cannot tolerate phlebotomy, iron chelating agents may be necessary. First-degree relatives of patients with hereditary hemochromatosis should be screened for hemochromatosis. Patients who are diagnosed with hemochromatosis can subsequently be monitored for the development of iron overload. If patients are diagnosed prior to the onset of cirrhosis, and if iron overload is normalized by phlebotomy or iron chelation, the life expectancy of patients with hemochromatosis is expected to be normal.

α_1-Antitrypsin Deficiency

α_1-Antitrypsin deficiency is a conformational protein disorder that results in the hepatic accumulation of variant protein inclusions. The risk of cirrhosis and hepatocellular cancer is well recognized. There is no specific treatment for liver disease associated with α_1-antitrypsin deficiency. If hepatic failure develops, liver transplantation may be considered.

α_1-Antitrypsin deficiency causes pulmonary disease as well as liver disease owing to the inability of the liver to excrete the variant α_1-antitrypsin protein into the circulation. This results in the unchecked actions of proteolytic enzymes leading to panacinar emphysema. Risk factors for the development of pulmonary complications of α_1-antitrypsin deficiency include age, tobacco use, and other underlying lung diseases. Patients with α_1-antitrypsin deficiency should be monitored

regularly with pulmonary function testing for the development of obstructive lung disease. Intravenous supplemental α_1-antitrypsin can be administered to patients with obstructive lung disease.

Wilson Disease

Wilson disease is an autosomal recessive disorder of copper transport that results in increased hepatic uptake and decreased biliary excretion of copper. Wilson disease is rare and affects 1 in 30,000 newborns.

Wilson disease may present as fulminant liver failure. Fulminant Wilson disease is characterized by abnormal hepatic aminotransferases, hemolytic anemia, and normal to decreased serum alkaline phosphatase levels (copper interferes with the synthesis of alkaline phosphatase enzymes). Fulminant Wilson disease is uniformly fatal without urgent liver transplantation.

Wilson disease is typically diagnosed in patients younger than 45 years. Wilson disease can be diagnosed prior to the development of fulminant liver failure and should always be excluded during the evaluation of abnormal liver tests in a young patient. The most common screening test for Wilson disease is serum ceruloplasmin, which is reduced; elevated urine excretion of copper is ascertained to verify the presumptive diagnosis of Wilson disease. In a young patient with elevated liver tests, a low ceruloplasmin level, and elevated urine copper excretion, liver biopsy is typically obtained to confirm the diagnosis of Wilson disease. Liver biopsy demonstrates excessive intrahepatic copper. Kayser-Fleischer rings, noted on ophthalmologic examination, indicate copper deposition in the Descemet membrane of the iris. A common extrahepatic manifestation of Wilson disease is neuropsychiatric abnormalities caused by accumulation of excess copper in the brain.

Patients with Wilson disease are treated with copper chelating agents (trientine, penicillamine) and are placed on a low-copper diet.

KEY POINTS

- Nonalcoholic fatty liver disease usually results from insulin resistance and the metabolic syndrome (obesity, diabetes mellitus, dyslipidemia, and hypertension); the mainstay of treatment is weight loss and management of comorbidities.

- Hereditary hemochromatosis is a common genetic disorder characterized by excessive iron deposition in various organs; iron overload can lead to cirrhosis and hepatocellular cancer.

- α_1-Antitrypsin deficiency causes liver disease (owing to intrahepatic accumulation of variant protein inclusions) and panacinar emphysema in the lungs in susceptible persons.

- Wilson disease is a rare hereditary disease characterized by increased hepatic uptake and decreased biliary excretion of copper.

Cholestatic Liver Disease

Primary Biliary Cirrhosis

Primary biliary cirrhosis (PBC) is a chronic cholestatic liver disease of unknown cause. PBC mainly affects middle-aged women, and the median age of disease onset is 50 years. The annual incidence of PBC ranges between 2 and 24 cases per million persons, while prevalence estimates range from 19 to 402 cases per million persons. Most patients (>60%) with PBC are asymptomatic at initial presentation, but most asymptomatic patients will develop symptoms of PBC within 10 years. Fatigue, dry eyes, dry mouth, and pruritus are the most common symptoms. Jaundice, cutaneous hyperpigmentation, hepatosplenomegaly, and xanthelasmas are rarely observed at diagnosis.

PBC is diagnosed by serum alkaline phosphatase levels greater than 1.5 times the upper limit of normal and typically normal serum total bilirubin levels. Increases in serum AST and ALT levels less than 5 times the upper limit of normal may be seen as well. Serum antimitochondrial antibody is present in 90% to 95% of patients with PBC at titers greater than 1:40. For patients with undetectable serum antimitochondrial antibody levels, a liver biopsy is required for diagnosis. Histology demonstrating focal duct obliteration with granuloma formation, known as the "florid duct lesion," is pathognomonic.

The treatment of PBC symptoms is empiric. Antihistamines and phenobarbital have marginal clinical efficacy for pruritus. Cholestyramine, sertraline, and rifampin are effective for many patients with moderate to severe pruritus. Artificial tears and oral sialagogues are recommended for keratoconjunctivitis sicca and xerostomia (dry mouth). Oral pilocarpine and cevimeline may also be effective agents for sicca symptoms.

Malabsorption of fat-soluble vitamins from cholestasis can be seen even in the absence of cirrhosis. Supplementation of fat-soluble vitamins in patients with PBC and cirrhosis is warranted if low levels are documented (they should not be replaced empirically). While the link between hypercholesterolemia and mortality from cardiovascular disease in this population has not been established, pharmacologic therapy with statins may have an important role in patients with significant risk factors for coronary artery disease. Metabolic bone disease in PBC is associated with age, low BMI, and advanced histologic disease. First-line therapies are weight-bearing exercise and oral calcium and vitamin D replacement. Intravenous bisphosphonate therapy should be considered in patients with esophageal varices.

Ursodeoxycholic acid (UDCA) offers a survival benefit for patients with PBC. However, approximately 50% to 60% of patients do not achieve a complete biochemical response to UDCA (defined as serum alkaline phosphatase and/or AST levels greater than 1.5 times normal). No effective salvage therapy is available for patients who have an incomplete response to UDCA. Liver transplantation is highly effective for end-stage PBC. PBC recurs in up to 30% of patients after liver transplantation.

Primary Sclerosing Cholangitis

Primary sclerosing cholangitis (PSC) is a chronic inflammatory disorder that affects the intra- and extrahepatic bile ducts. The mean age at diagnosis is 40 years, and approximately 60% of affected patients are men. Annual incidence rates are between 0.9 and 1.3 cases per 100,000 persons, with point prevalence rates of 8.5 and 13.6 cases per 100,000 persons. In European and North American populations, approximately 70% to 80% of patients with PSC have inflammatory bowel disease. Conversely, about 2% to 4% of patients with inflammatory bowel disease have or develop PSC. Most patients with PSC (40% to 60%) are asymptomatic at presentation. Pruritus, abdominal pain, and jaundice are common manifestations in symptomatic patients.

PSC is diagnosed by measuring liver enzymes and performing cholangiography. Serum alkaline phosphatase values are 3 to 10 times the upper limit of normal, and serum ALT and AST levels are two to three times the upper limit of normal. Serum total bilirubin levels may be normal in 60% of patients. Higher levels of total bilirubin are concerning for advanced disease, superimposed choledocholithiasis, or malignancy. Serum antinuclear and smooth muscle antibodies are present in 20% to 50% of patients, but antimitochondrial antibodies are rarely found in PSC. The gold standard for diagnosis of PSC is cholangiography. Diagnostic findings are segmental bile duct fibrosis with saccular dilatation of normal intervening areas, resulting in the characteristic "beads on a string" appearance. Magnetic resonance cholangiopancreatography (MRCP) has been increasingly used and has an overall diagnostic accuracy rate of 90% (**Figure 24**). MRCP should be performed when PSC is suspected. If common bile duct obstruction is observed based on clinical or conventional cross-sectional imaging, then endoscopic retrograde cholangiopancreatography is required for diagnosis and therapy. Liver biopsy is required for making a diagnosis of small-duct PSC when cholangiography is normal. Periductal fibrosis with inflammation, bile duct proliferation, and ductopenia are the main histologic findings. Fibro-obliterative cholangiopathy, the pathologic hallmark of PSC, is uncommonly observed (see Figure 24).

The approach for patients with PSC and fatigue, pruritus, and metabolic bone disease is similar to the approach for patients with PBC. Choledocholithiasis occurs in 10% to 25% of symptomatic patients, and dominant strictures occur in 5% to 10%. Manifestations of stricture include a sudden increase in serum alkaline phosphatase and/or bilirubin levels, progressive jaundice, and bacterial cholangitis. Both conditions are successfully treated endoscopically or percutaneously. Biliary reconstructive surgery is rarely required. Endoscopic brushings and biopsy are required to exclude malignancy when dominant strictures are identified.

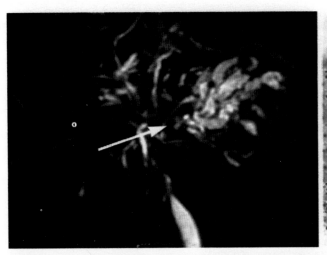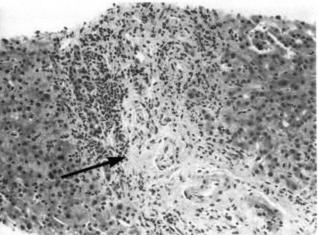

FIGURE 24. Magnetic resonance cholangiopancreatography (*left panel*) revealing upstream intrahepatic bile duct dilatation involving the left hepatic lobe (*arrow*) with stricturing of the left hepatic duct. Liver histology (*right panel*) demonstrates portal tract expansion, edema, and ductular proliferation with lymphocytic cholangitis (*arrow*) consistent with primary sclerosing cholangitis.

No effective medical therapy has been identified for PSC. Two randomized controlled trials of high-dose UDCA (greater than 25 mg/kg/d) failed to identify clinical and survival benefits compared with placebo. PSC remains a major indication for liver transplantation with excellent survival rates reported. Disease may recur in 10% to 20% of patients after transplantation.

PSC confers an estimated annual risk for cholangiocarcinoma of 0.5% to 1.5%, and the prevalence rate varies between 4% and 20%. In addition, 30% to 50% of patients are diagnosed with cholangiocarcinoma within 2 years of PSC diagnosis. Risk factors for cholangiocarcinoma in PSC are poorly understood. When patients with PSC are found to have acute worsening of liver tests, acute worsening of symptoms, or a new dominant stricture noted on cholangiography, the possibility of cholangiocarcinoma should be considered.

KEY POINTS

- Treatment of primary biliary cirrhosis consists of ursodeoxycholic acid and symptomatic treatment of dry eyes, dry mouth, and pruritus.

- The gold standard for diagnosis of primary sclerosing cholangitis is cholangiography.

- Primary sclerosing cholangitis confers a significant risk for cholangiocarcinoma.

Complications of Liver Disease

Portal Hypertension and Gastroesophageal Varices

Portal hypertension is associated with hemodynamic alterations in portal venous blood flow. Clinically significant portal hypertension occurs when portal vein pressure exceeds 8 to 10 mm Hg (normal is 3 to 5 mm Hg). The most common cause of portal hypertension is cirrhosis, and the most common clinical manifestations of portal hypertension are gastroesophageal varices, ascites, and hepatic encephalopathy.

Gastroesophageal varices are present in 30% to 60% of patients with cirrhosis at diagnosis. Over time, esophageal varices enlarge and may spontaneously rupture, leading to bleeding and possible death. Mortality rate for acute variceal hemorrhage has been significantly reduced to 15% to 20% with treatment. Supportive care, systemic pharmacologic therapies including antibiotics, and endoscopic therapy (variceal band ligation or sclerotherapy) are the standard of care (**Table 31**). Control of bleeding is achieved in almost 90% of patients with these techniques.

For patients with cirrhosis and no history of variceal hemorrhage, guidelines recommend screening with upper endoscopy to exclude large esophageal varices. Patients with large esophageal varices should receive prophylactic treatment with nonselective β-blockers (propranolol, nadolol) or endoscopic variceal band ligation (**Table 32**). Patients with contraindications to β-blocker therapy such as asthma, hypotension, or resting bradycardia can be offered endoscopic ligation therapy as alternative prophylactic therapy. Both strategies reduce the risk of variceal hemorrhage by 40%. Nonselective β-blockers should be titrated to attain a reduction in resting heart rate of 25% or 55 to 60/min. β-Blocker therapy eliminates the need for continued endoscopies. Surveillance endoscopy is required indefinitely after variceal band ligation. Patients with no esophageal varices require surveillance endoscopy every 2 to 3 years, whereas patients with small esophageal varices require surveillance annually to identify growth into large varices. In patients who survive variceal hemorrhage, the combination of nonselective β-blockers with endoscopic variceal band ligation is most effective as

TABLE 31. Treatment of Acute Variceal Hemorrhage[a]

Regimen	Dose	Duration	Follow-up	Comments
Vasoconstrictor				
Octreotide	Intravenous 50-µg bolus, followed by infusion of 50 µg/h	2-5 days	Bolus can be repeated in first hour if variceal hemorrhage uncontrolled; if rebleeding occurs during therapy, consider TIPS	Available in the United States
Terlipressin	2 mg given intravenously every 4 h for first 48 h, followed by 1 mg given intravenously every 4 h	2-5 days	If rebleeding occurs during therapy, consider TIPS	Not available in the United States
Somatostatin	Intravenous 250-mg bolus, followed by infusion of 250 mg/h	2-5 days	Bolus can be repeated in first hour if variceal hemorrhage uncontrolled; if rebleeding occurs during therapy, consider TIPS	Not available in the United States
Vapreotide[b]	Intravenous 50-µg bolus, followed by infusion of 50 µg/h	2-5 days	If rebleeding occurs during therapy, consider TIPS	Not available in the United States
Antibiotic				
Ceftriaxone	Intravenously at a dose of 1 g/d	5-7 days or until discharge	No long-term antibiotics unless spontaneous bacterial peritonitis develops	Used in patients with advanced liver disease, high probability of fluoroquinolone resistance, or both
Norfloxacin	400 mg orally twice a day	5-7 days or until discharge	No long-term antibiotics unless spontaneous bacterial peritonitis develops	Used in patients with low probability of fluoroquinolone-resistant organisms
Endoscopic therapy				
Endoscopic variceal ligation	Once, at time of diagnostic upper endoscopy	Until variceal obliteration achieved	If rebleeding occurs during therapy, consider TIPS	Requires endoscopist with special expertise
Endoscopic variceal sclerotherapy	Once, at time of diagnostic upper endoscopy	Only at diagnostic endoscopy	Continue with endoscopic variceal ligation until obliteration achieved	Used when endoscopic variceal ligation not possible; requires endoscopist with special expertise

[a]Only one vasoconstrictor plus one antibiotic plus endoscopic therapy should be used. Therapies that should not be used for first-line management of acute esophageal variceal hemorrhage are endoscopic variceal obturation (which is indicated in fundal gastric hemorrhage but not in esophageal variceal hemorrhage) and recombinant factor VIIa.

[b]Recommendations for vapreotide are based on findings from a single study (Calès P, Masliah C, Bernard B, et al; French Club for the Study of Portal Hypertension. Early administration of vapreotide for variceal bleeding in patients with cirrhosis. N Engl J Med. 2001;344(1):23-28. [PMID: 11136956])

TIPS = transjugular intrahepatic portosystemic shunt.

Source: Garcia-Tsao G, Bosch J. Management of varices and variceal hemorrhage in cirrhosis. N Engl J Med. 2010;362(9):823-832. [PMID: 20200386]. Copyright 2010, Massachusetts Medical Society.

secondary prophylaxis. Recurrent or refractory variceal hemorrhage may require transjugular intrahepatic portosystemic shunt (TIPS) insertion, which is highly effective.

Nonselective β-blockers and variceal band ligation are not as effective in patients with large gastric varices and no history of variceal hemorrhage. Bleeding from gastric varices is treated using endoscopic sclerotherapy or band ligation, but the risk of rebleeding is high. Secondary prophylaxis with TIPS is recommended in eligible patients. The safety and efficacy of glue injection as secondary prophylaxis for gastric variceal bleeding remains unknown.

Ascites

Ascites is the most frequent complication of portal hypertension. Approximately 50% of patients with compensated cirrhosis will develop ascites within 10 years. The diagnosis of new-onset ascites is usually confirmed by physical examination and/or ultrasound if occult ascites is present. Diagnostic paracentesis is typically performed when ascites develops. Ascitic fluid should be analyzed for cell count and differential, albumin, and total protein concentration. If infection is suspected, inoculation of bacteria culture bottles at the bedside is required. The serum-ascites albumin gradient (SAAG) is

TABLE 32. Primary Prophylaxis Against Variceal Hemorrhage[a]

Regimen[b]	Dose	Goal	Duration	Follow-up
Propranolol	Starting dose of 20 mg orally twice a day	Increase to maximally tolerated dose or until heart rate is approximately 55/min	Indefinite	Ensure heart-rate goals met at each clinic visit; no need for follow-up endoscopy
Nadolol	Starting dose of 40 mg orally twice a day	Increase to maximally tolerated dose or until heart rate is approximately 55/min	Indefinite	Ensure heart-rate goals met at each clinic visit; no need for follow-up endoscopy
Endoscopic variceal ligation	Every 2-4 weeks	Obliterate varices	Until variceal obliteration achieved (usually 2-4 sessions)	Perform first surveillance endoscopy 1-3 months after obliteration, then every 6-12 months indefinitely

[a]Therapies that should not be used as prophylaxis include nitrates alone, endoscopic variceal sclerotherapy, shunt therapy (either transjugular intrahepatic portosystemic shunt or surgical shunt), nonselective β-blockers plus endoscopic variceal ligation, and nonselective β-blockers plus nitrates.

[b]Only one of the three regimens should be used.

Source: Garcia-Tsao G, Bosch J. Management of varices and variceal hemorrhage in cirrhosis. N Engl J Med. 2010;362(9):823-32. [PMID: 20200386]. Copyright 2010, Massachusetts Medical Society.

calculated by subtracting the ascitic fluid albumin concentration from the serum albumin concentration. If the SAAG is 1.1 g/dL (11 g/L) or greater and total ascites protein is less than 2.5 g/dL (25 g/L), then portal hypertension is the cause of ascites. A SAAG value of 1.1 g/dL (11 g/L) or greater with total ascites protein greater than 2.5 g/dL (25 g/L) indicates cardiac disease such as chronic heart failure or constrictive pericarditis.

Treatment of uncomplicated ascites involves dietary sodium restriction (≤2000 mg/d) and oral diuretics. For patients with moderate to severe ascites, large-volume paracentesis with administration of intravenous albumin (8 g per L of fluid removed) may be necessary in conjunction with medical therapy. Refractory ascites occurs when there is resistance to sodium restriction and high-dose diuretic treatment or when side effects prevent maximizing oral diuretics. Treatment options for patients with refractory ascites are serial therapeutic paracentesis, TIPS, and liver transplantation.

Spontaneous Bacterial Peritonitis

The prevalence of spontaneous bacterial peritonitis (SBP) among hospitalized patients has remained stable while mortality rates have declined from 50% to 15%. SBP is diagnosed when ascitic fluid bacterial culture is positive and ascitic fluid absolute polymorphonuclear count is elevated (≥250 cells/microliter). A third-generation cephalosporin should be given until the culture report is finalized. In patients with SBP and evidence for significant liver and/or kidney dysfunction, the concomitant use of intravenous albumin is associated with a survival benefit compared with antibiotic therapy alone. Repeat paracentesis at 48 hours will reveal a drop in the polymorphonuclear count with effective medical therapy of SBP, but it will often rise despite therapy in patients with secondary peritonitis. Norfloxacin has been reported to successfully prevent recurrent SBP in patients with previous SBP. Trimethoprim-sulfamethoxazole can be used in patients who are allergic to fluoroquinolones. Primary prophylaxis against SBP with norfloxacin is warranted in patients with low-protein ascitic fluid (<1 g/dL [10 g/L]) and severe liver dysfunction, especially when they are hospitalized.

Hepatic Encephalopathy

Hepatic encephalopathy (HE) is a disturbance in central nervous system function caused by hepatic insufficiency and portosystemic shunting. Although the frequency of HE is unrelated to the cause of cirrhosis, increased frequency and severity of HE predict an increased risk of death. The classification of HE is based on West Haven criteria (**Table 33**). Stage 0 can apply to individuals with normal cognitive function as well as those with minimal HE. Distinguishing between stage 0 and stage I may be difficult because criteria for both stages may be found concomitantly in the same patient. Minimal HE is defined as cognitive dysfunction without clinical signs of overt HE. Minimal HE should be investigated in order to advise patients with cirrhosis who are at risk for accidents, such as active drivers; those with a decline in work performance; or those who have cognitive symptoms. Patients with stage II HE are generally confused and often require urgent medical evaluation and subsequent hospitalization.

HE diagnosis requires excluding other causes of encephalopathy including metabolic disorders, infectious diseases, medications, and intracranial lesions or events. Patients with cirrhosis may develop encephalopathy owing to recent

TABLE 33. West Haven Criteria for Classification of Hepatic Encephalopathy

Stage	Features
0	No abnormality detected
I	Trivial lack of awareness, euphoria or anxiety, shortened attention span, impairment of addition or subtraction
II	Lethargy or apathy, disorientation for time, obvious personality change, inappropriate behavior
III	Somnolence to semistupor, responsive to stimuli, confused, gross disorientation, bizarre behavior
IV	Coma, unable to test mental state

Reprinted from Hepatology. 50(6). Bajaj JS, Wade JB, Sanyal AJ. Spectrum of neurocognitive impairment in cirrhosis: Implications for the assessment of hepatic encephalopathy; 2014-2021. Copyright 2009, with permission from John Wiley and Sons.

TIPS placement or large spontaneous portosystemic shunts detected on CT imaging. Serum ammonia levels do not correlate with stage of HE but may be helpful in the initial evaluation of unexplained confusion in patients without a history of liver disease.

HE is managed by recognizing and treating precipitating factors such as gastrointestinal hemorrhage, infection, electrolyte disturbances (including intravascular volume depletion and overaggresive diuresis), analgesic and sedative medications, constipation, and superimposed acute liver injury (alcoholic hepatitis, hypotension, portal vein thrombosis, recent surgery). Treatment is focused on reducing excess nitrogen in the gut. Lactulose is a nonabsorbable disaccharide that decreases the absorption of ammonia. Patients on lactulose who have more than three to four bowel movements per day and/or watery diarrhea should have their dose and/or frequency decreased, but lactulose therapy should not be stopped. Oral antibiotics such as neomycin and rifaximin reduce the effects of colonic bacteria on ammonia production, but neomycin can have associated side effects with long-term use. The risk of an acute exacerbation of chronic HE is reduced by 60% with rifaximin compared with placebo, and it is well tolerated. Dietary protein restriction is no longer commonly recommended given its association with increased mortality risk.

Hepatorenal Syndrome

Hepatorenal syndrome (HRS) is characterized by renal vasoconstriction that leads to a severe reduction in glomerular function with minimal histologic abnormalities. Type I HRS is characterized by a rapidly progressive reduction in kidney function, defined by a doubling of the initial serum creatinine to greater than 2.5 mg/dL (221 micromoles/L) or a 50% reduction of the initial 24-hour creatinine clearance to a level less than 20 mL/min/1.73 m^2 in less than 2 weeks. Type II HRS does not have a rapidly progressive course and is commonly associated with refractory ascites. The major criteria for diagnosing HRS are serum creatinine greater than 1.5 mg/dL (132.6 micromoles/L); no improvement of serum creatinine (improvement is defined by a decrease to ≤1.5 mg/dL [132.6 micromoles/L]) after at least 2 days of diuretic withdrawal and volume expansion with albumin; the absence of septic shock or hypotension; no current or recent treatment with nephrotoxic drugs; and the absence of identifiable parenchymal kidney disease (no significant proteinuria [<500 mg/d], hematuria, findings of acute tubular necrosis [pigmented granular casts on urinalysis], or evidence of obstruction on ultrasound).

Several medical therapies are available for the treatment of type I HRS. Terlipressin has been shown to reverse both type I and II HRS in selected patients but is currently unavailable for use in the United States. The next most promising treatment is intravenous albumin, which has been shown in randomized trials to be associated with improvement in serum creatinine and urine output in patients with type I HRS. While reports exist supporting the use of octreotide with midodrine and intravenous albumin for type I HRS, the uncertain status of midodrine availability potentially eliminates this regimen as a realistic option. Furthermore, there is no evidence demonstrating clinical benefit with octreotide monotherapy. Liver (with or without kidney) transplantation is the most effective treatment for HRS.

Hepatopulmonary Syndrome

Hepatopulmonary syndrome (HPS) is characterized by a defect in arterial oxygenation induced by pulmonary vascular dilatation in the setting of cirrhosis and portal hypertension. The prevalence of HPS ranges from 5% to 30% in patients with cirrhosis. HPS should be suspected in patients with cirrhosis who develop hypoxemia in the absence of other causes such as hepatic hydrothorax, COPD, and chronic thromboembolic disease. Physical examination may reveal digital clubbing and cyanosis. Laboratory testing discloses hypoxemia on arterial blood gas measurement. Contrast-enhanced transthoracic echocardiography with agitated saline administration is the most effective screening tool for HPS. Microbubble visualization within the left atrium after three to six cardiac cycles is diagnostic for HPS. There are currently no effective medical therapies for HPS. Patients with HPS and an arterial Po$_2$ of 60 mm Hg or less are considered high-priority candidates for liver transplantation based on the progressive nature of HPS.

Portopulmonary Hypertension

Portopulmonary hypertension (POPH) is characterized by coexisting primary portal hypertension with pulmonary hypertension. The prevalence of POPH in patients with liver disease is 4% to 10%.

Patients with POPH may be asymptomatic or may have progressive exertional dyspnea. The diagnosis of POPH is suggested by estimated right ventricular systolic pressures of 50 mm Hg or higher on transthoracic Doppler echocardiography. POPH diagnosis is confirmed by right heart catheterization. Hemodynamic criteria for POPH are a mean pulmonary artery pressure of 25 mm Hg or greater, pulmonary vascular resistance of 240 dynes/s/cm^{-5} or greater, and pulmonary artery occlusion pressure less than 15 mm Hg.

POPH has a poor prognosis when mean pulmonary artery pressures exceed 35 mm Hg. There have been no controlled, randomized studies of medical treatment for POPH, but intravenous epoprostenol, oral sildenafil, and bosentan have been used with variable success. The 5-year survival of untreated patients with POPH is 15% but improves to 65% when medical treatment is provided. Survival is improved following liver transplantation for patients with mild to moderate POPH. Patients with mean pulmonary artery pressures above 35 to 50 mm Hg are not candidates for liver transplantation because of an increased risk for perioperative death. $\boxed{\text{H}}$

Hepatocellular Carcinoma

Hepatocellular carcinoma (HCC) is the third leading cause of cancer-related death worldwide. Incidence rates have been rising in Western countries. Nearly 80% of HCC cases occur in patients with cirrhosis. Major risk factors are male sex, chronic hepatitis B and C infection, hemochromatosis, and α_1-antitrypsin deficiency; however, cirrhosis from any cause can result in HCC. Screening and surveillance for HCC consists of cross-sectional imaging. Ultrasound is the most widely available and least expensive imaging modality. CT and MRI offer better resolution and detection of early-stage HCC. For patients with normal imaging at diagnosis, the recommended interval for surveillance imaging is 6 months. Serum α-fetoprotein measurement does not have sufficient diagnostic accuracy alone to be a valuable tool for early detection.

HCC lesions greater than 2 cm in diameter can be accurately diagnosed in patients with cirrhosis using contrast-enhanced CT, MRI, and angiography. The presence of arterial hypervascularization with delayed venous contrast washout on at least two imaging studies is required. When only a single imaging study documents these features, HCC can still be diagnosed if the serum α-fetoprotein level is 400 ng/mL (400 micrograms/L) or greater. Image-guided biopsy is reserved for patients in whom radiologic criteria are equivocal or inconsistent with HCC. A negative biopsy result in the setting of cirrhosis does not confidently exclude HCC. Tumor seeding from invasive biopsy has been described but appears to be rare. When solid or indeterminate lesions between 1 and 2 cm (or any lesion increasing in size over 3 to 6 months) are identified, enhanced follow-up with more frequent imaging is required.

Treatment for HCC is guided by the Barcelona Classification for Liver Cancer (BCLC) system (**Figure 25**).

For patients with early-stage disease, liver transplantation is the most effective therapy. Surgical resection is reserved for patients without advanced fibrosis or portal hypertension whose tumor location is amenable to operative therapy. Ablative treatments, including transarterial hepatic artery chemoembolization, radiofrequency ablation, and percutaneous ethanol injection, can prolong short-term survival in selected patients and are commonly used as a bridge to liver transplantation. For patients with advanced HCC and intact liver function, the use of sorafenib has been shown to improve survival as compared with standard therapy. Side effects, including hypertension and hand-foot syndrome, limit the effectiveness of this agent.

KEY POINTS

- The most common cause of portal hypertension is cirrhosis, and the most common clinical manifestations of portal hypertension are gastroesophageal varices, ascites, and hepatic encephalopathy.
- Treatment of uncomplicated ascites involves dietary sodium restriction and judicious use of oral diuretics.
- Hepatopulmonary syndrome should be suspected in patients with cirrhosis who develop hypoxemia in the absence of other causes such as hepatic hydrothorax, COPD, and chronic thromboembolic disease.
- Hepatocellular carcinoma is the third leading cause of cancer-related death worldwide; nearly 80% of hepatocellular carcinomas occur in patients with cirrhosis.

Fulminant Hepatic Failure $\boxed{\text{H}}$

Fulminant hepatic failure (FHF) is defined as hepatic encephalopathy in the setting of jaundice without preexisting liver disease. This is contrasted with liver injury, which is characterized by elevated liver tests and/or jaundice in the absence of evidence of failure of liver function. Liver failure is classified by the number of weeks after jaundice onset that encephalopathy appears; hyperacute liver failure is within 1 week, acute liver failure is between 1 and 4 weeks, and subacute liver failure is between 4 and 12 weeks. Patients with hyperacute liver failure have the best overall prognosis of these groups.

Causes of FHF are described in **Table 34**. The most common cause of FHF in the United States is acetaminophen overdose. In the presence of concurrent risk factors such as chronic alcohol ingestion, fasting, or malnutrition, even therapeutic doses of acetaminophen (<4 g/d) can cause significant hepatotoxicity. The treatment of acetaminophen toxicity is prompt initiation of N-acetylcysteine therapy. Acyclovir can be used to treat herpesvirus-induced hepatitis, and penicillin G or silymarin can be used for *Amanita* mushroom intoxication. Oral antiviral therapy with a nucleoside/nucleotide analogue may be beneficial in the setting of fulminant HBV infection.

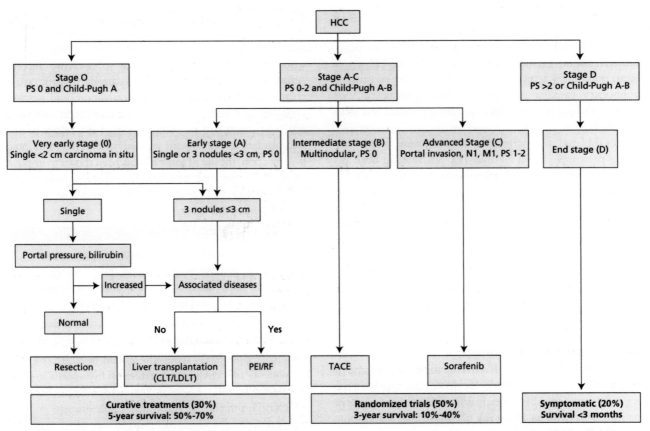

FIGURE 25. Barcelona Classification for Liver Cancer (BCLC) Treatment System. CLT = cadaveric liver transplantation; HCC = hepatocellular carcinoma; LDLT = living donor liver transplantation; PEI = percutaneous ethanol injection; PS = physical status; RF = radiofrequency (ablation); TACE = transarterial chemoembolization.

Figure credit: Llovet JM, Di Bisceglie AM, Bruix J, et al; Panel of Experts in HCC-Design Clinical Trials. Design and endpoints of clinical trials in hepatocellular carcinoma. J Natl Cancer Inst. 2008;100(10):698-711. [PMID: 18477802]

The recognition of FHF should prompt immediate referral to a liver transplantation center for intensive monitoring and consideration of liver transplantation. Between 5% and 12% of patients undergoing liver transplantation have FHF. Outcomes of liver transplantation for patients with FHF are not as good as those for patients with chronic liver disease; 1-year survival is 73%. Nonetheless, liver transplantation is the only treatment that has been shown to substantially improve mortality from FHF.

Supportive care is warranted for patients with FHF while arranging logistics of transfer to a liver transplant center. Significant complications of FHF are hypoglycemia, infection, cerebral edema, and coagulopathy. Coagulopathy of FHF, as measured by prothrombin time, is a useful marker of liver function; administration of fresh frozen plasma is not clinically indicated unless the patient is actively bleeding or if an invasive procedure is planned. Cerebral edema can develop quickly in patients with FHF, and altered mental status should prompt the measurement of intracerebral pressure by invasive monitoring. Mannitol therapy, induced hypothermia, and avoidance of overstimulation can help decrease intracerebral pressures.

KEY POINT

- The recognition of fulminant hepatic failure should prompt immediate referral to a liver transplantation center.

Liver Transplantation

Liver transplantation is often the only life-prolonging intervention available for patients with FHF or decompensated cirrhosis. Another indication for liver transplantation is HCC within the Milan criteria (one tumor that is 5 cm or smaller, or no more than three tumors 3 cm or smaller). When patients develop decompensated cirrhosis (manifested by the complications of ascites, hepatic encephalopathy, jaundice, or portal-hypertension–related bleeding), liver transplantation should be considered. One-year survival after liver transplantation is typically 80% to 90%.

Patients being considered for liver transplantation must be carefully assessed by the transplant center for potential contraindications to liver transplantation (**Table 35**). Medical comorbidities that often accompany end-stage liver disease

TABLE 34.	Causes of Fulminant Hepatic Failure
Drugs	
Acetaminophen	
Isoniazid	
Sulfonamides	
Tetracycline	
MDMA ("ecstasy")	
NSAIDs	
Herbal remedies (black cohosh, chaparral)	
Cocaine	
Viruses	
Hepatitis A	
Hepatitis B	
Hepatitis E	
Herpes simplex virus	
Cytomegalovirus	
Epstein-Barr virus	
Parvovirus B19	
Varicella zoster virus	
Other	
Amanita phalloides mushroom intoxication	
Bacillus cereus	
Budd-Chiari syndrome	
Acute fatty liver of pregnancy	
HELLP syndrome	
Autoimmune hepatitis	

HELLP = Hemolysis, Elevated Liver enzymes, and Low Platelets; MDMA = 3,4-methylene-dioxymethamphetamine.

TABLE 35.	Contraindications for Liver Transplantation
Severe cardiac and pulmonary disease	
Cholangiocarcinoma (with exception of clinical protocols)	
Hepatocellular carcinoma exceeding Milan criteria limits	
Active alcohol or substance abuse	
Extrahepatic malignancy	
Systemic infections without adequate treatment	
Morbid obesity	
Inability to comply with pre- and posttransplant regimens	
AIDS (HIV infection is a contraindication at some transplant centers)	
Advanced age is a relative contraindication	

CONT.

include obesity, substance use, diabetes mellitus, and vascular disease. These must be managed while the patient is awaiting liver transplantation to ensure that patients remain candidates for liver transplantation. ▣

Hepatic Tumors, Cysts, and Abscesses

Hepatic Cysts

Benign liver findings are commonly detected on liver imaging; hepatic cysts are noted most frequently. Simple hepatic cysts have a uniform, thin wall and no internal echoic structures. These occur more commonly in women and are typically asymptomatic. Incidental simple cysts of less than 4 cm are rarely of clinical significance.

A large cyst rarely produces symptoms such as nausea or abdominal discomfort. The preferred therapeutic approach to a large symptomatic simple cyst is laparoscopic fenestration, because simple needle aspiration is associated with high rates of cyst recurrence.

Because simple hepatic cysts are rarely symptomatic, the presence of symptoms with a hepatic cyst should raise suspicion for a cystadenoma. These lesions can be differentiated from simple cysts by ultrasonography; wall irregularity and internal echoes are consistent with cystadenoma. Cystadenomas have a risk of malignant transformation to cystadenocarcinoma and should be resected. It is difficult to differentiate a cystadenoma from a cystadenocarcinoma on clinical, radiologic, and even histologic appearance.

Focal Nodular Hyperplasia

Focal nodular hyperplasia (FNH) is a benign liver lesion that is thought to be a hypertrophic tissue reaction to an anomalous artery. FNH is more common in women than men, and most are found incidentally. The diagnosis of FNH is typically made radiographically; the appearance of the anomalous artery as a "central scar" on CT or MRI is characteristic. If a "central scar" is not identified, the differentiation between FNH and hepatic adenoma can be challenging, and liver biopsy is occasionally required. Commonly, a benign-appearing indeterminate lesion in a noncirrhotic liver that is less than 5 cm in diameter can be monitored by ultrasound every 6 months to confirm that it has not changed in size, without a liver biopsy being performed. FNH has no malignant potential and extremely low risk of rupture or other complications. The management of FNH is typically reassurance. FNH is not hormone responsive and, therefore, pregnancy and oral contraceptives are not contraindicated.

Hepatic Adenoma

The lesion most commonly confused with FNH is hepatic adenoma (HA). HAs are characterized histologically by sheets of benign hepatocytes without biliary structures or other nonparenchymal liver cells. HAs occur more commonly in women and are associated with the use of oral contraceptives. There is a risk of malignant transformation or spontaneous rupture with bleeding. Surgical resection is recommended for HAs greater than 5 cm in diameter or if pregnancy is being considered. HAs less than 5 cm in diameter can be managed with discontinuation of oral contraceptives and sequential imaging to determine if there is lesion regression.

Hepatic Hemangioma

Hepatic hemangiomas are common benign liver findings. They can range from less than 1 cm to greater than 20 cm in diameter. Hepatic hemangiomas greater than 5 cm are called giant hemangiomas. Symptoms of large hemangiomas are most commonly right upper quadrant fullness or discomfort. The diagnosis is most commonly made by contrast-enhanced CT or MRI, which shows peripheral nodular enhancement of the lesion followed by centripetal filling. The prognosis of patients with hepatic hemangiomas is excellent, and patients with small lesions can be reassured. Giant hemangiomas have a risk of bleeding that is too low to warrant prophylactic resection. If sequential imaging demonstrates growth or if symptoms develop, operative resection can be considered.

Liver Abscesses

Patients with liver abscesses typically have fever, dull abdominal pain, anorexia, and malaise. Most liver abscesses are found on abdominal imaging. Hepatic abscesses are believed to be caused by direct spreading from associated peritonitis or hematogenous seeding from abdominal infections such as appendicitis, diverticulitis, or cholangitis. Most hepatic abscesses are associated with enteric organisms such as *Escherichia coli* or anaerobic bacteria. The management of hepatic abscesses is by percutaneous drainage and antibiotics.

Amebiasis

Patients who have traveled to areas where amebiasis is endemic (such as tropical areas with poor sanitation) and present with symptoms of fever and right upper quadrant pain may have amebic liver abscesses. Amebic cysts migrate to the liver via the portal vein after invasion of the colonic wall. The interval between exposure and symptom onset is 2 to 4 months. Diagnosis is made by abdominal imaging in conjunction with serologic and stool testing for amebiasis. Amebic abscesses are treated with antibiotics to prevent potentially life-threatening rupture.

KEY POINTS

- Because simple hepatic cysts are rarely symptomatic, the presence of symptoms with a hepatic cyst should raise suspicion for a cystadenoma, which has a risk of malignant transformation.
- Hepatic adenomas are hormone responsive and oral contraceptives should be discontinued; resection is warranted for large adenomas owing to a risk of rupture or malignant transformation.

- Hepatic abscesses typically present with nonspecific symptoms such as fever, dull abdominal pain, anorexia, and malaise, and management consists of drainage and antibiotics.

Pregnancy-Related Liver Disease

Physiologic changes of pregnancy may mimic liver disease. Edema, palmar erythema, and spider angiomas may occur because of increased circulatory volumes and altered hormonal states. Chronic liver diseases unrelated to pregnancy can occur coincidentally with pregnancy and include viral, immune-mediated, and metabolic liver diseases.

Several diseases of the liver can complicate pregnancy (**Table 36**). Pregnancy-related liver disease can recur during subsequent pregnancies. During the first trimester, hyperemesis gravidarum occurs when prolonged vomiting results in fluid and electrolyte abnormalities. Elevated hepatic aminotransferases are seen in up to 50% of patients. Laboratory abnormalities remit with resolution of vomiting. Hyperemesis gravidarum is very rarely associated with liver failure.

Intrahepatic cholestasis of pregnancy (ICP) occurs in between 1:300 and 1:1000 pregnancies and is more common in women of Scandinavian, South American, or South Asian origin. ICP is presumed to result from cholestatic effects of increased pregnancy-related hormones; similar symptoms can sometimes be seen in nonpregnant women treated with supplemental estrogens and progesterones. ICP typically presents in the second to third trimesters of pregnancy. Symptoms include pruritus in most patients and jaundice in 10% to 25% of patients. Elevated serum bile acids are diagnostic of ICP. Ursodeoxycholic acid is effective for ICP. Fetal complications such as preterm labor, fetal distress, and intrauterine death are increased in ICP. Intrauterine deaths can occur late in gestation, and women with proven ICP typically are induced at 36 to 38 weeks of gestation.

HELLP (Hemolysis, Elevated Liver enzymes, and Low Platelets) syndrome presents during the third trimester and is an advanced complication of preeclampsia. HELLP syndrome typically presents with abdominal pain, new-onset nausea and vomiting, pruritus, and jaundice. Maternal mortality can be as high as 20% and perinatal mortality as high as 33%; therefore, patients with HELLP syndrome should be managed in high-risk obstetric care units. Careful monitoring of blood pressure, fluid and electrolyte balance, kidney function, and coagulopathy is required prior to delivery. Although delivery is the definitive therapy for HELLP syndrome, the mother's condition may continue to deteriorate in the immediate postpartum period. Resolution is typically seen within 4 to 6 days after delivery. Rarely, liver transplantation may be required if fulminant hepatic failure develops. HELLP syndrome can recur in up to 25% of subsequent pregnancies.

Acute fatty liver of pregnancy (AFLP) is a rare but dangerous condition that occurs during the third trimester.

TABLE 36. Characteristics of Pregnancy-Related Liver Diseases

Disease	Trimester	Hepatic Aminotransferases (units/L)	Bilirubin (mg/dL [µmol/L])	Other Laboratory Changes	Treatment	Prognosis
Hyperemesis gravidarum	First	<500	<4 (68.4)	Electrolyte abnormalities	Antiemetics, intravenous fluids	Good
Intrahepatic cholestasis of pregnancy	Second/third	<500	<6 (102.6)	Elevated serum bile acids	Ursodeoxycholic acid	Good
HELLP syndrome	Third	<500	Elevated, unconjugated	Low platelets, hemolytic anemia	Delivery	High maternal and fetal mortality; liver transplantation may be required
AFLP	Third	100-1000	Elevated	Hypoglycemia, coagulopathy	Delivery	High maternal and fetal mortality; liver transplantation may be required

AFLP = acute fatty liver of pregnancy; HELLP = Hemolysis, Elevated Liver enzymes, and Low Platelets.

CONT.

AFLP may be difficult to differentiate from HELLP syndrome. Indicators of hepatic failure, including hypoglycemia and coagulopathy, tend to be worse in AFLP. AFLP is a recognized cause of liver failure, and the care of patients with AFLP should involve a hepatologist to facilitate transfer to a liver transplant center. Prompt delivery once AFLP is recognized typically results in stabilization and improvement of the mother's medical condition over the subsequent 48 to 72 hours. AFLP can recur in subsequent pregnancies. AFLP is associated with long-chain 3-hydroxyacyl-CoA dehydrogenase deficiency, and affected women and their children should be screened for this deficiency. H

KEY POINTS

- The most serious pregnancy-related liver diseases are HELLP (Hemolysis, Elevated Liver enzymes, and Low Platelets) syndrome and acute fatty liver of pregnancy; both require urgent delivery.
- All causes of pregnancy-related liver disease can recur during subsequent pregnancies.

Health Care Maintenance of the Patient with Cirrhosis

Metabolic Bone Disease
Metabolic bone disease consists primarily of osteoporosis, osteopenia, and rarely osteomalacia. Osteoporosis is clinically important and common (10% to 50%) in patients with cirrhosis. Risk factors for osteoporosis (poor nutrition, excess alcohol intake, and hypogonadism) are frequently found in patients with cirrhosis. Approximately 30% of spinal fractures in patients with cirrhosis are asymptomatic and are identified only on radiology. In contrast, femoral

neck fractures are uncommon because they occur beyond the life expectancy of most patients with cirrhosis. Bone mineral density testing should be performed in patients with cirrhosis and risk factors for osteoporosis, especially for patients on long-term corticosteroids. In the absence of osteoporosis, surveillance bone mineral density testing every 2 to 3 years is sufficient. Treatment consists of weight-bearing exercises and pharmacologic therapy. Both calcium and vitamin D should be provided for patients with osteopenia and osteoporosis. There are no studies of the safety or efficacy of oral bisphosphonates or raloxifene for osteoporosis in patients with cirrhosis, but these agents appear to be well tolerated. Intravenous preparations should be considered for patients with large varices or recent esophageal banding/sclerotherapy. Male patients with hypogonadism and cirrhosis can be treated with transdermal testosterone; however, a theoretical risk for HCC is a concern.

Immunizations
Routine immunizations are safe in patients with cirrhosis with the exception of live attenuated vaccines. All eligible patients with cirrhosis should receive annual influenza vaccination. Pneumococcal vaccination can be given every 5 years and tetanus toxoid every 10 years. HAV and HBV vaccination is safe and recommended for patients with compensated cirrhosis or chronic liver disease. Response rates in terms of adequate serum titer formation are between 90% and 95% after both vaccine series are completed. Booster inoculation for HBV may be necessary if titers become undetectable. Prior to vaccination, serologic testing for previous exposure to HAV and HBV is warranted. The presence of serum antibody titers from previous exposure is sufficient to declare an immunized state in these patients.

Medications to Avoid

Patients with cirrhosis should be cautioned about the use of medications because of the potential for drug-related adverse events. Regular NSAID and aspirin use should be avoided in patients with esophageal varices to minimize ulceration and in patients with ascites to prevent kidney dysfunction. The occasional use of acetaminophen is likely to be safe and a better alternative than NSAIDs unless the patient continues to drink alcohol. Tramadol does not appear to have a significant increased risk for hepatotoxicity. Benzodiazepines that are metabolized in the liver (such as diazepam and chlordiazepoxide) may result in increased accumulation of metabolites and excessive sedation. In contrast, lorazepam and oxazepam are excreted by the kidneys and may be more suitable for use in patients with cirrhosis. Opioids should be used with caution in patients with cirrhosis, and patients often require reduced doses and prolonged intervals of administration. The safety and effectiveness of zolpidem, ramelteon, and eszopiclone in patients with cirrhosis are unknown, but they are used commonly in patients with compensated disease.

Antibiotics associated with drug-induced liver injury (amoxicillin-clavulanate, isoniazid) should be avoided. Fluoroquinolones and cephalosporins are safe in this population. Trimethoprim-sulfamethoxazole may be useful but has been rarely associated with cholestasis. Statins do not appear to increase the risk of hepatotoxicity in patients with cirrhosis, but close monitoring of liver enzymes is required. Patients with cirrhosis and diabetes mellitus can be managed with usual oral hypoglycemic therapy. While some of these patients will go on to require insulin, anecdotal experience suggests that oral agents may be continued safely as long as they are effective.

Nutrition

Appropriate nutrition is essential to avoid the catabolic effects associated with cirrhosis. Many patients are at risk for developing protein-calorie malnutrition, resulting in further muscle wasting and greater risk for infection. Gastric accommodation may also be impaired, resulting in early satiety and reduced intake. A strategy of eating smaller portions more frequently (4 to 6 times per day) can minimize symptoms and allow the daily caloric requirement to be met. Enteral supplements are high-calorie, low-volume products that can also be used to sustain nutrition. Eating a snack prior to bedtime may also blunt the catabolic response, which intensifies overnight during the fasting state. Serum levels of fat-soluble vitamins (A, D, and E) and zinc should be checked and replaced by oral supplementation when deficiency occurs.

KEY POINTS

- Bone mineral density testing should be performed in patients with cirrhosis and risk factors for osteoporosis, especially for patients taking long-term corticosteroids.

- Routine immunizations are safe in patients with cirrhosis with the exception of live attenuated vaccines.

- Patients with cirrhosis should be cautioned about the use of medications because of the increased potential for drug-related adverse events.

- Appropriate nutrition is essential to avoid the catabolic effects associated with cirrhosis.

Vascular Disorders of the Liver

Budd-Chiari Syndrome

Budd-Chiari syndrome (BCS) is characterized by hepatic venous outflow tract obstruction (including the suprahepatic inferior vena cava) in the absence of right-sided heart failure or constrictive pericarditis. When obstruction is caused by invasion or compression from a malignancy, BCS is considered secondary. An underlying risk factor for thrombosis is found in up to 80% of patients with BCS, with myeloproliferative diseases accounting for about 50% of cases. Other causes include Behçet syndrome, antiphospholipid antibody syndrome, and oral contraceptive use.

BCS may be asymptomatic in 15% of patients; preservation of some hepatic veins with large intrahepatic or extrahepatic collaterals is seen incidentally on cross-sectional imaging. Abdominal pain, ascites, liver and spleen enlargement, and portal hypertension occur with symptomatic BCS. Marked dilation of subcutaneous veins on the trunk is suggestive of inferior vena cava obstruction. Liver chemistry testing is not helpful in diagnosis. Ascites protein content greater than 2.5 g/dL (25 g/L) and SAAG of 1.1 g/dL (11 g/L) or more suggest BCS and cardiac disease. BCS is diagnosed by an obstructed hepatic venous outflow tract on Doppler ultrasonography, triphasic CT, or MRI. Hepatic venography is necessary for diagnosis in difficult cases or when precise delineation of venous stenoses is required.

Patients with symptomatic BCS have a poor prognosis if untreated, with an estimated 90% mortality rate within 3 years largely from complications of end-stage liver disease. Anticoagulation therapy is recommended for all patients with BCS regardless of whether an underlying prothrombotic disorder is discovered. Oral contraceptives are contraindicated in patients with BCS. Hepatic vein or inferior vena cava angioplasty with or without stenting is also recommended in patients with symptomatic BCS refractory to anticoagulation. Complications of portal hypertension are managed similarly to other liver diseases. When disease is not fully controlled by medical management, the next step is TIPS insertion. For patients unresponsive to TIPS, liver transplantation is the only remaining therapeutic option, with 5-year survival rates of 70%. Lifelong anticoagulation is required after liver transplantation.

Portal Vein Thrombosis

Acute portal vein thrombosis (PVT) is characterized by the sudden formation of thrombus within the portal vein. The thrombus can also involve segments of the mesenteric veins and/or the splenic vein. Acute PVT usually presents with fever and abdominal pain of sudden onset when there is mesenteric extension; intestinal ischemia and eventually infarction can develop. Doppler ultrasound or contrast-enhanced CT demonstrates hyperechoic material in the vessel lumen with distention of the portal vein and its tributaries. Treatment consists of anticoagulation and surgery to rule out intestinal infarction. Data on use of thrombolytic therapy are lacking.

Chronic PVT is often identified incidentally and is commonly associated with cirrhosis and portal hypertension. Stasis from reduced blood flow is believed to be the cause of chronic PVT. The development of cavernous transformation with portosystemic collaterals is often observed by imaging studies. While anticoagulation has been suggested for chronic PVT by some authorities, its safety and efficacy have not been proved. Expectant management is recommended. ▣

KEY POINTS

- Budd-Chiari syndrome is characterized by hepatic venous outflow tract obstruction (including the suprahepatic inferior vena cava) in the absence of right heart failure or constrictive pericarditis.

- Portal vein thrombosis is characterized by the formation of thrombus within the portal vein and may be acute or chronic.

Disorders of the Gallbladder and Bile Ducts

Asymptomatic Gallstones

Approximately 90% of gallstones are of the cholesterol or mixed (cholesterol and bilirubin) type. Black-pigmented stones are associated with chronic hemolytic disease and cirrhosis. Brown-pigmented stones are associated with biliary tract infection. Gallstones are twice as common in women than in men; the incidence is 0.5% to 3% in men and 1.5% to 4% in women. There is a genetic predisposition in persons of Pima Indian and Scandinavian descent. Other risk factors are obesity, dyslipidemia, pregnancy, diabetes mellitus, cirrhosis, Crohn disease, resection of the terminal ileum, and gastric bypass surgery.

An estimated 60% to 80% of gallstones are asymptomatic. Over a 20-year period, 50% of patients remain asymptomatic, 30% have biliary colic, and 20% have more important complications.

Observation is recommended for adult patients with asymptomatic gallstones. The possible exceptions to this recommendation are groups at higher risk for gallbladder carcinoma, such as patients with a calcified (porcelain) gallbladder, certain American Indians, and patients with gallstones larger than 3 cm. Prophylactic cholecystectomy is currently not recommended for asymptomatic patients with diabetes.

Biliary Colic and Acute Cholecystitis

Epidemiology and Clinical Manifestations

Biliary colic is the most common clinical presentation in patients with symptomatic gallstones. The usual presentation of biliary colic is episodic, severe abdominal pain typically in the epigastrium and/or right upper quadrant but occasionally in the right lower or mid abdomen. The pain rapidly intensifies over a 15-minute interval to a steady plateau that lasts as long as 3 hours and resolves slowly. The pain is often associated with nausea or vomiting, and there is no jaundice. Pain may radiate to the interscapular region or right shoulder. Biliary colic may not always be precipitated by a large or fatty meal; attacks can occur after periods of fasting. Pain that lasts more than 6 hours suggests cholecystitis. Once an episode of biliary colic has occurred, repeated episodes are highly likely. Greater than 90% of more important complications, such as cholecystitis, cholangitis, or pancreatitis, are preceded by attacks of biliary colic. After 5 years without symptoms, however, the risk of biliary colic and complications appears to be as low as that of patients with asymptomatic stones.

Approximately 90% of cases of acute cholecystitis are caused by obstruction of the cystic duct by gallstones. Most patients with acute cholecystitis have had previous attacks of biliary colic. The pain of acute cholecystitis typically lasts longer than 3 hours and shifts to the right upper quadrant, causing localized tenderness. The pain is due to gallbladder distention, ongoing gallbladder contraction against the obstructed outlet, and occasionally bacterial infection, leading to inflammation of the gallbladder wall. Fever, nausea, and vomiting are frequent, but jaundice is unusual. Patients who are elderly or immunosuppressed or have diabetes may be remarkably asymptomatic, without fever or pain. Physical examination may disclose Murphy sign (an arrest in inspiration during direct palpation of the right upper quadrant) in 30% to 40% of patients.

Diagnosis

Ultrasonography has high sensitivity and specificity for gallstones (84% and 99% respectively) and should be routinely performed when there are features of biliary colic or a diagnosis of cholecystitis is suspected. The sensitivity of ultrasound for acute cholecystitis is 88% and the specificity is 80%. Findings of gallbladder inflammation may include thickening of the gallbladder wall (>2 mm), intramural gas,

CONT.

and pericholecystic fluid. Hepatobiliary scintigraphy (hepatobiliary iminodiacetic acid [HIDA] scan) is indicated to confirm or exclude the diagnosis of acute cholecystitis when the initial ultrasound is indeterminate, because it has high sensitivity (97%) and specificity (90%) except in the presence of acalculous cholecystitis, prolonged fasting, and chronic alcoholism.

Management

Laparoscopic cholecystectomy is the treatment of choice for symptomatic biliary colic and acute cholecystitis. Mortality rates following laparoscopic cholecystectomy are less than 0.7%, and complication rates (including bile duct injuries) do not differ between laparoscopic and open cholecystectomy. For acute cholecystitis, initial treatment is with intravenous fluids and antibiotics, followed by laparoscopic cholecystectomy within 48 to 96 hours of hospitalization. **H**

KEY POINTS

- Asymptomatic gallstone disease has a benign course and can be managed with observation.
- Biliary colic is the most common clinical presentation in patients with symptomatic gallstones.
- Laparoscopic cholecystectomy is the treatment of choice for biliary colic and acute cholecystitis.

H Acalculous Cholecystitis

Acute acalculous cholecystitis is gallbladder inflammation in the absence of obstructive cholelithiasis. Predisposing factors are hospitalization for critical illness, burns, advanced age, atherosclerotic vascular disease, AIDS, infection with *Salmonella* or cytomegalovirus, polyarteritis nodosa, and systemic lupus erythematosus. Unexplained fever and/or hyperamylasemia in patients with predisposing factors should raise suspicion for acalculous cholecystitis. Approximately 50% of these high-risk patients will develop cholangitis, empyema, gangrene, or gallbladder perforation during their hospitalization. Abdominal ultrasonography demonstrates significant gallbladder wall thickening and/or distention. Supportive treatment with intravenous antibiotic coverage of anaerobic and gram-negative bacteria is required. Definitive therapy with cholecystectomy is preferred but may be contraindicated in severely ill patients. Therapeutic decompression can be achieved with image-guided percutaneous cholecystostomy tube placement. The mortality rate for acute acalculous cholecystitis is between 10% and 50%. **H**

KEY POINT

- Acute acalculous cholecystitis is gallbladder inflammation in the absence of obstructive cholelithiasis.

Common Bile Duct Stones and Cholangitis **H**

Choledocholithiasis (common bile duct stones) is a leading cause of obstructive jaundice. Although complications are more common than with symptomatic gallstones, less than 50% of patients with choledocholithiasis develop symptoms, and 20% spontaneously pass stones from the common bile duct.

Symptomatic choledocholithiasis usually presents with jaundice, abdominal discomfort, and pruritus. Dark urine or light-colored stools may be observed.

Dilation of the extrahepatic and intrahepatic bile ducts on abdominal ultrasound or noncontrast CT scan is consistent with a diagnosis of choledocholithiasis, but these studies lack sufficient sensitivity to rule out the diagnosis. Biliary and pancreatic ducts can be better imaged using magnetic resonance cholangiopancreatography (MRCP), which has 95% to 100% sensitivity and 75% to 95% specificity for common bile duct stones. Endoscopic ultrasound has similar test characteristics as MRCP and is less invasive than endoscopic retrograde cholangiopancreatography (ERCP). It also has the benefit of being more sensitive for identifying sludge and smaller stones.

ERCP is the preferred therapeutic method for relieving obstruction due to choledocholithiasis, with or without acute cholangitis. After endoscopic treatment of choledocholithiasis, elective cholecystectomy should be performed within 6 weeks in eligible patients. In patients who are not candidates for surgery, endoscopic sphincterotomy should be performed to allow the passage of stones.

Fever suggests the development of cholangitis, which is potentially life threatening. Cholangitis typically presents with fever, jaundice, and pain in the right upper quadrant (Charcot triad). Most patients will have cholelithiasis, elevated aminotransferase levels, and hyperbilirubinemia. Ultrasonography may show a dilated common bile duct. MRCP is a more sensitive study than ultrasonography. Acute cholangitis is usually caused by *Escherichia coli*, *Klebsiella* species, *Pseudomonas* species, and enterococci and can progress to septic shock with or without liver abscess formation. Empiric antibiotics targeting these likely organisms should be administered immediately when cholangitis is suspected, and urgent biliary decompression, typically with ERCP, is indicated. **H**

KEY POINTS

- Choledocholithiasis, or common bile duct stones, is a leading cause of obstructive jaundice.
- Endoscopic retrograde cholangiopancreatography is the preferred therapeutic method for choledocholithiasis.

Biliary Neoplasms

Gallbladder Cancer

The most common cancer of the biliary tree is gallbladder cancer. Risk factors for gallbladder cancer are age greater than 50 years, female sex, gallstones, obesity, gallbladder polyps larger than 1 cm, chronic infection with *Salmonella typhi*, and porcelain gallbladder. Prophylactic cholecystectomy should be considered in patients with gallbladder polyps larger than 1 cm, gallstones larger than 3 cm, or porcelain gallbladder to prevent gallbladder cancer. Gallbladder cancer is uncommon, but it is often fatal because it is typically diagnosed at an advanced stage.

Symptoms of gallbladder cancer are nonspecific and include abdominal discomfort, nausea, anorexia, and weight loss. Laboratory findings are often normal until obstructive jaundice develops. Gallbladder cancer is often diagnosed intraoperatively (during cholecystectomy for gallbladder symptoms) or on abdominal imaging (ultrasound, CT, or MRI may reveal abnormalities of the gallbladder wall).

The management of gallbladder cancer depends on the stage of disease. Open cholecystectomy should be performed if cancer is localized to the gallbladder mucosa. Radical cholecystectomy may be curative in patients with advanced disease but limited extension into adjacent organs. In advanced tumors, curative therapy is not possible; palliative management consists of operative diversion of bile flow or endoscopic stenting of the bile ducts. The utility of chemotherapy and radiation for gallbladder cancer has not been definitively demonstrated.

Cholangiocarcinoma

Cholangiocarcinoma is cancer derived from the biliary tree exclusive of the gallbladder or the ampulla. Risk factors for cholangiocarcinoma are primary sclerosing cholangitis, biliary atresia, chronic infection with liver flukes, and biliary cysts. Screening for cholangiocarcinoma in high-risk patients, such as those with primary sclerosing cholangitis, has been a clinical challenge. There is no evidence that serial abdominal imaging with or without serum tumor markers is a useful and cost-effective screening strategy. Cholangiocarcinoma should be suspected in patients with primary sclerosing cholangitis who develop signs of clinical decompensation.

Cholangiocarcinoma is classified by location as intrahepatic and hilar/extrahepatic. Intrahepatic cholangiocarcinoma is typically asymptomatic until the tumor is advanced, at which time right upper quadrant discomfort, weight loss, and fever may be the only symptoms. An elevated serum alkaline phosphatase level may be noted. Advanced intrahepatic cholangiocarcinoma has a poor prognosis. Curative resection is not commonly possible. Radiation and chemotherapy are of undefined benefit in cholangiocarcinoma.

Cholangiocarcinoma of the hilum (Klatskin tumor) or distal bile duct commonly presents with jaundice caused by complete obstruction of the biliary tree. The diagnosis should be suspected when abdominal imaging demonstrates bile duct dilatation and an obstructing lesion. Endoscopic cholangiography with brushings or biopsies of the involved lesion is the best test to diagnose malignant changes of the bile duct. For extrahepatic tumors, operative resection would be required for potential curative management. Hilar cholangiocarcinoma can be resected if the tumor does not extend into both intrahepatic bile ducts. However, survival is poor even with successful resection. Although some centers now perform liver transplantation for selected patients, the role of liver transplantation is not yet fully defined.

Ampullary Adenocarcinoma

Ampullary adenocarcinoma is a rare cancer that occurs most often in hereditary polyposis syndromes such as familial adenomatous polyposis or Peutz-Jeghers syndrome. Patients with these syndromes should undergo regular surveillance endoscopy. Obstructive jaundice is the most common presenting symptom. Ampullary adenocarcinoma is diagnosed by endoscopic biopsy and abdominal imaging with CT. Endoscopic ultrasound is also used to diagnose and stage ampullary adenocarcinoma. Most ampullary adenocarcinomas are resectable, and prognosis is good. Excision by pancreaticoduodenectomy (Whipple procedure) is the recommended therapeutic management of ampullary adenocarcinoma.

Biliary Cysts

The diagnosis of a biliary cyst should be considered when dilatation of the bile duct is found without evidence of an obstructing lesion. Symptoms of biliary cysts include chronic, intermittent abdominal pain and recurrent bouts of cholangitis or jaundice. When abdominal ultrasound or CT suggests a biliary cyst, MR cholangiography, endoscopic cholangiography, or endoscopic ultrasound can be used to define cystic dilatation of the bile ducts and the absence of obstruction. There is a 20-fold increased risk of cholangiocarcinoma in patients with biliary cysts. Therefore, surgical excision of the entire cyst with formation of a hepaticojejunostomy is indicated. Operative resection of biliary cysts not only reduces risks of malignancy but can also alleviate development of further bouts of cholangitis.

KEY POINTS

- Prophylactic cholecystectomy should be performed in patients with gallbladder polyps larger than 1 cm, gallstones larger than 3 cm, or porcelain gallbladder to prevent gallbladder cancer.
- Gallbladder cancer is often advanced at the time of diagnosis and has a very poor prognosis.
- Cholangiocarcinoma has a poor prognosis, and there is no defined screening protocol.

- Patients with hereditary polyposis syndromes should undergo regular surveillance endoscopy to monitor for ampullary adenocarcinoma.

- Biliary cysts have a risk of malignancy and should be resected.

Gastrointestinal Bleeding

Overview

Bleeding from the gastrointestinal tract is common and causes more than one million hospital admissions in the United States yearly. Between 1998 and 2006, hospitalizations for all-cause gastrointestinal bleeding decreased by 4% and inpatient death rates decreased by 23%; these improvements may be a result of treatment of *Helicobacter pylori* infection and the use of proton pump inhibitors (PPIs). Mortality is highly dependent on age, comorbid illness, and source of bleeding.

Severe gastrointestinal bleeding is characterized by orthostatic hypotension, shock, hemoglobin level decreased more than 2 g/dL (20 g/L) from baseline, hematocrit level decreased more than 6% from baseline, or the need for more than two units of packed red blood cells. Presenting symptoms may provide clues to the cause. Hematemesis is vomiting of bright red blood (fresh blood) or coffee-ground material (altered blood) and is most commonly related to bleeding from the esophagus, stomach, or duodenum. Melena (black, tarry-appearing stool) occurs when as little as 50 to 100 mL of blood enters the gastrointestinal tract; it can originate from the esophagus, stomach, small intestine, or proximal colon. Hematochezia (bright red blood per rectum) is most commonly caused by a lower gastrointestinal source of bleeding. Hematochezia from an upper gastrointestinal source often leads to hemodynamic instability, but distal colon or rectal bleeding rarely does.

Assessment of the patient with acute gastrointestinal hemorrhage should begin with prompt attention to hemodynamic status, risk stratification, and consideration of the origin of blood loss. In many cases, the assessment of hemodynamic status and management with intravenous fluids or blood products are simultaneous.

Upper Gastrointestinal Bleeding

Upper gastrointestinal bleeding is the most common type of gastrointestinal bleeding. It is defined as intraluminal blood loss proximal to the ligament of Treitz. Upper gastrointestinal bleeding causes approximately 500,000 hospital admissions in the United States yearly and has a mortality rate of 5% to 10%. Eighty percent of upper gastrointestinal bleeding episodes stop spontaneously, but patients with continued bleeding or rebleeding are at high risk of death. Adverse prognostic indicators are advanced age, variceal bleeding, comorbid conditions (organ failure or disseminated malignancy), shock, hematemesis, increasing number of erythrocyte transfusions, active bleeding, and a visible vessel or clot in an ulcer base on endoscopy. The goal is to identify patients at highest risk of mortality so that the adequate level of in-hospital care can be provided.

Causes

The most common causes of upper gastrointestinal bleeding are peptic ulcer disease (38%), esophageal varices (16%), esophagitis (13%), malignancy (7%), angioectasia (6%), Mallory-Weiss tear (4%), and Dieulafoy lesions (2%). Dieulafoy lesions are submucosal arterioles that intermittently protrude through the mucosa and cause hemorrhage. Other important but less common lesions are cancer, portal hypertensive gastropathy (PHG), gastric antral vascular ectasias (GAVE), Cameron lesions, hemobilia, proximal Crohn disease, and gastrointestinal telangiectasias.

Upper gastrointestinal cancers rarely result in severe bleeding (1%) and may arise from esophageal or gastric cancer or gastrointestinal stromal tumors (GIST). Cameron lesions are erosions found on the crest of gastric folds within a large hiatal hernia and are thought to be caused by mechanical trauma as the hiatal hernia slides up and down. Up to 5% of patients with known hiatal hernias may have Cameron lesions. GAVE (or "watermelon stomach") can be seen in cirrhosis and connective tissue diseases; it has a characteristic endoscopic appearance with linear ectatic vessels (that resemble erythematous stripes) that arise from the pylorus. PHG is commonly seen with cirrhosis and has a characteristic mosaic appearance at endoscopy, most often seen in the body and fundus; it is classified as mild or severe depending on the absence or presence of red spots, respectively. Bleeding from PHG, GAVE, and Cameron lesions is typically chronic rather than acute. Hemobilia is a rare cause of acute gastrointestinal bleeding from the biliary tree that can occur after liver biopsy, endoscopic retrograde cholangiopancreatography (ERCP), or transjugular intrahepatic portosystemic shunt and may present with the triad of biliary colic, obstructive jaundice (from clotted blood), and melena. Telangiectasias can be seen in the stomach and proximal small bowel in patients with the rare disease hereditary hemorrhagic telangiectasia (HHT, also called Osler-Weber-Rendu disease), which results in acute or chronic gastrointestinal blood loss. These lesions most typically occur in the setting of recurrent epistaxis, mucocutaneous telangiectasia, other visceral involvement (lung, liver, brain), and a family history of HHT.

There are a few diagnoses that should not be overlooked because bleeding can be brisk and mortality high. These include bleeding from varices, pseudoaneurysms, and aortoenteric fistulas. Liver disease is common, and up to one third of patients with cirrhosis will have bleeding from esophageal varices with resultant 15% to 20% mortality. Variceal bleeding may be the first presentation of cirrhosis, and therefore a high index of suspicion is needed (see Disorders of the Liver). Acute or chronic pancreatitis can be associated with pseudocyst formation, which can erode into an adjacent artery (pseudoaneurysm). A pseudoaneurysm, while rare, can cause very brisk gastrointestinal bleeding (hemosuccus pancreaticus). A repaired abdominal aortic aneurysm (especially endovascular repair) can lead to the rare complication of an aortoenteric fistula, often as a result of graft infection or inflammation. An aortoenteric fistula can present with a minor herald bleed, followed by a torrential, life-threatening gastrointestinal bleed.

Evaluation

Evaluation of the patient with suspected upper gastrointestinal bleeding should focus on history and physical examination clues to the origin of bleeding, attention to hemodynamic status to quantify the amount of blood loss, and stratification of risk for ongoing or recurrent gastrointestinal bleeding.

The type of blood loss—hematemesis, coffee grounds, melena, or hematochezia—can suggest the origin. Slow or intermittent upper gastrointestinal bleeding usually presents with iron deficiency anemia. Brisk upper gastrointestinal bleeding presents with hematemesis or coffee-ground emesis. Hematemesis may indicate variceal bleeding. Coffee-ground emesis is more typical of gastritis or peptic ulcer disease (PUD). Historical features such as a history of PUD or NSAID use, chronic alcohol consumption or liver disease, recent history of pancreatitis, or chronic gastroesophageal reflux disease symptoms can point to PUD, variceal bleeding, pseudoaneurysmal bleeding, or esophagitis, respectively. A history of aortic endovascular stent placement, biliary manipulation, or radiation therapy may indicate bleeding from an aortoenteric fistula, hemobilia, or radiation-related gastrointestinal bleeding, respectively.

The most important components of the physical examination are routine and orthostatic vital signs. Tachycardia indicates a 15% to 30% blood loss, and hypotension indicates greater than 30% blood loss. Orthostasis indicates large-volume bleeding when routine vital signs are normal. The remainder of the physical examination should focus on identifying signs of chronic liver disease such as scleral icterus, spider angiomata, gynecomastia, and ascites.

Laboratory studies should include a complete blood count, INR, blood urea nitrogen (BUN), and serum creatinine. The hemoglobin and hematocrit are not accurate measurements of blood loss during the acute phase of bleeding but may aid decisions on erythrocyte transfusion requirements. Macrocytosis and an elevated INR are clues for underlying liver disease, and microcytosis can indicate chronic bleeding. An elevated BUN to creatinine ratio may suggest an upper gastrointestinal source.

There are several prognostic scoring systems to quantitate the risk of needing endoscopic intervention, but these are not widely used in clinical practice. The Blatchford Score can be used to predict patients with signs of upper gastrointestinal bleeding who can be managed as outpatients if all of the following are present: BUN less than 18 mg/dL (6.4 mmol/L); normal hemoglobin; systolic blood pressure greater than 109 mm Hg; pulse rate less than 100/min; and absence of melena, syncope, and hepatic and cardiac disease.

Management

Variceal bleeding is managed differently than nonvariceal bleeding, but the initial management is the same until upper endoscopy can be performed to verify the cause of bleeding. The initial management should consist of airway protection, placement of two large-bore intravenous catheters, and resuscitation with intravenous crystalloids and packed red blood cell infusions. Continuous hemodynamic monitoring is more helpful than hemoglobin and hematocrit in guiding resuscitation, but a hemoglobin level less than 7.0 g/dL (70 g/L) is an absolute indication for packed red blood cell transfusion.

For suspected nonvariceal bleeding, an intravenous PPI is often initiated before endoscopy. Nasogastric tubes are not routinely recommended. Erythromycin and metoclopramide (motility agents) should not be used routinely because they have not been shown to alter the need for erythrocyte transfusion or surgery or shorten hospital stay. However, motility agents may decrease the need for repeat endoscopy owing to improved visibility at the initial endoscopy. Patients on anticoagulation with a supratherapeutic INR should receive fresh frozen plasma. Clinical guidelines state that the risk of continued bleeding on warfarin therapy must be weighed against the risk of stopping anticoagulation. The guidelines further state that endoscopy should not be delayed for anticoagulation reversal unless the INR is supratherapeutic (INR >3.0). If a variceal bleed is suspected, octreotide and antibiotics should be administered as soon as possible. Upper endoscopy should be performed after hemodynamic stabilization of the patient but within 24 hours of presentation and within 12 hours for suspected variceal bleeding.

Endoscopic treatment of a bleeding ulcer depends on the ulcer characteristics, which are important predictors of recurrent bleeding. Patients with low-risk stigmata (a clean-based ulcer [rebleeding risk with medical therapy 3%-5%] or a nonprotuberant pigmented spot in an ulcer bed [rebleeding risk with medical therapy 5%-10%]) can be fed within 24 hours, should receive oral PPI therapy, and can undergo early hospital discharge (**Figure 26** and **Figure 27**). Duration of PPI therapy depends on the underlying cause of the ulcer and future need for NSAIDs. Ulcers with adherent clots (rebleeding risk with medical therapy 25%-30%) can be irrigated to disrupt the clot, and endoscopic treatment can be provided thereafter (**Figure 28**). Patients with high-risk stigmata (active arterial spurting [rebleeding risk with medical therapy

80%-90%] or a nonbleeding visible vessel in an ulcer base [rebleeding risk with medical therapy 40%-50%]) should be treated with epinephrine injection plus one of the following: hemoclips, thermocoagulation, or a sclerosant (**Figure 29** and **Figure 30**). Bolus followed by maintenance intravenous PPI for 72 hours is recommended for patients at high risk to decrease the risk of rebleeding, followed by oral PPI therapy. Patients at high risk require hospitalization for at least 72 hours after intervention. Surgery or interventional radiology (for embolization) is reserved for refractory bleeding or rebleeding despite endoscopic therapy.

Routine second-look endoscopy (within 24 hours) is not recommended, but it should be performed if visualization or endoscopic treatment during the initial examination was suboptimal. A repeat endoscopy should be performed for rebleeding prior to considering surgery or interventional radiology. Surveillance endoscopy for gastric ulcers to rule out malignancy (6-8 weeks later) is recommended when biopsies of the ulcer were not performed during the initial endoscopy, which is generally the case in the context of a bleeding event. Further management of PUD should focus

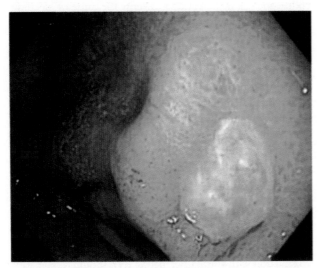

FIGURE 26. Clean-based gastric ulcer with no blood vessels, pigmented spots/protuberances, or clots noted in the base of this ulcer. This ulcer is at low risk for rebleeding; endoscopic therapy is not indicated.

Courtesy of Louis M. Wong Kee Song M.D., Mayo Clinic

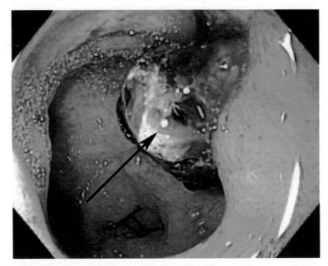

FIGURE 28. Duodenal ulcer with adherent clot (*arrow*) that is at risk for rebleeding. This can be treated medically or by clot removal and endoscopic therapy in addition to standard medical therapy.

Courtesy of Louis M. Wong Kee Song M.D., Mayo Clinic

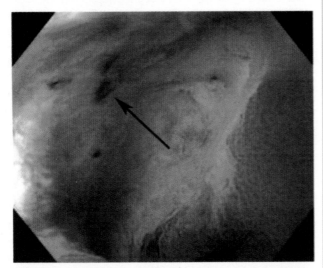

FIGURE 27. Nonprotuberant pigmented spot (*arrow*) in a duodenal ulcer bed. This ulcer is at low risk for rebleeding; endoscopic treatment is not indicated.

Courtesy of Louis M. Wong Kee Song M.D., Mayo Clinic

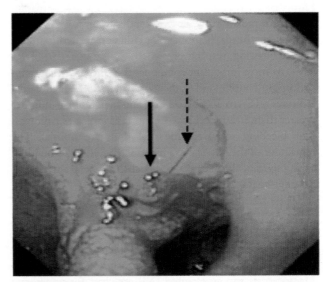

FIGURE 29. Active arterial spurting (*dotted arrow*) from a duodenal ulcer (*solid arrow*). This lesion is at the highest risk of rebleeding and must be treated endoscopically.

Courtesy of Louis M. Wong Kee Song M.D., Mayo Clinic

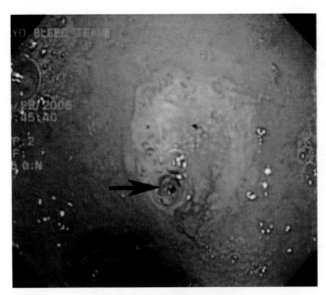

FIGURE 30. Duodenal ulcer with nonbleeding visible vessel (*arrow*) that is at high risk for rebleeding and must be treated endoscopically

Courtesy of Louis M. Wong Kee Song M.D., Mayo Clinic

on the cause, with treatment and confirmation of eradication of *Helicobacter pylori* when present and counseling regarding cessation of NSAIDs when they are causative. For patients who require aspirin for cardiovascular prophylaxis, aspirin should be restarted while continuing PPI therapy when the benefit outweighs the risk of bleeding. For further discussion of ulcers caused by NSAIDs and *H. pylori*, see Disorders of the Stomach and Duodenum. **H**

KEY POINTS

- The most common causes of upper gastrointestinal bleeding are peptic ulcer disease and esophageal varices.

- In patients with upper gastrointestinal bleeding, upper endoscopy should be performed after hemodynamic stabilization but within 24 hours of presentation (sooner if variceal bleeding is suspected).

- Endoscopy is essential for estimating risk of rebleeding and for guiding therapy in patients with upper gastrointestinal bleeding.

Lower Gastrointestinal Bleeding

Lower gastrointestinal bleeding is bleeding distal to the ligament of Treitz, typically from the colon or anorectum. It presents with bright red blood per rectum or red/maroon-colored stool (hematochezia) that is acute in onset, usually without significant abdominal pain. Patients typically have evidence of anemia but less commonly have hemodynamic instability. Although significant hypotension can result from a lower gastrointestinal source of bleeding, it should prompt

consideration of a briskly bleeding upper gastrointestinal source. The risk of lower gastrointestinal bleeding increases with age; affected patients are typically in their seventh or eighth decade of life.

Causes

The majority of patients with hematochezia (75%) have a colonic source of bleeding (**Figure 31**). Fifteen to twenty percent of patients with hematochezia have bleeding from the upper gastrointestinal tract, and 5% have bleeding from the small bowel. A source is not identified in approximately 3% of patients. When bleeding is from the colon, the most frequent source is diverticula. Colonic diverticula (actually pseudodiverticula because the outpouching occurs between the muscle fibers) occur when increased intraluminal pressure causes herniation of the colonic mucosa and submucosa through the muscular layers of the colon; they occur at points of relative weakness of the colon wall. Diverticula tend to occur at the site of entry of the small arteries (vasa recta), and these vessels may bleed at the base of the diverticular neck. Diverticulosis is most common in the left colon, but right-sided diverticula are more likely to bleed. Approximately 3% to 5% of patients with diverticulosis experience diverticular bleeding at some time.

The second most common colonic cause of lower gastrointestinal bleeding is internal hemorrhoids. Hemorrhoidal bleeding is characterized by bright red blood on the outside of the stool, on the toilet paper, or in the toilet bowl. Occasionally, hemorrhoidal bleeding can present with a large amount of fresh blood in the toilet water, and some patients can pass clots.

Bleeding can occur following colonoscopy with polypectomy and may account for up to 13% of cases of lower gastrointestinal bleeding. Postpolypectomy bleeding may occur immediately following polyp removal and is typically caused by vascular injury at the base of the polyp stalk; bleeding may also be delayed for several days, resulting from ulceration of the colon from electrocautery used for polyp removal.

Angioectasias (also called angiodysplasia, but often incorrectly referred to as arteriovenous malformations) occur less frequently than diverticular or hemorrhoidal bleeding but are an important cause of lower gastrointestinal bleeding, and their frequency increases with age. These lesions can be numerous yet subtle and can be easily missed on colonoscopy if not actively bleeding. Other causes of lower gastrointestinal bleeding are noted in Figure 31.

Evaluation

The first step in the evaluation of lower gastrointestinal bleeding is to consider whether the bleeding source could be from the upper gastrointestinal tract. Upper gastrointestinal bleeding typically presents with melena; however, it may present with hematochezia when brisk and can be life threatening if not treated early. Although placement of a nasogastric tube

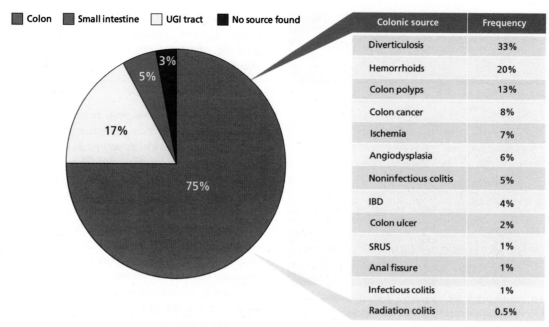

Legend: ■ Colon ■ Small intestine □ UGI tract ■ No source found

Pie graph values: 3%, 5%, 17%, 75%

Colonic source	Frequency
Diverticulosis	33%
Hemorrhoids	20%
Colon polyps	13%
Colon cancer	8%
Ischemia	7%
Angiodysplasia	6%
Noninfectious colitis	5%
IBD	4%
Colon ulcer	2%
SRUS	1%
Anal fissure	1%
Infectious colitis	1%
Radiation colitis	0.5%

FIGURE 31. The causes of hematochezia are shown in the pie graph. The most common site is the colon. The source and frequency of colonic bleeding are displayed to the right of the graph. IBD = inflammatory bowel disease; SRUS = solitary rectal ulcer syndrome; UGI = upper gastrointestinal.

Figure and data adapted/reprinted from Savides TJ, Jensen DM. Gastrointestinal bleeding. In: Feldman M, Friedman LS, Brandt LJ, eds. Sleisenger and Fordtran's Gastrointestinal and Liver Disease. Volume 1. 9th ed. Philadelphia: Saunders Elsevier, 2010:285-322. AND Reprinted/adapted from Clinical Gastroenterology and Hepatology. 6(9). Strate LL, Ayanian JZ, Kotler G, Syngal S. Risk factors for mortality in lower intestinal bleeding. 1004-1010. [PMID: 18558513] Copyright 2008, with permission from Elsevier.

had previously been standard to rule out upper gastrointestinal bleeding, it can miss up to 15% of actively bleeding lesions. Even a bile-stained nasogastric tube aspirate cannot rule out a postpyloric bleeding source, as this can be incorrect up to 50% of the time. Therefore, if an upper gastrointestinal source is suspected, upper endoscopy is the most appropriate diagnostic procedure. If an upper source is not a consideration or the patient has had a negative upper endoscopy, the next step in evaluation is colonoscopy. Anoscopy or sigmoidoscopy could be considered as alternatives if there is a high suspicion of hemorrhoids or left-sided bleeding, respectively, but the majority of patients will require a complete colonoscopy. Colonoscopy identifies a presumed or definite cause of lower gastrointestinal bleeding approximately two thirds of the time. The optimal timing of when to perform colonoscopy is not clear. The sooner the colonoscopy is performed, the more likely it is to identify a source; however, colonoscopy is typically performed on the second day of hospitalization to allow for resuscitation and a proper bowel preparation.

If colonoscopy does not identify the site of bleeding and the patient has ongoing bleeding, the next step is to evaluate for obscure gastrointestinal bleeding (see Obscure Gastrointestinal Bleeding).

Management

At presentation and throughout the evaluation, patients should be medically resuscitated and two large-bore intravenous lines should be operational at all times. Patients should be hospitalized if they have predictors of severe bleeding (defined as orthostatic vital signs, bleeding in the first 4 hours of evaluation, use of anticoagulants including aspirin, or multiple comorbidities). Most lower gastrointestinal bleeding stops without direct intervention within 24 hours, but early rebleeding is common. In one study, a therapeutic intervention was required to control continued bleeding or rebleeding in approximately two thirds of cases. Basic endoscopic therapies for bleeding due to diverticular disease or angioectasias consist of multipolar electrocoagulation, epinephrine injection, and hemoclips. If endoscopic therapy is not successful, angiographic intervention with embolization is typically the next step. However, major complications (such as bowel ischemia, femoral artery thrombosis, contrast dye reactions, and acute kidney failure) occur in up to 3% of angiographic interventions. For patients at significant risk with angiography or who have persistent bleeding despite radiographic intervention, surgery may be required to identify and treat the bleeding site. The mortality rate of lower gastrointestinal bleeding is low (<5%), but it is highest in patients who experience bleeding while already hospitalized for another indication. ⊞

KEY POINTS

- Lower gastrointestinal bleeding presents with bright red blood per rectum or red/maroon-colored stool (hematochezia) that is acute in onset, usually without significant abdominal pain.

- Colonoscopy identifies the cause of lower gastrointestinal bleeding two thirds of the time; colonic diverticula and internal hemorrhoids are the two most common sources of lower gastrointestinal bleeding.
- Most lower gastrointestinal bleeding stops without direct intervention, but early rebleeding is common.

Obscure Gastrointestinal Bleeding

Obscure gastrointestinal bleeding is recurrent bleeding without a defined source following standard upper endoscopy and colonoscopy. Obscure bleeding in which blood is clinically apparent (such as melena) is known as overt bleeding. Occult bleeding is defined as clinically suspected bleeding without overt signs of blood loss (for example, in the setting of anemia and positive fecal occult blood testing). Obscure bleeding is present in 5% of patients admitted to the hospital with gastrointestinal hemorrhage.

Causes

Causes of obscure/occult bleeding include but are not limited to angioectasias, Cameron erosions (in the context of a large hiatal hernia), NSAID-induced ulcers, or malignancy. Causes of obscure/overt bleeding include angioectasias, Dieulafoy lesions, colonic diverticula, and Meckel diverticula (**Table 37**).

Evaluation

Patients with obscure gastrointestinal bleeding should undergo repeat colonoscopy and/or upper endoscopy (depending on the suspected site of bleeding). Approximately 30% to 50% of lesions can be detected using this approach. If the site of bleeding is still not known, then the diagnostic evaluations described below can be performed, guided by the suspected site of bleeding, level of urgency, and local expertise.

Angiography

Angiography should only be performed in patients with active overt bleeding, as it requires a bleeding rate greater than 1 mL/min. It allows for immediate therapy with arterial embolization. However, the sensitivity of angiography is generally poor (only about 40%) and is operator dependent. Complications such as kidney failure, organ necrosis, and vascular dissection/aneurysm can occur.

Technetium-Labeled Nuclear Scan

Technetium-labeled nuclear scans provide the best sensitivity for actively bleeding lesions; a technetium-99m (^{99m}Tc) radiolabeled red blood cell scan requires a flow rate of only 0.1 to 0.5 mL/min. However, technetium scans are nonspecific (they often do not disclose a specific site of bleeding), and they do not allow for diagnostic intervention.

The two primary types of nuclear scans are ^{99m}Tc pertechnetate red blood cell and ^{99m}Tc sulfur colloid. Red blood cell scanning is positive in 45% of patients with an active

TABLE 37. Causes of Obscure Gastrointestinal Bleeding			
Location	**Differential Diagnosis**	**Age (Years)**	**Clinical Clues**
Proximal to the ligament of Treitz	Cameron erosion	20-60	Large hiatal hernia
	NSAID ulcerations	>20	Medication review
	Dieulafoy lesion	>40	Intermittent large-volume bleeding
	Crohn disease	20-60	Family history, extraintestinal manifestations; may also occur in small bowel and colon
	Gastric antral vascular ectasia	20-60	Female, autoimmune disease
Small bowel	Angioectasias	>60	Intermittent, usually occult bleeding; may also occur in colon
	Peutz-Jeghers syndrome	<20	Perioral pigmentation, obstructive symptoms
	Meckel diverticulum	20-60	Possible abdominal pain
	Hemangioma	<20	Possible cutaneous hemangiomas
	Malignancy	>50	Weight loss, abdominal pain
	Hereditary hemorrhagic telangiectasia	>50	Facial telangiectasias
Colon	Diverticulosis	>50	Intermittent, painless bleeding
	Malignancy	>50	Weight loss, family history

bleed and has an overall accuracy for localizing the bleeding of 78%. This scan is more sensitive than angiography and is often the first radiologic test performed.

Wireless Capsule Endoscopy

Wireless capsule endoscopy is a relatively new but effective technology that allows excellent visualization of the small bowel. Unlike angiography and technetium scans, wireless capsule endoscopy is effective even in the absence of active bleeding. Wireless capsule endoscopy detects the source of occult bleeding in 50% to 75% of patients. In patients with iron deficiency anemia, in whom bleeding can be episodic, capsule endoscopy is another way to investigate potential sources of blood loss after other investigations have been unrevealing. Capsules can become obstructed at the site of small-bowel tumors or stenoses, so it is important to counsel patients about this complication. Wireless capsule endoscopy has generally replaced push enteroscopy as the test of choice following negative upper endoscopy/colonoscopy in patients with occult bleeding.

Push Enteroscopy

Push enteroscopy is performed with a dedicated enteroscope or pediatric colonoscope and allows visualization of the distal duodenum and jejunum up to 80 cm beyond the ligament of Treitz. This technique has been used less often since the refinement of wireless capsule endoscopy. However, push enteroscopy allows for therapeutic intervention (such as coagulation of angioectasias), and therefore still has a prominent role in management of obscure bleeding. Complications of push enteroscopy are rare but include perforation, mucosal avulsion, and bleeding. The diagnostic effectiveness of enteroscopy, including the depth of insertion, is operator dependent.

Spiral Enteroscopy

Spiral enteroscopy is a new technique that allows deep bowel penetration using a spiral-shaped overtube that fits over a standard colonoscope or enteroscope. Using a "corkscrew" motion allows the endoscope to visualize deep into the distal jejunum and ileum. Spiral enteroscopy has both diagnostic and therapeutic capabilities. For example, the spiral overtube can deliver a duodenoscope to the ampulla in a patient needing endoscopic retrograde cholangiopancreatography who has previously undergone Roux-en-Y surgery. Preliminary data comparing spiral enteroscopy to wireless capsule endoscopy and push enteroscopy are lacking. The major complication of spiral enteroscopy is perforation secondary to the increased torque on the small bowel.

Single- and Double-Balloon Enteroscopy

Single- or double-balloon enteroscopy is used similarly to spiral enteroscopy to visualize the small bowel. Latex balloons are mounted on an overtube that can deliver the enteroscope into the small bowel through successive inflation and deflation. Balloon enteroscopes can deliver the enteroscope orally or rectally and can be used for diagnosis and therapy. Complications of balloon enteroscopy are perforation and bleeding via avulsion of the bowel. Contraindications are radiation enteritis, severe ulceration, and recent bowel surgery.

Small-Bowel Radiography

Small-bowel radiography is used less frequently, because newer techniques provide both imaging and localized therapy. Small-bowel barium studies and enteroclysis (small-bowel barium enema) are generally not first-line diagnostic tests for obscure bleeding. Although these examinations can visualize luminal masses and diverticula, they cannot adequately assess for conditions such as angioectasias. Their role is extremely limited in patients with gastrointestinal bleeding.

Intraoperative Endoscopy

Intraoperative endoscopy is generally employed only as a last resort for the evaluation of obscure gastrointestinal bleeding. The patient undergoes laparotomy or laparoscopy, and the bowel is evaluated with a colonoscope following surgical enterotomy. This technique should only be used if other less invasive options have been exhausted or if a patient has unexplained, life-threatening bleeding. In addition, the yield is somewhat low (approximately 25%).

Treatment

Treatment of obscure gastrointestinal bleeding depends on the source and site of pathology. Luminal tumors should generally be excised surgically, as should focal lesions such as Meckel diverticulum. Angioectasias, Dieulafoy lesions, and GAVE lesions can generally be treated endoscopically with electrocautery and/or argon plasma coagulation. Angiography can be used in patients with brisk bleeding that cannot be managed or localized endoscopically, followed by intraoperative endoscopy if angiography is unsuccessful. In patients with NSAID-induced lesions, removal of the causative agent is usually effective. In patients with angioectasias associated with aortic stenosis (Heyde syndrome), valve replacement is usually successful. Patients with von Willebrand disease and recurrent bleeding can often be treated with desmopressin or replacement of deficient factor. In patients with diffuse angioectasias not amenable to localized therapy, treatment with estrogens, octreotide, or thalidomide has had some success. **H**

KEY POINTS

- In patients with obscure gastrointestinal bleeding, repeat upper endoscopy and/or colonoscopy often identifies the cause of bleeding and should be the first step.

- Angiography (diagnostic and therapeutic) and technetium-labeled nuclear scans (diagnostic only) are only helpful in patients with active bleeding.

- Capsule endoscopy allows for diagnostic imaging of the small bowel in patients with obscure gastrointestinal bleeding and does not require active bleeding, while push, balloon, and spiral enteroscopy provide the opportunity for therapeutic intervention.

- Therapy for obscure gastrointestinal bleeding is generally directed at local control of the bleeding lesion.

Bibliography

Disorders of the Esophagus

El-Serag HB. Time trends of gastroesophageal reflux disease: a systematic review. Clin Gastroenterol Hepatol. 2007;5(1):17-26. [PMID: 17142109]

Francis DL, Katzka DA. Achalasia: update on the disease and its treatment. Gastroenterology. 2010;139(2):369-374. [PMID: 20600038]

Kahrilas PJ, Shaheen NJ, Vaezi MF, et al; American Gastroenterological Association. American Gastroenterological Association Medical Position Statement on the management of gastroesophageal reflux disease. Gastroenterology. 2008;135(4):1383-1391. [PMID: 18789939]

Pandolfino JE, Kahrilas PJ; American Gastroenterological Association. AGA technical review on the clinical use of esophageal manometry. Gastroenterology. 2005;128(1):209-224. [PMID: 15633138]

Prasad GA, Talley NJ. Eosinophilic esophagitis in adults. Gastroenterol Clin North Am. 2008;37(2):349-368. [PMID: 18499024]

Shaheen NJ, Richter JE. Barrett's oesophagus. Lancet. 2009;373(9666):850-861. [PMID: 19269522]

Tran T, Lowry AM, El-Serag HB. Meta-analysis: the efficacy of over-the-counter gastro-oesophageal reflux disease therapies. Aliment Pharmacol Ther. 2007;25(2):143-153. [PMID: 17229239]

Wang KK, Sampliner RE; Practice Parameters Committee of the American College of Gastroenterology. Updated guidelines 2008 for the diagnosis, surveillance and therapy of Barrett's esophagus. Am J Gastroenterol. 2008;103(3):788-797. [PMID: 18341497]

Disorders of the Stomach and Duodenum

Abell TL, Camilleri M, Donohoe K, et al; American Neurogastroenterology and Motility Society and the Society of Nuclear Medicine. Consensus recommendations for gastric emptying scintigraphy: a joint report of the American Neurogastroenterology and Motility Society and the Society of Nuclear Medicine. Am J Gastroenterol. 2008;103(3):753-763. [PMID: 18028513]

Chey WD, Wong BC; Practice Parameters Committee of the American College of Gastroenterology. American College of Gastroenterology guideline on the management of Helicobacter pylori infection. Am J Gastroenterol. 2007;102(8):1808-1825. [PMID: 17608775]

Frank P, Crookes PF. Short- and long-term surgical follow-up of the postbariatric surgery patient. Gastroenterol Clin North Am. 2010;39(1):135-146. [PMID: 20202586]

Hirota WK, Zuckerman MJ, Adler DG, et al; Standards of Practice Committee, American Society for Gastrointestinal Endoscopy. ASGE guideline: the role of endoscopy in the surveillance of premalignant conditions of the upper GI tract. Gastrointest Endosc. 2006;63(4):570-580. [PMID: 16564854]

Hwang JH, Rulyak SD, Kimmey MB; American Gastroenterological Association Institute. American Gastroenterological Association Institute technical review on the management of gastric subepithelial masses. Gastroenterology. 2006;130(7):2217-2228. [PMID: 16762644]

Jemal A, Siegel R, Xu J, Ward E. Cancer statistics, 2010. CA Cancer J Clin. 2010;60(5):277-300. [PMID: 20610543]

Lanza FL, Chan FK, Quigley EM; Practice Parameters Committee of the American College of Gastroenterology. Guidelines for prevention of NSAID-related ulcer complications. Am J Gastroenterol. 2009;104(3):728-738. [PMID: 19240698]

Malfertheiner P, Chan FK, McColl KE. Peptic ulcer disease. Lancet. 2009;374(9699):1449-1461. [PMID: 19683340]

McColl KE. Clinical practice. Helicobacter pylori infection. N Engl J Med. 2010;362(17):1597-1604. [PMID: 20427808]

Park do Y, Lauwers GY. Gastric polyps: classification and management. Arch Pathol Lab Med. 2008;132(4):633-640. [PMID: 18384215]

Shankar P, Boylan M, Sriram K. Micronutrient deficiencies after bariatric surgery. Nutrition. 2010;26(11-12):1031-1037. [PMID: 20363593]

Tack J, Talley NJ. Gastroduodenal disorders. Am J Gastroenterol. 2010;105(4):757-763. [PMID: 20372127]

Disorders of the Pancreas

Banks PA, Freeman ML; Practice Parameters Committee of the American College of Gastroenterology. Practice guidelines in acute pancreatitis. Am J Gastroenterol. 2006;101(10):2379-2400. [PMID: 17032204]

Cahen DL, Gouma DJ, Nio Y, et al. Endoscopic versus surgical drainage of the pancreatic duct in chronic pancreatitis. N Engl J Med. 2007;356(7):676-684. [PMID: 17301298]

Davies K, Conlon KC. Neuroendocrine tumors of the pancreas. Curr Gastroenterol Rep. 2009;11(2):119-127. [PMID: 19281699]

Ferrone CR, Correa-Gallego C, Warshaw AL, et al. Current trends in pancreatic cystic neoplasms. Arch Surg. 2009;144(5):448-454. [PMID: 19451487]

Hidalgo M. Pancreatic cancer. N Engl J Med. 2010;362(17):1605-1617. [PMID: 20427809]

Leib JG 2nd, Forsmark CE. Review article: pain and chronic pancreatitis. Aliment Pharmacol Ther. 2009;29(7):706-719. [PMID: 19284407]

Sah RP, Chari ST, Pannala R, et al. Differences in clinical profile and relapse rate of type 1 versus type 2 autoimmune pancreatitis. Gastroenterology. 2010;139(1):140-148. [PMID: 20353791]

Weinberg BM, Spiegel BM, Tomlinson JS, Farrell JJ. Asymptomatic pancreatic cystic neoplasms: maximizing survival and quality of life using Markov-based clinical nomograms. Gastroenterology. 2010;138(2):531-540. [PMID: 19818780]

Disorders of the Small and Large Bowel

American College of Gastroenterology Task Force on Irritable Bowel Syndrome, Brandt LJ, Chey WD, Foxx-Orenstein AE, et al. An evidence-based position statement on the management of irritable bowel syndrome. Am J Gastroenterol. 2009;104 Suppl 1:S1-S35. [PMID: 19521341]

Bharucha AE, Wald AM. Anorectal disorders. Am J Gastroenterol. 2010;105(4):786-794. [PMID: 20372131]

Brandt LJ, Boley SJ. AGA technical review on intestinal ischemia. American Gastrointestinal Association. Gastroenterology. 2000;118(5):954-968. [PMID: 10784596]

Bures J, Cyrany J, Kohoutova D, et al. Small intestinal bacterial overgrowth syndrome. World J Gastroenterol. 2010;16(24):2978-2990. [PMID: 20572300]

Donohoe CL, Reynolds JV. Short bowel syndrome. Surgeon. 2010;8(5):270-279. [PMID: 20709285]

Kornbluth A, Sachar DB; Practice Parameters Committee of the American College of Gastroenterology. Ulcerative colitis practice guidelines in adults: American College Of Gastroenterology, Practice Parameters Committee. Am J Gastroenterol. 2010;105(3):501-523. [PMID: 20068560]

Lichtenstein GR, Hanauer SB, Sandborn WJ; Practice Parameters Committee of American College of Gastroenterology. Management of Crohn's disease in adults. Am J Gastroenterol. 2009;104(2):465-483. [PMID: 19174807]

Rao SS, Go JT. Update on the management of constipation in the elderly: new treatment options. Clin Interv Aging. 2010;5:163-171. [PMID: 20711435]

Rubio-Tapia A, Murray JA. Celiac disease. Curr Opin Gastroenterol. 2010;26(2):116-122. [PMID: 20040864]

Shaukat A, Levitt MD, Taylor BC, et al. Systematic review: effective management strategies for lactose intolerance. Ann Intern Med. 2010;152(12):797-803. [PMID: 20404262]

Spiller RC, Thompson WG. Bowel disorders. Am J Gastroenterol. 2010;105(4):775-785. [PMID: 20372130]

Touzios JG, Dozois EJ. Diverticulosis and acute diverticulitis. Gastroenterol Clin North Am. 2009;38(3):513-525. [PMID: 19699411]

Colorectal Neoplasia

Beggs AD, Latchford AR, Vasen HF, et al. Peutz-Jeghers syndrome: a systematic review and recommendations for management. Gut. 2010;59(7):975-986. [PMID: 20581245]

East JE, Saunders BP, Jass JR. Sporadic and syndromic hyperplastic polyps and serrated adenomas of the colon: classification, molecular genetics, natural history, and clinical management. Gastroenterol Clin North Am. 2008;37(1):25-46. [PMID: 18313538]

Farraye FA, Odze RD, Eaden J, et al; AGA Institute Medical Position Panel on Diagnosis and Management of Colorectal Neoplasia in Inflammatory Bowel Disease. AGA medical position statement on the diagnosis and management of colorectal neoplasia in inflammatory bowel disease. Gastroenterology. 2010;138(2):738-745. [PMID: 20141808]

Huxley RR, Ansary-Moghaddam A, Clifton P, Czernichow S, Parr CL, Woodward M. The impact of dietary and lifestyle risk factors on risk of colorectal cancer: a quantitative overview of the epidemiological evidence. Int J Cancer. 2009;125(1):171-180. [PMID: 19350627]

Levin B, Lieberman DA, McFarland B, et al; American Cancer Society Colorectal Cancer Advisory Group; US Multi-Society Task Force; American College of Radiology Colon Cancer Committee. Screening and surveillance for the early detection of colorectal cancer and adenomatous polyps, 2008: a joint guideline from the American Cancer Society, the US Multi-Society Task Force on Colorectal Cancer, and the American College of Radiology. Gastroenterology. 2008;134(5):1570-1595. [PMID: 18384785]

Lieberman D. Progress and challenges in colorectal cancer screening and surveillance. Gastroenterology. 2010;138(6):2115-2126. [PMID: 20167216]

Lindor NM, McMaster ML, Lindor CJ, Greene MH; National Cancer Institute, Division of Cancer Prevention, Community Oncology and Prevention Trials Research Group. Concise handbook of familial cancer susceptibility syndromes - second edition. J Natl Cancer Inst Monogr. 2008;(38):1-93. [PMID: 18559331]

Qaseem A, Denberg TD, Hopkins RH Jr, et al; for the Clinical Guidelines Committee of the American College of Physicians. Screening for Colorectal Cancer: A Guidance Statement From the American College of Physicians. Ann Intern Med. 2012;156(5):378-386. [PMID: 22393133]

Umar A, Boland CR, Terdiman JP, et al. Revised Bethesda Guidelines for hereditary nonpolyposis colorectal cancer (Lynch syndrome) and microsatellite instability. J Natl Cancer Inst. 2004;96(4):261-268. [PMID: 14970275]

Vasen HF, Watson P, Mecklin JP, Lynch HT. New clinical criteria for hereditary nonpolyposis colorectal cancer (HNPCC, Lynch syndrome) proposed by the International Collaborative group on HNPCC. Gastroenterology. 1999;116(6):1453-1456. [PMID: 10348829]

Whitlock EP, Lin JS, Liles E, Beil TL, Fu R. Screening for colorectal cancer: a targeted, updated systematic review for the U.S. Preventive Services Task Force. Ann Intern Med. 2008;149(9):638-658. [PMID: 18838718]

Disorders of the Liver

Bruix J, Sherman M; Practice Guidelines Committee, American Association for the Study of Liver Diseases. Management of hepatocellular carcinoma. Hepatology. 2005;42(5):1208-1236. [PMID: 16250051]

Chapman R, Fevery J, Kalloo A, et al; American Association for the Study of Liver Diseases. Diagnosis and management of primary sclerosing cholangitis. Hepatology. 2010;51(2):660-678. [PMID: 20101749]

Cheung O, Sanyal AJ. Recent advances in nonalcoholic fatty liver disease. Curr Opin Gastroenterol. 2010;26(3):202-208. [PMID: 20168226]

Córdoba J, Mínguez B. Hepatic encephalopathy. Semin Liver Dis. 2008;28(1):70-80. [PMID: 18293278]

DeLeve LD, Valla DC, Garcia-Tsao G; American Association for the Study Liver Diseases. Vascular disorders of the liver. Hepatology. 2009;49(5):1729-1764. [PMID: 19399912]

Garcia-Tsao G, Bosch J. Management of varices and variceal hemorrhage in cirrhosis. N Engl J Med. 2010;362(9):823-832. [PMID: 20200386]

Ghany MG, Strader DB, Thomas DL, Seeff LB; American Association for the Study of Liver Diseases. Diagnosis, management, and treatment of hepatitis C: an update. Hepatology. 2009;49(4):1335-1374. [PMID: 19330875]

Hoeper MM, Krowka MJ, Strassburg CP. Portopulmonary hypertension and hepatopulmonary syndrome. Lancet. 2004;363(9419):1461-1468. [PMID: 15121411]

Ichai P, Samuel D. Etiology and prognosis of fulminant hepatitis in adults. Liver Transpl. 2008;14(Suppl 2):S67-S79. [PMID: 18825677]

Lindor KD, Gershwin ME, Poupon R, Kaplan M, Bergasa NV, Heathcote EJ; American Association for Study of Liver Diseases. Primary biliary cirrhosis. Hepatology. 2009;50(1):291-308. [PMID: 19554543]

Lok AS, McMahon BJ. Chronic hepatitis B. Hepatology. 2007;45(2):507-539. [PMID: 17256718]

Manns MP, Czaja AJ, Gorham JD, et al; American Association for the Study of Liver Diseases. Diagnosis and management of autoimmune hepatitis. Hepatology. 2010;51(6):2193-2213. [PMID: 20513004]

Navarro VJ, Senior JR. Drug-related hepatotoxicity. N Engl J Med. 2006;354(7):731-739. [PMID: 16481640]

O'Shea RS, Dasarathy S, McCullough AJ; Practice Guideline Committee of the American Association for the Study of Liver Diseases; Practice Parameters Committee of the American College of Gastroenterology. Alcoholic liver disease. Hepatology. 2010;51(1):307-328. [PMID: 20034030]

Pietrangelo A. Inherited metabolic disease of the liver. Curr Opin Gastroenterol. 2009;25(3):209-214 [PMID: 19342951]

Runyon, BA; AASLD Practice Guidelines Committee. Management of adult patients with ascites due to cirrhosis: an update. Hepatology. 2009;49(6):2087-2107. [PMID: 19475696]

Disorders of the Gallbladder and Bile Ducts

Eslick GD. Epidemiology of gallbladder cancer. Gastroenterol Clin North Am. 2010;39(2):307-330. [PMID: 20478488]

Gatto M, Alvaro D. Cholangiocarcinoma: risk factors and clinical presentation. Eur Rev Med Pharmacol Sci. 2010;14(4):363-367. [PMID: 20496549]

Lammert F, Miquel JF. Gallstone disease: from genes to evidence-based therapy. J Hepatol. 2008;48(Suppl 1):S124-S135. [PMID: 18308417]

Wittenburg H. Hereditary liver disease: gallstones. Best Pract Res Clin Gastroenterol. 2010;24(5):747-756. [PMID: 20955975]

Gastrointestinal Bleeding

Akerman PA, Agrawal D, Chen W, Cantero D, Avila J, Pangtay J. Spiral enteroscopy: a novel method of enteroscopy by using the Endo-Ease Discovery SB overtube and a pediatric colonoscope. Gastrointest Endosc. 2009;69(2):327-332. [PMID: 19100974]

ASGE Standards of Practice Committee, Banerjee S, Cash BD, Dominitz JA, et al. The role of endoscopy in the management of patients with peptic ulcer disease. Gastrointest Endosc. 2010;71(4): 663-668. [PMID: 20363407]

Barkun AN, Bardou M, Kuipers EJ; International Consensus Upper Gastrointestinal Bleeding Conference Group. International consensus recommendations on the management of patients with nonvariceal upper gastrointestinal bleeding. Ann Intern Med. 2010;152(2):101-113. [PMID: 20083829]

Davila RE, Rajan E, Adler DG, et al; Standards of Practice Committee. ASGE Guideline: the role of endoscopy in the patient with lower-GI bleeding. Gastrointest Endosc. 2005;62(5):656-660. [PMID: 16246674]

de Leusse A, Vahedi K, Edery J, et al. Capsule endoscopy or push enteroscopy for first-line exploration of obscure gastrointestinal bleeding? Gastroenterology. 2007;132(3):855-862. [PMID: 17324401]

Junquera F, Feu F, Papo M, et al. A multicenter, randomized, clinical trial of hormonal therapy in the prevention of rebleeding from gastrointestinal angiodysplasia. Gastroenterology. 2001;121(5):1073-1079. [PMID: 11677198]

Raju GS, Gerson L, Das A, Lewis B; American Gastroenterological Association. American Gastroenterological Association (AGA) Institute technical review on obscure gastrointestinal bleeding. Gastroenterology. 2007;133(5):1697-1717. [PMID: 17983812]

Shinozaki S, Yamamoto H, Yano T, et al. Long-term outcome of patients with obscure gastrointestinal bleeding investigated by double-balloon endoscopy. Clin Gastroenterol Hepatol. 2010;8(2):151-158. [PMID: 19879968]

Strate LL, Ayanian JZ, Kotler G, Syngal S. Risk factors for mortality in lower intestinal bleeding. Clin Gastroenterol Hepatol. 2008;6(9): 1004-1010. [PMID: 18558513]

Gastroenterology and Hepatology Self-Assessment Test

This self-assessment test contains one-best-answer multiple-choice questions. Please read these directions carefully before answering the questions. Answers, critiques, and bibliographies immediately follow these multiple-choice questions. The American College of Physicians is accredited by the Accreditation Council for Continuing Medical Education (ACCME) to provide continuing medical education for physicians.

The American College of Physicians designates MKSAP 16 Gastroenterology and Hepatology for a maximum of 14 *AMA PRA Category 1 Credits*™. Physicians should claim only the credit commensurate with the extent of their participation in the activity.

Earn "Same-Day" CME Credits Online

For the first time, print subscribers can enter their answers online to earn CME credits in 24 hours or less. You can submit your answers using online answer sheets that are provided at mksap.acponline.org, where a record of your MKSAP 16 credits will be available. To earn CME credits, you need to answer all of the questions in a test and earn a score of at least 50% correct (number of correct answers divided by the total number of questions). Take any of the following approaches:

> ➤ Use the printed answer sheet at the back of this book to record your answers. Go to mksap.acponline.org, access the appropriate online answer sheet, transcribe your answers, and submit your test for same-day CME credits. There is no additional fee for this service.

> ➤ Go to mksap.acponline.org, access the appropriate online answer sheet, directly enter your answers, and submit your test for same-day CME credits. There is no additional fee for this service.

> ➤ Pay a $10 processing fee per answer sheet and submit the printed answer sheet at the back of this book by mail or fax, as instructed on the answer sheet. Make sure you calculate your score and fax the answer sheet to 215-351-2799 or mail the answer sheet to Member and Customer Service, American College of Physicians, 190 N. Independence Mall West, Philadelphia, PA 19106-1572, using the courtesy envelope provided in your MKSAP 16 slipcase. You will need your 10-digit order number and 8-digit ACP ID number, which are printed on your packing slip. Please allow 4 to 6 weeks for your score report to be emailed back to you. Be sure to include your email address for a response.

If you do not have a 10-digit order number and 8-digit ACP ID number or if you need help creating a username and password to access the MKSAP 16 online answer sheets, go to mksap.acponline.org or email custserv@acponline.org.

CME credit is available from the publication date of July 31, 2012, until July 31, 2015. You may submit your answer sheets at any time during this period.

Directions

*Each of the numbered items is followed by lettered answers. Select the **ONE** lettered answer that is **BEST** in each case.*

Self-Assessment Test

Item 1

A 36-year-old woman is evaluated during a routine examination. She is generally healthy and has no gastrointestinal problems. She would like to discuss colorectal cancer screening recommendations. Her family history is as follows:

Father	Colorectal cancer, age 52 years
Mother	No known cancers or precancerous lesions
Paternal aunt	Endometrial cancer, age 37 years
Paternal uncle	Large (2.5-cm) colorectal adenoma (ascending colon), age 42 years
Brother	Colorectal cancer, age 48 years

Physical examination, including cardiopulmonary examination, is normal.

Which of the following is the most appropriate management strategy?

(A) Colonoscopy now
(B) Colonoscopy at age 40 years
(C) Colonoscopy at age 50 years
(D) CT colonography at age 40 years
(E) Stool DNA test at age 40 years

Item 2

A 42-year-old man is evaluated in follow-up for elevated liver chemistry tests. He is asymptomatic. He has a 6-year history of type 2 diabetes mellitus, hyperlipidemia, and hypertension. His current medications are metformin, simvastatin, and lisinopril. He does not drink alcohol.

On physical examination, temperature is 37.0 °C (98.6 °F), blood pressure is 130/74 mm Hg, pulse rate is 82/min, and respiration rate is 14/min. BMI is 32. Abdominal examination discloses mild hepatomegaly and active bowel sounds.

Laboratory studies:

Alkaline phosphatase	90 units/L
Alanine aminotransferase	120 units/L
Aspartate aminotransferase	85 units/L
Total bilirubin	1.1 mg/dL (18.8 µmol/L)
LDL cholesterol	100 mg/dL (2.59 mmol/L)
Hemoglobin A_{1c}	7.2%
Iron	75 µg/dL (13 µmol/L)
Total iron-binding capacity	300 µg/dL (54 µmol/L)
Hepatitis B surface antigen	Negative
Antibody to hepatitis B surface antigen	Positive
Hepatitis C virus antibody	Negative

Abdominal ultrasound reveals increased hepatic echotexture consistent with hepatic steatosis. Hepatic configuration is otherwise normal.

In addition to weight loss, which of the following is the most appropriate management?

(A) Discontinue simvastatin
(B) Initiate entecavir
(C) Phlebotomy
(D) Serial monitoring of aminotransferases

Item 3

A 45-year-old man is admitted to the hospital for a 2-day history of fever and abdominal pain. His medical history is notable for cirrhosis due to chronic hepatitis C, esophageal varices, ascites, and minimal hepatic encephalopathy. His medications are furosemide, spironolactone, nadolol, lactulose, zinc, vitamin A, and vitamin D.

On physical examination, temperature is 36.5 °C (97.7 °F), blood pressure is 100/50 mm Hg, pulse rate is 84/min, and respiration rate is 20/min. BMI is 28. Abdominal examination discloses distention consistent with ascites. The abdomen is nontender to palpation.

Laboratory studies:

Hemoglobin	10 g/dL (100 g/L)
Leukocyte count	3500/µL (3.5×10^9/L)
Platelet count	70,000/µL (70×10^9/L)
INR	1.5 (normal range, 0.8-1.2)
Albumin	2.5 g/dL (25 g/L)
Alkaline phosphatase	220 units/L
Alanine aminotransferase	30 units/L
Aspartate aminotransferase	40 units/L
Total bilirubin	4 mg/dL (68.4 µmol/L)
Creatinine	1.8 mg/dL (159 µmol/L)
Urinalysis	Normal

Abdominal ultrasound discloses cirrhosis, splenomegaly, and ascites. The portal and hepatic veins are patent, and there is no hydronephrosis. Diagnostic paracentesis discloses a cell count of 2000/µL with 20% neutrophils, a total protein level of 1 g/dL (10 g/L), and an albumin level of 0.7 g/dL (7 g/L), consistent with spontaneous bacterial peritonitis.

Which of the following is the most appropriate treatment?

(A) Cefotaxime
(B) Cefotaxime and albumin
(C) Furosemide and spironolactone
(D) Large-volume paracentesis

Item 4

A 34-year-old woman is evaluated in an urgent care clinic for a 1-day history of watery diarrhea and mild abdominal cramps. She is having four watery stools per day. She has not had fever or blood in her stool. Although she has felt mildly nauseated, she has been able to stay hydrated with oral intake. She works as a banker, and colleagues at work have had similar gastrointestinal symptoms over recent weeks. She has no history of recent hospitalization, antibiotic use, or medication changes. She has no risk factors for HIV infection.

On physical examination, temperature is 36.1 °C (97.0 °F), blood pressure is 110/75 mm Hg, pulse rate is 86/min, and respiration rate is normal. BMI is 24. The mucous membranes are moist, and there is no skin tenting. Abdominal examination reveals mild abdominal tenderness but normal bowel sounds. There is no guarding or rebound. A urine pregnancy test is negative.

Which of the following is the most appropriate diagnostic test?

(A) *Clostridium difficile* polymerase chain reaction
(B) Fecal leukocyte testing
(C) Flexible sigmoidoscopy with biopsies
(D) General stool bacterial cultures
(E) No additional studies

Item 5

A 32-year-old woman is evaluated for a 10-day history of malaise, right upper quadrant discomfort, and progressive jaundice. She has had no recent travel outside of the United States, does not drink alcohol, and has no recent ingestions of drugs, including acetaminophen or herbal remedies. Up until this time, she has been healthy. She has a history of type 1 diabetes mellitus for which she takes insulin glargine and insulin detemir. She has no other medical problems.

On physical examination, temperature is 37.5 °C (99.5 °F), blood pressure is 106/68 mm Hg, pulse rate is 90/min, and respiration rate is 18/min. BMI is 24. Mental status is normal. Jaundice and scleral icterus are noted. Abdominal examination reveals tender hepatomegaly.

Laboratory studies:

INR	0.9 (normal range, 0.8-1.2)
Albumin	3.8 g/dL (38 g/L)
Alkaline phosphatase	220 units/L
Alanine aminotransferase	920 units/L
Aspartate aminotransferase	850 units/L
Total bilirubin	14.4 mg/dL (246.2 µmol/L)
Direct bilirubin	10.6 mg/dL (181.3 µmol/L)

Abdominal ultrasound demonstrates hepatic enlargement with edema surrounding the gallbladder. There is no biliary ductal dilatation. The portal vein and spleen are normal.

Which of the following is the most likely diagnosis?

(A) Acute viral hepatitis
(B) Fulminant liver failure
(C) Hemochromatosis
(D) Primary biliary cirrhosis

Item 6

A 52-year-old woman is evaluated during a routine examination. Although her mother was diagnosed with colorectal cancer at age 74 years, the patient herself has not been previously screened. She inquires about initiating colorectal cancer risk reduction strategies, including nutritional and pharmacologic interventions. She is postmenopausal, is otherwise healthy, and takes no medications.

Physical examination is normal.

In addition to colonoscopy, which of the following should be recommended?

(A) Aspirin
(B) Celecoxib
(C) Estrogen replacement
(D) No specific medications

Item 7

A 67-year-old man is evaluated in the emergency department for the acute onset of severe diffuse abdominal pain that began 1 hour ago. He has a history of arteriosclerotic cardiovascular disease, and he underwent three-vessel bypass surgery 2 years ago. His current medications are lisinopril, atenolol, simvastatin, and aspirin.

On physical examination, temperature is 36.8 °C (98.2 °F), blood pressure is 78/56 mm Hg, pulse rate is 142/min, and respiration rate is 29/min. Abdominal examination discloses diffuse mild abdominal tenderness to palpation with no guarding or rebound and no masses.

Laboratory studies reveal a leukocyte count of 14,000/µL (14×10^9/L), a bicarbonate level of 14 meq/L (14 mmol/L), and an elevated serum lactate level. CT scan shows small-bowel wall thickening and intestinal pneumatosis.

Which of the following is the most likely diagnosis?

(A) Acute mesenteric ischemia
(B) Crohn disease
(C) Intussusception
(D) Pancreatitis

Item 8

A 50-year-old man is evaluated during a routine visit for alcoholic cirrhosis. He has a 3-month history of hepatic encephalopathy, characterized by forgetfulness and personality changes, that is well controlled with lactulose. He has not consumed alcohol in the last 2 years. One year ago he developed ascites that required diuretics. At that time a screening upper endoscopy revealed no varices. His current medications are lactulose, spironolactone, and furosemide.

On physical examination, he is alert and in no distress. He is oriented but has mild psychomotor slowing. Vital signs are normal. Scleral icterus, temporal muscle wasting, and spider angiomata are noted. Neurologic examination reveals mild asterixis. On the Mini–Mental State Examination, he scores 28 out of 30, failing to recall one out of three objects and missing the day of the week.

Laboratory studies:

Hematocrit	33%
Platelet count	75,000/µL (75×10^9/L)
INR	1.4 (normal range, 0.8-1.2)
Albumin	2.9 g/dL (29 g/L)
Alanine aminotransferase	32 units/L
Aspartate aminotransferase	45 units/L
Total bilirubin	4 mg/dL (68.4 µmol/L)
Creatinine	1.3 mg/dL (115 µmol/L)
Electrolytes	Normal

Which of the following is the most appropriate management?

(A) Add nadolol
(B) Begin a low-protein diet
(C) Continue medical treatment without changes
(D) Refer for liver transplantation

Item 9

A 38-year-old man is evaluated during a routine examination. He was diagnosed with ulcerative colitis 10 years ago and is currently asymptomatic. His last colonoscopy, performed at the time of diagnosis, showed mildly active extensive colitis extending to the hepatic flexure. There is no family history of colon cancer or colon polyps. His only medication is mesalamine.

On physical examination, vital signs are normal. Abdominal examination is normal. Laboratory studies, including a complete blood count, liver chemistry studies, and C-reactive protein, are normal.

Which of the following is the most appropriate colonoscopy interval for this patient?

(A) Colonoscopy now and every 1 to 2 years
(B) Colonoscopy now and every 5 years
(C) Colonoscopy every 5 years starting at age 40
(D) Colonoscopy every 10 years starting at age 40

Item 10

A 42-year-old woman is evaluated for an 8-month history of crampy abdominal pain and three loose bowel movements per day. The pain is relieved by a bowel movement. There are no nocturnal bowel movements, and there is no blood or dark tarry material in the stool. She has not had fever, night sweats, or weight loss. She has a history of Hashimoto disease and is treated with levothyroxine.

On physical examination, temperature is 36.8 °C (98.2 °F), blood pressure is 128/84 mm Hg, pulse rate is 64/min, and respiration rate is 16/min; BMI is 23. No rash is noted. There is mild diffuse abdominal tenderness without peritoneal signs and no abdominal masses. Rectal examination is normal. Complete blood count and thyroid-stimulating hormone level are normal.

Which of the following is the most appropriate next step in management?

(A) Breath test for bacterial overgrowth
(B) Colonoscopy with random biopsies
(C) Stool culture
(D) Tissue transglutaminase antibody testing

Item 11

A 26-year-old woman is evaluated for intractable pruritus that keeps her awake at night. She is pregnant at 25 weeks' gestation. Her only medication is a prenatal vitamin and folic acid.

On physical examination, temperature is 36.7 °C (98.1 °F), blood pressure is 110/65 mm Hg, pulse rate is 88/min, and respiration rate is 14/min. BMI is 27. Mental status is normal. Scleral icterus is noted, and there are scattered excoriations on the arms, chest, and legs. There are no petechiae or ecchymoses.

Laboratory studies:

Hematocrit	36%
Leukocyte count	4500/µL (4.5 × 10⁹/L)
Platelet count	350,000/µL (350 × 10⁹/L)
INR	1.1 (normal range, 0.8-1.2)
Albumin	3.4 g/dL (34 g/L)
Alkaline phosphatase	160 units/L
Alanine aminotransferase	32 units/L
Aspartate aminotransferase	32 units/L
Total bilirubin	2.2 mg/dL (37.6 µmol/L)

Abdominal ultrasound is normal with a 25-week gravid uterus. There is no free abdominal fluid and no organomegaly.

Which of the following is the most likely diagnosis?

(A) Acute fatty liver of pregnancy
(B) HELLP (Hemolysis, Elevated Liver enzymes, and Low Platelets) syndrome
(C) Hyperemesis gravidarum
(D) Intrahepatic cholestasis of pregnancy

Item 12

A 72-year-old man is evaluated in the emergency department for a 2-week history of gnawing epigastric pain followed by one episode of coffee-ground emesis 6 hours ago. He has a history of prosthetic mitral valve replacement and chronic atrial fibrillation, and he had a transient ischemic attack 1 year ago. He has no history of liver disease. His current medications are warfarin and metoprolol. He is started on intravenous omeprazole.

On physical examination, blood pressure is 120/85 mm Hg (no orthostatic changes), pulse rate is 90/min, and respiration rate is 16/min. The abdomen is tender to palpation in the epigastrium. There are no stigmata of chronic liver disease.

Laboratory studies:

Hemoglobin	12.5 g/dL (125 g/L)
INR	2.3 (normal range, 0.8-1.2)
Blood urea nitrogen	46 mg/dL (16.4 mmol/L)
Creatinine	1.0 mg/dL (88.4 µmol/L)

Which of the following is the most appropriate management?

(A) Fresh frozen plasma
(B) Intravenous vitamin K
(C) Oral vitamin K
(D) Upper endoscopy

Item 13

A 57-year-old woman is evaluated in follow-up 6 weeks after hospitalization for uncomplicated acute diverticulitis in the sigmoid colon. Her inpatient treatment included intravenous antibiotics, which resulted in defervescence, symptom improvement, and resumption of oral diet within 72 hours. She was then discharged from the hospital on a 7-day course of oral antibiotics. She is doing well and is currently asymptomatic.

Which of the following is the most appropriate next step in management?

(A) Colonoscopy
(B) Elective segmental colon resection
(C) Probiotic therapy
(D) No additional testing or therapy

Item 14

A 35-year-old man is evaluated for a 2-year history of intermittent chest pain. The pain is retrosternal, lasts for seconds to minutes, is unrelated to exertion, and does not radiate. It is occasionally associated with swallowing. He reports intermittent dysphagia to solids and liquids. He denies any reflux symptoms or weight loss. He does not have any risk factors for cardiac disease.

Physical examination is unremarkable. Upper endoscopy is normal. A barium swallow is shown.

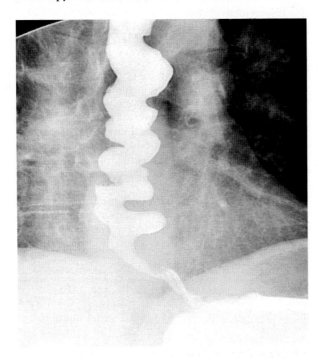

Which of the following is the most likely diagnosis?

(A) Achalasia
(B) Diffuse esophageal spasm
(C) Eosinophilic esophagitis
(D) Schatzki ring

Item 15

A 35-year-old woman is evaluated for a 6-month history of an upset stomach that usually occurs after meals. She also has heartburn symptoms after meals at least four times per week. She reports no difficulty or pain with swallowing and no vomiting, weight loss, altered stool habits, or blood in the stool. There is no family history of gastrointestinal malignancy.

On physical examination, vital signs are normal. Abdominal examination discloses a nontender epigastrium and no masses or lymphadenopathy. A complete blood count is normal.

Which of the following is the most appropriate management?

(A) Proton pump inhibitor
(B) Sucralfate
(C) Test for *Helicobacter pylori* and treat if positive
(D) Upper endoscopy

Item 16

A 58-year-old man is evaluated in the emergency department for painless bright red blood per rectum that began 3 hours ago. The bleeding was accompanied by a syncopal episode. He has a history of rheumatoid arthritis. His current medications are adalimumab, methotrexate, and ibuprofen.

On physical examination, temperature is 37.2 °C (99.0 °F), blood pressure is 88/58 mm Hg, pulse rate is 132/min, and respiration rate is 24/min. Abdominal examination is normal. Rectal examination discloses bright red blood in the rectal vault. Nasogastric tube aspirate shows no evidence of blood or coffee-ground material.

Laboratory studies reveal a hemoglobin level of 7.3 g/dL (73 g/L).

Emergency intravenous fluid resuscitation is begun.

Which of the following is the most appropriate diagnostic test to perform next?

(A) Colonoscopy
(B) Tagged red blood cell scan
(C) Upper endoscopy
(D) Video capsule endoscopy

Item 17

A 19-year-old woman is evaluated for a 3-month history of progressively worsening diarrhea, abdominal pain, and weight loss. Her brother was diagnosed with Crohn disease at age 16 years.

On physical examination, temperature is 37.4 °C (99.3 °F), blood pressure is 110/65 mm Hg, pulse rate is 90/min, and respiration rate is 20/min. Abdominal examination reveals tenderness to palpation in the right lower quadrant with no guarding or rebound tenderness. Perianal and rectal examinations are normal.

Colonoscopy discloses evidence of moderately to severely active Crohn disease involving the terminal ileum; the diagnosis is confirmed histologically. Magnetic resonance enterography shows active inflammation involving the distal 20 cm of the ileum without other bowel inflammation or obstruction. There is no evidence of abscess or phlegmon.

Which of the following is the most effective maintenance treatment?

(A) Ciprofloxacin and metronidazole
(B) Infliximab
(C) Mesalamine
(D) Prednisone
(E) Surgical resection

Item 18

A 45-year-old man is admitted to the hospital for new-onset right upper quadrant pain, ascites, fever, and anorexia. His medical history is notable for hypertension and alcoholism. His only medication is hydrochlorothiazide.

On physical examination, temperature is 38.1 °C (100.6 °F), blood pressure is 110/50 mm Hg, pulse rate is 92/min, and respiration rate is 16/min. BMI is 24. Spider angiomata are noted on the chest and neck. The liver edge is palpable and tender. There is abdominal distention with flank dullness to percussion.

Laboratory studies:

Alkaline phosphatase	210 units/L
Alanine aminotransferase	60 units/L
Aspartate aminotransferase	125 units/L
Total bilirubin	6.5 mg/dL (111.2 μmol/L)
Creatinine	1.8 mg/dL (159 μmol/L)

The Maddrey discriminant function score is 36. Ultrasound discloses coarsened hepatic echotexture, splenomegaly, and a moderate to large amount of ascites. Diagnostic paracentesis reveals spontaneous bacterial peritonitis, and intravenous ceftriaxone is administered. Upper endoscopy is notable for small esophageal varices without red wale signs and no evidence of recent bleeding.

In addition to continuing ceftriaxone and starting albumin, which of the following is the most appropriate treatment?

(A) Etanercept
(B) Infliximab
(C) Pentoxifylline
(D) Prednisolone

Item 19

A 55-year-old man is admitted to the hospital for epigastric pain and melena. He works as a carpenter and injured his back approximately 3 weeks ago while working. Since the injury, he has been taking ibuprofen.

On physical examination, blood pressure is 104/62 mm Hg and pulse rate is 110/min. Other than tachycardia, the general physical examination is normal.

Hemoglobin level is 10.2 g/dL (102 g/L). He is given appropriate resuscitation and stabilization. Upper endoscopy shows a 1-cm antral ulcer with a nonbleeding visible vessel. Endoscopic treatment with epinephrine injection and heater probe is performed. A proton pump inhibitor is started, and his hospital course is unremarkable.

Assuming the patient remains asymptomatic, how long should this patient be observed in the hospital after endoscopic treatment?

(A) 12 hours
(B) 24 hours
(C) 48 hours
(D) 72 hours

Item 20

A 76-year-old woman is admitted to the hospital for melena that has been recurrent over the past several weeks. She has not used NSAIDs. She recently had an upper endoscopy that demonstrated multiple bleeding angioectasias within the proximal duodenum. She has a history of aortic stenosis and has symptoms of lightheadedness and dyspnea with exertion. There is no family history of bleeding diathesis. She takes no medications.

On physical examination, vital signs are normal. There are no cutaneous signs of angioectasias. Cardiopulmonary examination discloses pulsus tardus and an early systolic murmur heard most profoundly at the right upper sternal border. Abdominal examination discloses no tenderness, masses, or hepatosplenomegaly.

Laboratory studies reveal a hemoglobin level of 7.2 g/dL (72 g/L) and a normal INR. A comprehensive metabolic panel is also normal.

Transthoracic echocardiogram demonstrates severe aortic stenosis and normal left ventricular size and function.

Which of the following is the best long-term management for this patient's gastrointestinal bleeding?

(A) Aortic valve replacement
(B) Endoscopic treatment of angioectasias
(C) Proton pump inhibitor
(D) Systemic estrogen therapy

Item 21

A 23-year-old man is evaluated in follow-up for familial adenomatous polyposis that was diagnosed 3 months ago after colonoscopy. He underwent complete colectomy and is now asymptomatic.

Physical examination is normal with the exception of well-healed scars from his colectomy.

Laboratory studies:

Hematocrit	42%
Alkaline phosphatase	80 units/L
Alanine aminotransferase	18 units/L
Aspartate aminotransferase	14 units/L
Total bilirubin	1.1 mg/dL (18.8 μmol/L)
Direct bilirubin	0.2 mg/dL (3.4 μmol/L)

Which of the following periodic surveillance procedures should be performed?

(A) Abdominal ultrasound
(B) Serial monitoring of aminotransferases
(C) Upper endoscopy
(D) No follow-up surveillance required

Item 22

A 42-year-old woman is evaluated following hospitalization for acute pancreatitis due to gallstone disease that occurred 8 weeks ago. An admission CT scan demonstrated no evidence of fluid collection or necrosis, and she had an uncomplicated cholecystectomy prior to discharge. She has no pain, nausea, or anorexia. However, 2 weeks ago she was evaluated for nephrolithiasis following an episode of renal colic and underwent a CT scan. The CT scan demonstrated a 4-mm stone in the right ureter and a 6-cm fluid collection adjacent to the pancreatic tail. There was no evidence of solid debris, and it did not communicate with the main pancreatic duct. There were no mass lesions in the liver and no pancreatic necrosis. She has since passed the kidney stone and is asymptomatic.

On physical examination, temperature is 37.2 °C (99.0 °F), blood pressure is 112/72 mm Hg, pulse rate is 66/min, and respiration rate is 18/min. BMI is 25. Abdominal examination discloses a nondistended abdomen and active bowel sounds. There is no tenderness to palpation, hepatosplenomegaly, or masses.

Laboratory studies, including complete blood count, liver chemistry tests, CA 19-9, and alkaline phosphatase, are normal.

Which of the following is the most appropriate next step in management?

(A) Endoscopic ultrasonography
(B) Magnetic resonance cholangiopancreatography
(C) Percutaneous drainage
(D) Surgical drainage
(E) No further diagnostic testing or therapy

Item 23

A 60-year-old woman is evaluated for a 1-month history of increasing abdominal distention. She has gained 6.8 kg (15.0 lb) over that time. Her medical history is significant for obesity and type 2 diabetes mellitus. Her current medications are metformin and aspirin.

On physical examination, temperature is 36.5 °C (97.7 °F), blood pressure is 100/50 mm Hg, pulse rate is 72/min, and respiration rate is 16/min. BMI is 31. Jugular venous distention is present and increases with inspiration. Cardiac sounds are normal with a loud S_3; no murmur is present. Lungs are clear to auscultation. Abdominal examination is notable for a tense abdomen with shifting dullness consistent with ascites. The spleen tip is not palpable.

Laboratory studies:

Hemoglobin	11.5 g/dL (115 g/L)
Leukocyte count	7000/µL (7 × 10⁹/L)
Platelet count	170,000/µL (170 × 10⁹/L)
INR	1.1 (normal range, 0.8-1.2)
Albumin	3.5 g/dL (35 g/L)
Alkaline phosphatase	100 units/L
Alanine aminotransferase	30 units/L
Aspartate aminotransferase	40 units/L
Total bilirubin	0.9 mg/dL (15.4 µmol/L)
Creatinine	0.9 mg/dL (79.6 µmol/L)
Urinalysis	Normal

Abdominal ultrasound shows a normal-appearing liver and ascites. Spleen size is normal. The portal and hepatic veins are patent. There is no hydronephrosis. Diagnostic paracentesis reveals a cell count of 300/µL with 20% neutrophils, a total protein level of 3 g/dL (30 g/L), and an ascites fluid albumin level of 2.2 g/dL (22 g/L).

Which of the following is the most appropriate diagnostic test to perform next?

(A) Echocardiography
(B) Hepatic venous pressure gradient measurement
(C) Serum CA-125
(D) 24-Hour urine total protein

Item 24

A 55-year-old man is evaluated during a routine follow-up visit for compensated cirrhosis. He is currently asymptomatic. His medical history is significant for chronic hepatitis B infection and esophageal varices. He currently takes nadolol.

On physical examination, temperature is 37.6 °C (99.7 °F), blood pressure is 120/70 mm Hg, pulse rate is 68/min, and respiration rate is 16/min. BMI is 31. Spider angiomata are noted on the neck and upper chest. The spleen tip is palpable.

Screening abdominal ultrasound discloses a nodular-appearing liver, splenomegaly, and intra-abdominal venous collaterals consistent with portal hypertension. A 1.6-cm lesion is noted in the right hepatic lobe; the lesion was not present in an ultrasound done 6 months ago.

Which of the following is the most appropriate diagnostic test to perform next?

(A) Contrast-enhanced CT
(B) Liver biopsy
(C) Repeat ultrasound in 6 months
(D) Serum carcinoembryonic antigen level

Item 25

A 40-year-old woman is evaluated for a 1-year history of reflux symptoms. She has heartburn and regurgitation of gastric contents several times a week. She was placed on lifestyle modification and an empiric trial of a once-daily proton pump inhibitor (PPI) 12 weeks ago with minimal relief of symptoms. For the past 6 weeks she has taken the PPI twice daily, also with minimal relief. She has had intermittent solid-food dysphagia. She appears to be adherent to her lifestyle and medical therapy.

Physical examination discloses normal vital signs and a BMI of 35.

Which of the following is the most appropriate next step in management?

(A) Add an H_2 blocker at night
(B) Ambulatory esophageal pH study
(C) Endoscopy
(D) Fundoplication

Item 26

A 52-year-old man is evaluated for a 3-day history of left lower quadrant abdominal pain. He rates the pain as 6 on a scale of 1 to 10. He has not needed any analgesic medications. His appetite is decreased, but he is able to tolerate oral intake. He is otherwise healthy and had no previous gastrointestinal problems.

On physical examination, temperature is 38.2 °C (100.8 °F), pulse rate is 103/min, and respiration rate is 14/min. Abdominal examination discloses focal tenderness in the left lower quadrant. There is perirectal fullness.

Laboratory studies reveal a hemoglobin level of 13.5 g/dL (135 g/L) and a leukocyte count of 14,000/µL (14×10^9/L). Urinalysis is unremarkable, and a Gram stain is negative. CT scan of the abdomen and pelvis discloses moderately dense diverticula in the descending colon and proximal sigmoid colon; focal bowel wall thickening (5 mm) in the midsigmoid colon with associated inflammation of the pericolic fat; and no evidence of ileus, obstruction, abscess, or perforation.

Which of the following is the most appropriate initial management strategy for this patient?

(A) Colonoscopy
(B) CT-guided percutaneous drainage
(C) Intravenous metronidazole and ciprofloxacin
(D) Oral metronidazole and ciprofloxacin
(E) Surgical consultation for segmental colectomy

Item 27

A 45-year-old man is evaluated for a 2-month history of progressive dyspnea on exertion. He has not had chest pain, palpitations, or orthopnea. His medical history is significant for chronic hepatitis C infection. He takes no medications.

On physical examination, temperature is 37.2 °C (99.0 °F), blood pressure is 115/60 mm Hg, pulse rate is 82/min, and respiration rate is 20/min. BMI is 27. Cardiopulmonary examination is normal. Spider angiomata are seen on the neck and upper chest. The spleen tip is palpable. There is no clubbing, cyanosis, or edema.

Laboratory studies show an albumin level of 3.6 g/dL (36 g/L), a total bilirubin level of 0.9 mg/dL (15.4 µmol/L), and an INR of 0.9 (normal range, 0.8-1.2).

Abdominal ultrasound discloses a nodular-appearing liver, splenomegaly, and intra-abdominal venous collaterals consistent with portal hypertension. No ascites is noted. A chest radiograph and electrocardiogram are normal. Arterial blood gas studies with the patient breathing ambient air show a P_{O_2} of 62 mm Hg (8.2 kPa) and oxygen saturation of 90%. Echocardiogram discloses normal left ventricular size and function. Estimated right ventricular systolic pressure is 24 mm Hg.

Which of the following is the most likely diagnosis?

(A) Deconditioning
(B) Hepatopulmonary syndrome
(C) Ischemic heart disease
(D) Portopulmonary hypertension

Item 28

A 65-year-old woman is evaluated for occasional epigastric pain following meals. She has not had dysphagia, odynophagia, reflux, fevers, or weight loss. She has no other medical problems, and her family history is noncontributory.

On physical examination, vital signs are normal, and BMI is 23. Abdominal examination discloses mild tenderness in the epigastric region without palpable masses. Bowel sounds are normal. There is no skin rash. Endoscopy reveals loss of rugal folds in the proximal stomach with visible submucosal vessels. Random biopsies from the body and fundus reveal chronic inflammation, glandular atrophy, and epithelial metaplasia. Two nodules (4 mm and 8 mm in diameter) were removed from the gastric body, and pathology reveals carcinoid tumors. The serum gastrin level is 550 pg/mL (550 ng/L) (normal, <100 pg/mL [100 ng/L]). CT of the abdomen and pelvis is unremarkable.

Which of the following is the most appropriate management?

(A) Antrectomy
(B) Begin octreotide
(C) Repeat endoscopy in 6 months
(D) Total gastrectomy

Item 29

A 45-year-old man is evaluated for a 1-week history of non-bloody diarrhea that occurs ten times per day and is accompanied by mild abdominal cramping. He has a 5-year history of ulcerative colitis for which he takes mesalamine.

On physical examination, temperature is 37.9 °C (100.2 °F), blood pressure is 110/80 mm Hg (no orthostatic changes), and pulse rate is 100/min. Abdominal examination discloses hyperactive bowel sounds and mild diffuse tenderness but no peritoneal signs.

Laboratory studies:

Hemoglobin	Normal
Leukocyte count	23,000/µL (23×10^9/L)
Platelet count	Normal
Blood urea nitrogen	15 mg/dL (5.4 mmol/L)
C-reactive protein	32 mg/dL (320 mg/L)
Creatinine	1.0 mg/dL (88.4 µmol/L)
Potassium	2.9 meq/L (2.9 mmol/L)

An acute abdominal radiograph series is normal.

Which of the following is the most appropriate diagnostic test to perform next?

(A) Abdominal CT
(B) Colonoscopy
(C) Right upper quadrant ultrasound
(D) Stool studies for *Clostridium difficile*

Item 30

A 24-year-old woman is evaluated during a routine examination in November. She has ulcerative colitis, which was diagnosed 10 years ago. Her last menstrual period was 5 weeks ago. She currently takes 6-mercaptopurine.

On physical examination, vital signs are normal. Abdominal examination is normal.

Laboratory studies, including a complete blood count, liver chemistry studies, and C-reactive protein, are normal. Pregnancy test is negative.

Which of the following vaccinations is contraindicated for this patient?

(A) Hepatitis B
(B) Human papillomavirus
(C) Pneumococcal polysaccharide vaccine
(D) Trivalent inactivated influenza
(E) Varicella (chickenpox)

Item 31

A 50-year-old woman is evaluated during a routine examination. She is in excellent health and has no gastrointestinal symptoms. She has no history of colorectal neoplasia.

Physical examination is normal. She is sent home with high-sensitivity guaiac fecal occult blood test (gFOBT) cards and is asked to collect two specimens each from three consecutive stools. One of the six samples is positive.

Which of the following is the most appropriate management for this patient?

(A) Colonoscopy now
(B) Fecal immunochemical test in 1 year
(C) Flexible sigmoidoscopy now
(D) gFOBT in 1 year
(E) Repeat gFOBT now

Item 32

A 55-year-old man is evaluated for chronic hepatitis C infection. He takes no medications.

On physical examination, temperature is 36.8 °C (98.2 °F), blood pressure is 135/82 mm Hg, pulse rate is 66/min, and respiration rate is 16/min. BMI is 30.

Abdominal ultrasound demonstrates cholelithiasis but is otherwise normal. Liver biopsy demonstrates mild inflammation and advanced fibrosis without established cirrhosis.

Which of the following is the most appropriate management?

(A) Corticosteroids
(B) Initiation of antiviral therapy
(C) Referral for liver transplantation
(D) Repeat liver biopsy in 6 months
(E) Serial aminotransferase monitoring

⊞ Item 33

A 55-year-old woman who underwent kidney transplantation 6 months ago is admitted to the hospital for dehydration. She has had odynophagia for the last week that has significantly reduced her oral intake of both solids and liquids. She also has had intermittent nausea and diarrhea. Her current medications are prednisone and tacrolimus.

On physical examination, temperature is 37.8 °C (100.0 °F). Other vital signs are normal. Oropharyngeal examination is normal. Endoscopy reveals two 1-cm ulcers in the midesophagus with biopsy showing inclusion bodies consistent with cytomegalovirus infection.

Which of the following is the most appropriate treatment?

(A) Acyclovir
(B) Fluconazole
(C) Ganciclovir
(D) Swallowed aerosolized fluticasone

⊞ Item 34

A 37-year-old woman is evaluated in the emergency department for the acute onset of pain after 2 weeks of bloody diarrhea. The diarrhea has escalated to 15 times per day. She has ulcerative colitis that was diagnosed 2 years ago. She currently takes azathioprine.

On physical examination, she appears ill. Following aggressive fluid resuscitation, temperature is 38.9 °C (102.0 °F), blood pressure is 70/40 mm Hg, pulse rate is 148/min, and respiration rate is 35/min. Abdominal examination discloses absent bowel sounds, distention, and diffuse marked tenderness with mild palpation.

Laboratory studies reveal a leukocyte count of 16,800/µL (16.8×10^9/L). Abdominal radiograph is shown.

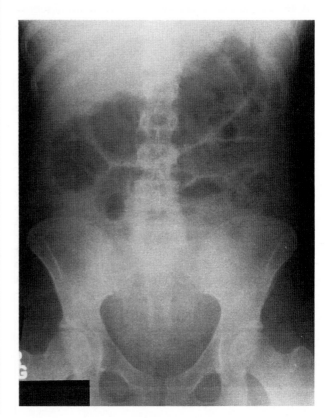

Which of the following is the most appropriate management?

(A) CT scan
(B) Immediate surgery
(C) Start infliximab
(D) Start intravenous hydrocortisone

Item 35

An 81-year-old man is evaluated for a 2-week history of painless jaundice and pruritus. He has had no weight loss, fever, chills, or nausea. He has no other medical problems and takes no medications.

On physical examination, temperature is 36.0 °C (96.8 °F), blood pressure is 122/76 mm Hg, pulse rate is 72/min, and respiration rate is 18/min. BMI is 31. There is scleral icterus. There are no cutaneous signs of cirrhosis. Active bowel sounds are noted. The abdomen is not distended, the gallbladder is not palpable, and there is no hepatosplenomegaly.

Laboratory studies:

Alkaline phosphatase	343 units/L
Alanine aminotransferase	172 units/L
Aspartate aminotransferase	181 units/L
Total bilirubin	14.1 mg/dL (241.1 µmol/L)
Direct bilirubin	9.8 mg/dL (167.6 µmol/L)
IgG4	576 mg/dL (5.8 g/L) (normal, <135 mg/dL [1.35 g/L])
CA 19-9	12.1 units/mL (12.1 kU/L) (normal, <39 units/mL [39 kU/L])

Contrast-enhanced CT scan demonstrates a diffusely enlarged (sausage-shaped) pancreas with a narrowed pancreatic duct. The extrahepatic bile duct is dilated to 10 mm with narrowing within the peripancreatic segment. CT and endoscopic ultrasound demonstrate no evidence of mass lesion.

Which of the following is the most appropriate treatment?

(A) Broad-spectrum antibiotics
(B) Corticosteroids
(C) Endoscopic retrograde cholangiopancreatography with biliary stent placement
(D) Pancreaticoduodenectomy

Item 36

An 82-year-old man is evaluated for recurrent obscure gastrointestinal bleeding. He has experienced four episodes of melena in the past 6 months. Results of a colonoscopy and upper endoscopy 3 months ago were unremarkable. There is no family history of bleeding diathesis. His only medication is iron sulfate for anemia.

On physical examination, vital signs are normal. BMI is 32. There is no abdominal tenderness. Digital rectal examination is normal.

Laboratory studies reveal a hemoglobin level of 10.1 g/dL (101 g/L); platelet count, complete metabolic panel, and INR are normal.

Which of the following is the most appropriate diagnostic test to perform next?

(A) Intraoperative endoscopy
(B) Repeat upper endoscopy
(C) Single-balloon enteroscopy
(D) Wireless capsule endoscopy

Item 37

A 75-year-old man is evaluated in follow-up after recent surveillance endoscopy for Barrett esophagus. Biopsy from the salmon-colored columnar segment shows high-grade dysplasia. His gastroesophageal reflux disease symptoms are well controlled with proton pump inhibitor therapy. His medical history is significant for New York Heart Association functional class III heart failure (ejection fraction, 30%). His medications are pantoprazole, furosemide, digoxin, metoprolol, enalapril, and spironolactone.

On physical examination, he is afebrile, blood pressure is 100/50 mm Hg, pulse rate is 62/min, and respiration rate is 12/min; BMI is 35. There is no evidence of jugular venous distention. Cardiac rhythm is regular, with a soft S_3 at the cardiac apex. The lungs are clear. No peripheral edema is present.

Which of the following is the most appropriate management?

(A) Endoscopic ablation
(B) Esophagectomy
(C) Fundoplication
(D) Repeat endoscopic surveillance in 3 years

Item 38

A 52-year-old woman is evaluated for a 9-year history of intermittent rectal bleeding with associated mucus. She has an average of four small-volume bowel movements per day. Over the past several weeks, she has noticed increased fecal urgency and tenesmus with associated rectal bleeding, prompting the current visit. She is otherwise healthy. There is no history of inflammatory bowel disease or colorectal cancer among her first- and second-degree relatives.

On physical examination, vital signs are normal. There is mild lower abdominal tenderness to palpation. Colonoscopy discloses normal endoscopic appearance of the entire colon. Random biopsies show no evidence of inflammation and no dysplasia. Rectal mucosa shows loss of vascular markings, erythema, and friability; biopsies show chronic inflammatory changes including crypt distortion and crypt atrophy, consistent with ulcerative proctitis. No dysplasia is noted.

Which of the following is the most appropriate approach to colorectal cancer surveillance for this patient?

(A) Colonoscopy in 1 year
(B) Colonoscopy in 3 years
(C) Colonoscopy in 5 years
(D) Colonoscopy in 10 years

Item 39

A 64-year-old man was admitted to the hospital 4 days ago for severe, acute abdominal pain and was found to have acute mesenteric ischemia. He underwent massive small-bowel resection, with 180 cm of small bowel remaining, and his colon was able to be salvaged. Over the past 4 days since surgery, he has been on parenteral nutrition with gradual progression of oral intake. He has significant diarrhea that wakes him up at night. He has been afebrile and has not had recurrent or worsening abdominal pain. His medications are low-dose low-molecular-weight heparin, ciprofloxacin, and metronidazole. He is also taking loperamide four times daily.

On physical examination, temperature is 36.2 °C (97.2 °F), blood pressure is 118/60 mm Hg, pulse rate is 68/min and regular, and respiration rate is 12/min. BMI is 25. Abdominal examination discloses a large scar from his recent surgery that is healing well. Bowel sounds are very active and there is mild tenderness throughout, as is expected postoperatively.

Laboratory studies, including serum electrolyte, glucose, and thyroid-stimulating hormone levels, are normal. Stool cultures and *Clostridium difficile* polymerase chain reaction are normal.

Which of the following is the most appropriate management?

(A) Decrease the lipids in his parenteral nutrition
(B) Increase the loperamide
(C) Initiate cholestyramine
(D) Initiate omeprazole
(E) Stop oral intake

Item 40

A 37-year-old man is evaluated during a routine examination. He has no gastrointestinal problems. He has had no previous colorectal cancer screening evaluation. His mother was diagnosed with colon cancer at age 54 years. Other than his mother, there is no additional history of familial polyps, colon cancer, or other cancer diagnoses.

Physical examination is normal.

Which of the following is the most appropriate management?

(A) Colonoscopy now
(B) Colonoscopy at age 40 years
(C) Colonoscopy at age 44 years
(D) Fecal occult blood test at age 40 years

Item 41

A 42-year-old woman is evaluated for new-onset constipation that has progressively worsened over the last 3 months. She previously had normal bowel habits, with an average of one bowel movement per day. She now has one bowel movement every 4 to 5 days with decreased stool caliber. She has not had problems with hemorrhoids before, but she has noticed blood on the stool in the last month. She denies pain with defecation. She has had no change in her diet and has not started on any new medications. She has not had weight loss. She has a history of hypothyroidism for which she takes levothyroxine. There is no family history of colorectal cancer or polyps.

On physical examination, blood pressure is 110/70 mm Hg and pulse rate is 72/min. Abdominal examination is normal. External anal inspection reveals no hemorrhoids or fissures. On digital rectal examination, resting and squeeze tone are normal, with normal relaxation of the puborectalis with simulated defecation. No masses are palpable. The examination finger reveals blood streaking. Laboratory studies, including a complete blood count and glucose, calcium, and thyroid-stimulating hormone levels, are all within normal limits.

Which of the following is the most appropriate management?

(A) Begin fiber supplementation
(B) Check serum free thyroxine level
(C) Perform anorectal manometry
(D) Perform colonoscopy
(E) Perform stool guaiac testing

Item 42

A 70-year-old man is referred for abdominal aortic aneurysm (AAA) screening. He is asymptomatic and takes no medications. He has a 50-pack-year smoking history.

On physical examination, temperature is 37.5 °C (99.5 °F), blood pressure is 125/60 mm Hg, pulse rate is 72/min, and respiration rate is 16/min. BMI is 30. Abdominal examination discloses mild tenderness to palpation over the epigastrium and no rebound tenderness or guarding.

Abdominal ultrasound discloses a normal-appearing liver without splenomegaly or liver masses. Numerous gallstones are noted. There is no evidence of AAA.

Which of the following is the most appropriate management?

(A) Abdominal CT scan
(B) Laparoscopic cholecystectomy
(C) Ursodeoxycholic acid
(D) Observation

Item 43

A 60-year-old man is evaluated for a long-standing history of osteoarthritis that primarily causes pain in the base of the thumbs, fingers, and left knee. He had balloon angioplasty after a myocardial infarction 10 years ago. His medications are high-dose naproxen, non–enteric-coated aspirin, lisinopril, and atorvastatin. He has tried other medications for his joint disease, including acetaminophen and other NSAIDs, but has not had significant relief. He tried tramadol for his joint pain but stopped because of nausea.

The physical examination is unremarkable except for findings consistent with osteoarthritis. Laboratory studies reveal a normal complete blood count and serum creatinine level.

Which of the following is the most appropriate treatment?

(A) Change aspirin to an enteric-coated aspirin
(B) Change naproxen to low-dose celecoxib
(C) Discontinue aspirin
(D) Initiate omeprazole

Item 44

A 48-year-old woman is evaluated for constipation-predominant irritable bowel syndrome that was diagnosed 1 year ago. She has tried multiple over-the-counter laxative products and is currently taking a fiber supplement (with adequate water intake) and polyethylene glycol twice daily. Despite her current medications, she remains symptomatic with abdominal cramping and infrequent bowel movements. She has no family history of gastrointestinal conditions or malignancy. A colonoscopy performed 6 months ago was normal.

On physical examination, vital signs are normal. Abdominal examination discloses mild tenderness to palpation in the right and left lower quadrants without peritoneal signs. No masses are noted. Anal tone is normal at rest and with simulated evacuation.

Which of the following is the most appropriate treatment?

(A) Hyoscyamine
(B) Lubiprostone
(C) Metoclopramide
(D) Tricyclic antidepressant

Item 45

A 68-year-old man is evaluated during a routine examination. He is generally healthy and has no gastrointestinal symptoms. His last screening colonoscopy 10 years ago was normal. His mother was diagnosed with colorectal cancer at age 65 years.

Physical examination is normal. Colonoscopy to the terminal ileum discloses a 1.5-cm polyp in the ascending colon (villous adenoma, low-grade dysplasia) and a 6-mm polyp in the sigmoid colon (tubular adenoma, low-grade dysplasia). The polyps are completely removed.

Which of the following is the most appropriate management for this patient?

(A) Colonoscopy in 2 to 6 months
(B) Colonoscopy in 1 year
(C) Colonoscopy in 3 years
(D) Colonoscopy in 10 years

Item 46

A 50-year-old woman is evaluated for a 2-day history of constant right upper quadrant abdominal pain. She has not

had nausea or vomiting. Her medical history is notable for polycythemia vera.

On physical examination, vital signs are normal. Cardiac examination discloses a normal S_1 and S_2 without extra sounds or murmurs. On abdominal examination, the liver edge is 3 cm below the right costal margin and is tender to palpation. The spleen tip is not palpable.

Laboratory studies:

Hematocrit	50%
Leukocyte count	7500/µL (7.5 × 10⁹/L)
Platelet count	300,000/µL (300 × 10⁹/L)
INR	0.9 (normal range, 0.8-1.2)
Alkaline phosphatase	120 units/L
Alanine aminotransferase	85 units/L
Aspartate aminotransferase	75 units/L
Total bilirubin	1.2 mg/dL (20.5 µmol/L)
Creatinine	0.9 mg/dL (79.6 µmol/L)

Abdominal ultrasound discloses hepatomegaly with splenomegaly and ascites. Doppler studies do not show evidence of blood flow in the hepatic veins, but the portal vein is patent. The gallbladder and pancreas are normal.

Which of the following is the most likely diagnosis?

(A) Budd-Chiari syndrome
(B) Constrictive pericarditis
(C) Fulminant hepatic failure
(D) Splenic vein thrombosis

Item 47

A 37-year-old woman is evaluated in the emergency department for a 1-day history of generalized abdominal pain. She has had no nausea, vomiting, diarrhea, melena, or hematochezia. She denies dyspnea or cough. One week ago she underwent laparoscopic Roux-en-Y gastric bypass for obesity, and she had an uncomplicated cholecystectomy 2 years ago. Her medications are vitamin B₁₂ injections, oral iron, and a multivitamin that contains folate.

On physical examination, she is afebrile. Blood pressure is 110/75 mm Hg (without orthostatic changes), pulse rate is 130/min, and respiration rate is 12/min; BMI is 46. Cardiac examination reveals tachycardia. Bowel sounds are normal. There is diffuse abdominal tenderness but no guarding or rebound. There are well-healing trocar sites from her recent surgery. Rectal examination reveals normal-colored stool that is guaiac negative.

Laboratory studies, including a complete blood count, liver chemistry studies, and pancreatic enzymes, are normal. An electrocardiogram shows sinus tachycardia. A plain radiograph of the abdomen is normal.

Which of the following is the most appropriate next step in management?

(A) CT angiography of the chest
(B) Emergent surgical exploration
(C) Upper endoscopy
(D) Upper gastrointestinal oral contrast radiograph

Item 48

A 23-year-old woman is evaluated in the hospital for recurrent episodes of hypoglycemia. During hospitalization, she developed neuroglycopenic symptoms after 8 hours of fasting associated with a plasma glucose level of 30 mg/dL (1.7 mmol/L) and a corresponding insulin level of 8 µU/mL (58 pmol/L). She does not have diabetes mellitus and does not take oral hypoglycemic agents or insulin.

On physical examination, temperature is 37.0 °C (98.6 °F), blood pressure is 90/56 mm Hg, pulse rate is 110/min, and respiration rate is 22/min. BMI is 22. No tenderness, masses, or hepatosplenomegaly is found on abdominal examination.

A contrast-enhanced CT scan demonstrates no evidence of a pancreatic mass.

Which of the following is the most appropriate diagnostic test to perform next?

(A) Endoscopic ultrasound
(B) MRI
(C) Operative pancreatic exploration
(D) Pentetreotide scintigraphy

Item 49

A 40-year-old woman is evaluated for mild right upper quadrant abdominal discomfort that has persisted for the last 3 months. She has a history of irritable bowel syndrome, but the current pain seems more persistent and different in quality than her usual pain associated with irritable bowel syndrome. Her medications are a multivitamin and hyoscyamine as necessary for abdominal pain.

On physical examination, vital signs are normal. Abdominal examination discloses mild tenderness to palpation of the right upper quadrant but no organomegaly.

Laboratory studies, including a complete blood count, liver chemistry studies, and basic metabolic panel, are normal. Abdominal ultrasound discloses a 4-cm cyst in the liver with wall irregularity and thin septations.

Which of the following is the most appropriate management?

(A) Cyst aspiration
(B) Referral for surgical resection
(C) Repeat ultrasound in 6 months
(D) Reassurance

Item 50

A 75-year-old man is evaluated for a 2-month history of progressive solid-food dysphagia. He has transitioned from solid to puréed foods and has been able to maintain his weight. He has a 40-pack-year history of cigarette smoking and a history of alcohol abuse.

On physical examination, vital signs are normal. BMI is 35. There is no evidence of supraclavicular lymphadenopathy. Cardiopulmonary examination is normal.

On abdominal examination, there is no evidence of mass, tenderness, or hepatomegaly.

A complete blood count reveals a hemoglobin level of 10.9 g/dL (109 g/L). Endoscopy reveals an obstructive mass in the distal esophagus, and biopsies show invasive adenocarcinoma.

Which of the following is the most appropriate management?

(A) CT/PET and endoscopic ultrasonography
(B) Esophagectomy
(C) Feeding tube placement
(D) Radiation therapy

Item 51

A 37-year-old woman is evaluated for diarrhea that has been present since a presumed food-borne illness 1 month ago. She reports that, at that time, she had 2 days of nausea, vomiting, and watery diarrhea. Although her symptoms improved after several days, she continued to have episodic diarrhea. She has three to four watery stools per day, often following meals. She has had excessive flatus and bloating over the past month. She has not had nocturnal stools, weight loss, fever, or obvious blood in her stool. She has not recently used antibiotics. Her medical history is notable for a cholecystectomy 2 years ago.

On physical examination, vital signs are normal. There is no wheezing. Abdominal examination discloses normal bowel sounds and a nontender abdomen. Rectal examination is normal. A complete blood count with differential is normal. Fecal leukocytes, general stool studies (including *Clostridium difficile*, ova, and parasites), and *Giardia* antigen are all negative. Stool sodium is 40 meq/L (40 mmol/L); stool potassium is 20 meq/L (20 mmol/L).

Which of the following is the most likely diagnosis?

(A) Bile-salt–induced diarrhea
(B) Eosinophilic gastroenteritis
(C) Irritable bowel syndrome
(D) Lactose malabsorption
(E) Microscopic colitis

Item 52

A 50-year-old man is evaluated for persistent heartburn and regurgitation despite taking a high-dose proton pump inhibitor twice a day for 6 months. His symptoms have improved, but he continues to have symptoms many times a week. He has not had dysphagia, chest pain, or weight loss. He has significantly modified his diet. His only medication is esomeprazole, 40 mg twice a day, which he takes as directed.

Physical examination is notable for a BMI of 34. The remainder of the physical examination is normal.

Endoscopy reveals persistent esophagitis and a moderately large hiatal hernia.

Which of the following is the most appropriate next step in treatment?

(A) Add twice-daily sucralfate
(B) Fundoplication
(C) Increase dose of esomeprazole
(D) Radiofrequency ablation

Item 53

A 37-year-old man is evaluated for a 1-month history of stool leakage. In the past week he has developed perianal pain and low-grade fevers. He was diagnosed 4 years ago with Crohn disease involving the small bowel and colon. He takes 6-mercaptopurine.

On physical examination, temperature is 37.9 °C (100.2 °F), blood pressure is 140/90 mm Hg, pulse rate is 88/min, and respiration rate is 20/min. Abdominal examination is normal. Perianal examination discloses two fistula orifices right anterolateral to the anus with expression of white material with gentle palpation. A fluctuant, tender region that is 1.5 cm in diameter is noted left posterolateral to the anus.

In addition to examination under anesthesia and appropriate surgical treatment of abscess cavities and fistula tracts, which of the following is the most appropriate management?

(A) Ciprofloxacin
(B) Corticosteroids
(C) Infliximab
(D) Metronidazole

Item 54

A 63-year-old woman is evaluated in the emergency department for an 8-hour history of abdominal pain in the epigastrium that radiates to the back. The patient is nauseated, anorexic, tachypneic, and in moderate distress. She has no other medical problems and takes no medications.

On physical examination, temperature is 39.1 °C (102.4 °F), blood pressure is 166/98 mm Hg, pulse rate is 102/min, and respiration rate is 26/min. BMI is 33. Breath sounds are decreased at the left lung base. The abdomen is distended, and there is tenderness with palpation in the epigastrium. No masses or peritoneal signs are noted.

Laboratory studies:

Hemoglobin	15 g/dL (150 g/L)
Leukocyte count	16,300/µL (16.3 × 10⁹/L)
Amylase	35,312 units/L
Blood urea nitrogen	64 mg/dL (22.8 mmol/L)
Creatinine	2.4 mg/dL (212 µmol/L)
Lipase	12,642 units/L

Contrast-enhanced CT scan demonstrates pancreatic and peripancreatic edema without evidence of necrosis. There is no evidence of mass lesions in the liver or pancreatic fluid collections.

Which of the following most accurately predicts a severe clinical course for this patient?

(A) Amylase and lipase levels
(B) Blood urea nitrogen level
(C) Peripancreatic edema on CT scan
(D) Temperature

Item 55

A 51-year-old woman is evaluated for a 6-month history of diarrhea and bloating. She reports four to six loose stools per day, with occasional nocturnal stools. She has had a few episodes of incontinence secondary to urgency. She has not had melena or hematochezia but notes an occasional oily appearance to the stool. She has lost 6.8 kg (15.0 lb) during this time period. Results of a colonoscopy 1 year ago were normal. She has not had recent travel, antibiotic use, or medication changes. She does not think consumption of dairy products alters her symptoms. She has a history of systemic sclerosis for which she takes omeprazole for symptoms of gastroesophageal reflux disease.

On physical examination, vital signs are normal. BMI is 22. Facial telangiectasias are present, and there is bilateral skin thickening of the hands. The abdomen is mildly distended, and bowel sounds are normal. Rectal examination is normal, with normal resting and squeeze tone. There are no palpable mass lesions.

Laboratory studies:

Hemoglobin	10.8 g/dL (108 g/L)
Mean corpuscular volume	104 fL
Serum electrolytes	Normal
Folate	63 ng/mL (143 nmol/L)
Glucose	Normal
Thyroid-stimulating hormone	Normal
Vitamin B₁₂	118 pg/mL (87 pmol/L)
Tissue transglutaminase antibody	Normal

Stool cultures, including an ova and parasite examination, are normal.

Which of the following is the most likely diagnosis?

(A) Celiac disease
(B) Irritable bowel syndrome
(C) Lactose malabsorption
(D) Microscopic colitis
(E) Small intestinal bacterial overgrowth

Item 56

A 26-year-old woman is evaluated after recently undergoing community screening for viral hepatitis. She is currently asymptomatic. She is of Laotian descent, and she has two older siblings with hepatitis B virus (HBV) infection. There is no family history of malignancies. She takes no medications.

On physical examination, vital signs are normal. BMI is 22.

Laboratory studies:

INR	0.9 (normal range, 0.8-1.2)
Alkaline phosphatase	90 units/L
Alanine aminotransferase	18 units/L
Aspartate aminotransferase	14 units/L
Albumin	4.2 g/dL (42 g/L)
Total bilirubin	2.2 mg/dL (37.6 µmol/L)
Direct bilirubin	0.2 mg/dL (3.4 µmol/L)

HBV serology:

Hepatitis B surface antigen	Positive
Antibody to hepatitis B surface antigen	Negative
Hepatitis B core antibody	Positive
Hepatitis B e antigen	Positive
Antibody to hepatitis B e antigen	Negative
HBV DNA	>200,000 units/mL

Which of the following is the most appropriate next step in management?

(A) Immunization against hepatitis B virus
(B) Liver biopsy
(C) Serial monitoring of aminotransferases
(D) Tenofovir

Item 57

A 50-year-old woman is evaluated for a 1-year history of recurrent left-sided chest pain. The pain is poorly localized, nonexertional, and occurs in 1-minute episodes. There is no dyspnea, nausea, or diaphoresis associated with these episodes. She has not had dysphagia, heartburn, weight change, or other gastrointestinal symptoms. She has no other medical problems and does not smoke cigarettes. Family history is noncontributory.

On physical examination, vital signs are normal and BMI is 30. The patient's chest pain is not reproducible with palpation. The cardiac examination reveals normal heart sounds without murmurs or extracardiac sounds. The remainder of the physical examination is normal.

A lipid panel, fasting plasma glucose test, and chest radiograph are normal. An echocardiogram shows a normal ejection fraction with no wall motion abnormalities.

An exercise stress test is normal.

Which of the following is the most appropriate management?

(A) Ambulatory pH study
(B) Begin an NSAID
(C) Endoscopy
(D) Trial of a proton pump inhibitor

Item 58

An 83-year-old woman is admitted from the emergency department to the intensive care unit for hematemesis. The patient was hypotensive and tachycardic in the emergency department. Two 16-gauge intravenous catheters were placed, and intravenous resuscitation was initiated with bolus administration of 2 L of normal saline and two units of packed red blood cells. Intravenous omeprazole was begun. She has no history of gastrointestinal bleeding or liver disease. She has osteoarthritis for which she takes daily aspirin.

Two hours later, the blood pressure is 87/58 mm Hg, pulse rate is 112/min, and respiration rate is 12/min. Abdominal examination discloses hyperactive bowel sounds. The abdomen is nontender and there is no organomegaly. There are no stigmata of liver disease. Hemoglobin level is 7.0 g/dL (70 g/L).

Which of the following is the most appropriate next step in management?

(A) Continue fluid and erythrocyte resuscitation
(B) Initiate octreotide
(C) Perform immediate upper endoscopy
(D) Place a diagnostic nasogastric tube

Item 59

A 25-year-old man is evaluated for a 5-year history of slowly progressive solid-food dysphagia that is accompanied by a sensation of food sticking in his lower retrosternal area. He has compensated by modifying his diet and avoiding fibrous meats. He has not lost weight, and he has not had trouble drinking liquids. He has had episodes of food impaction that he manages by inducing vomiting. He has had no difficulty initiating a swallow and has not had chest pain, odynophagia, reflux symptoms, or aspiration of food while swallowing. He has seasonal allergies that are treated with antihistamines and asthma that is treated with inhaled albuterol.

Physical examination is normal.

Which of the following is the most likely diagnosis?

(A) Achalasia
(B) Eosinophilic esophagitis
(C) Esophageal candidiasis
(D) Esophageal malignancy
(E) Oropharyngeal dysphagia

Item 60

A 24-year-old man is evaluated for a 2-month history of new-onset jaundice and worsening pruritus. He has a history of primary sclerosing cholangitis, which was diagnosed at age 20 years when he presented with pruritus. His only medication is diphenhydramine as needed for pruritus; he takes no herbal or over-the-counter medications.

On physical examination, vital signs are normal. Scleral icterus and jaundice are noted. There are multiple excoriations on the extremities and torso. Abdominal examination is unremarkable.

Laboratory studies:

Alkaline phosphatase	350 units/L
Alanine aminotransferase	110 units/L
Aspartate aminotransferase	85 units/L
Total bilirubin	8.0 mg/dL (136.8 µmol/L)
Direct bilirubin	6.5 mg/dL (111.2 µmol/L)

Magnetic resonance cholangiopancreatography reveals a new dominant stricture of the mid common bile duct with dilatation of the common bile duct and common hepatic duct proximal to the stricture. The intrahepatic bile ducts are diffusely diseased consistent with primary sclerosing cholangitis and are unchanged from previous evaluations.

Which of the following is the most appropriate next step in management?

(A) Abdominal ultrasonography
(B) CA 19-9 measurement
(C) Endoscopic retrograde cholangiography
(D) Serial monitoring of aminotransferases

Item 61

A 60-year-old woman who was hospitalized for spontaneous bacterial peritonitis 4 days ago is now evaluated for an increase in serum creatinine level. Her medical history is notable for cirrhosis due to primary biliary cirrhosis. She also has esophageal varices, ascites, and minimal hepatic encephalopathy. Her medications are furosemide, spironolactone, nadolol, ceftriaxone, and ursodeoxycholic acid. Furosemide, spironolactone, and nadolol were stopped on admission.

On physical examination, temperature is 36.5 °C (97.7 °F), blood pressure is 100/50 mm Hg, pulse rate is 96/min, and respiration rate is 28/min. BMI is 32. Pulmonary examination discloses crackles at the right lung base. Abdominal examination discloses distention consistent with ascites. The abdomen is nontender to palpation.

Laboratory studies:

INR	1.8 (normal range, 0.8-1.2)
Albumin	2.5 g/dL (25 g/L)
Alkaline phosphatase	205 units/L
Alanine aminotransferase	50 units/L
Aspartate aminotransferase	60 units/L
Total bilirubin	7 mg/dL (119.7 µmol/L)
Creatinine	3.0 mg/dL (265 µmol/L), increased from an initial admission value of 0.9 mg/dL (79.6 µmol/L)
Urinalysis	1-3 erythrocytes, no leukocytes, no renal epithelial cells, no hyaline casts
Urine sodium	<10 meq/L (10 mmol/L)

Abdominal ultrasound discloses cirrhosis, splenomegaly, and ascites. The portal and hepatic veins are patent. There is no hydronephrosis. Urine output has decreased over the 4 days of her hospitalization.

Which of the following is the most appropriate treatment?

(A) Albumin
(B) Dopamine
(C) Octreotide
(D) Vasopressin

Item 62

A 36-year-old man is evaluated in the emergency department for melena. He began taking an over-the-counter proton pump inhibitor (PPI) 7 days ago for epigastric pain. He has no previous history of gastrointestinal illnesses.

On physical examination, vital signs are normal. BMI is 21. Abdominal palpation discloses epigastric tenderness without rebound; no masses are present. The remainder of the physical examination is normal. Hemoglobin level is 10.4 g/dL (104 g/L). Endoscopy shows a 1-cm, clean-based duodenal ulcer. Histologic examination for *Helicobacter pylori* is negative.

Which of the following is the most appropriate management?

(A) Continue the PPI with no further testing for *H. pylori*
(B) *H. pylori* serology
(C) *H. pylori* stool antigen test
(D) Urea breath test

Item 63

A 44-year-old woman is evaluated for a 1-year history of vague upper abdominal discomfort that occurs after eating. She is from a rural area in a developing country. She has not had nausea, vomiting, dysphagia, odynophagia, weight loss, or black or bloody stools. She is otherwise healthy. She has no personal history of peptic ulcer disease and no family history of gastrointestinal malignancy. Her only medication is a multivitamin.

On physical examination, temperature is 36.8 °C (98.2 °F), blood pressure is 127/82 mm Hg, pulse rate is 72/min, and respiration rate is 16/min. BMI is 27. There is epigastric tenderness with moderate palpation but no masses or lymphadenopathy. Complete blood count is normal.

Which of the following is the most appropriate management?

(A) *Helicobacter pylori* stool antigen testing
(B) Initiate an H_2 blocker
(C) Initiate empiric treatment for *H. pylori* infection
(D) Perform endoscopy

Item 64

A 26-year-old man is evaluated for a 16-month history of intermittent episodes of abdominal discomfort, nausea, and vomiting. He is relatively asymptomatic between episodes, which occur every 4 to 6 weeks. Episodes consist of vomiting once every 2 to 4 hours for about 48 hours. The only relieving factor is hot baths. He currently feels well, but it has been 5 weeks since his last episode. His medical history is notable for daily marijuana use for the past 2 years.

On physical examination, vital signs are normal. BMI is 25. Abdominal examination is normal.

Laboratory studies reveal a normal complete blood count and normal plasma glucose and thyroid-stimulating hormone levels. An abdominal radiograph is normal.

Which of the following is the most likely diagnosis?

(A) Cannabinoid hyperemesis syndrome
(B) Chronic intestinal pseudo-obstruction
(C) Cyclic vomiting syndrome
(D) Gastroparesis

Item 65

A 68-year-old woman is hospitalized for anemia and persistently melenic stools (fecal occult blood testing is positive). She is hemodynamically stable but is dependent on a transfusion of one unit of blood every 3 days to keep her hemoglobin level above 10 g/dL (100 g/L).

On physical examination, temperature is 37.3 °C (99.1 °F), blood pressure is 134/78 mm Hg, pulse rate is 88/min, and respiration rate is 18/min. Abdominal examination is normal.

Laboratory studies reveal a hemoglobin level of 8.9 g/dL (89 g/L) and an INR of 1.2 (normal range, 0.8-1.2). A peripheral blood smear is normal. Two upper endoscopies and colonoscopies performed within the past 2 weeks show no evidence of a bleeding source. A video capsule endoscopy was nondiagnostic. On the second colonoscopy, dark blood was noted in the terminal ileum.

Which of the following tests should be done next?

(A) Angiography
(B) MR enterography
(C) Nuclear scintigraphy
(D) Small-bowel barium examination

Item 66

A 45-year-old man is evaluated in follow-up for elevated liver chemistry studies that were discovered during an evaluation for life insurance. He is otherwise healthy and takes no medications.

On physical examination, temperature is 36.9 °C (98.4 °F), blood pressure is 124/82 mm Hg, pulse rate is 88/min, and respiration rate is 14/min. BMI is 26. Increased skin pigmentation is noted. The abdomen is soft and nontender, and there is no organomegaly. Bowel sounds are active.

Laboratory studies:

Hematocrit	48%
Alanine aminotransferase	60 units/L
Aspartate aminotransferase	80 units/L
Total bilirubin	1.2 mg/dL (20.5 µmol/L)
Ferritin	1100 ng/mL (1100 µg/L)
Iron	200 µg/dL (36 µmol/L)
Total iron-binding capacity	240 µg/dL (43 µmol/L)

HFE genotype is homozygous for two copies of the *C282Y* mutation. Abdominal ultrasound is normal.

Which of the following is the most appropriate next step in management?

(A) Iron chelation therapy
(B) Liver biopsy
(C) Phlebotomy
(D) Observation

Item 67

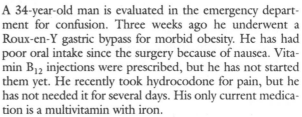

A 34-year-old man is evaluated in the emergency department for confusion. Three weeks ago he underwent a Roux-en-Y gastric bypass for morbid obesity. He has had poor oral intake since the surgery because of nausea. Vitamin B_{12} injections were prescribed, but he has not started them yet. He recently took hydrocodone for pain, but he has not needed it for several days. His only current medication is a multivitamin with iron.

On physical examination, he is afebrile. Blood pressure is 115/80 mm Hg (no orthostatic changes), and pulse rate is 85/min. The mucous membranes are moist, and there is no skin tenting. He has an ataxic gait, nystagmus, and a disconjugate gaze. The remainder of the neurologic examination is normal.

Laboratory studies, including a complete blood count, glucose, and electrolytes, are normal.

Which of the following is the most appropriate next step in management?

(A) CT of the head
(B) Glucose infusion
(C) Intravenous naloxone
(D) Intravenous thiamine
(E) Subcutaneous vitamin B_{12}

Item 68

A 24-year-old woman is evaluated for an 8-month history of daily vomiting. She describes passive movement of undigested stomach contents into the mouth without active retching, which she normally spits out or swallows. She has a history of type 1 diabetes mellitus diagnosed 2 years ago and depression that has been treated with cognitive behavioral therapy for the past year. Her medications are insulin glargine and insulin aspart. She takes no other medications or illicit drugs.

On physical examination, temperature is 36.8 °C (98.2 °F), blood pressure is 135/87 mm Hg, pulse rate is 80/min, and respiration rate is 16/min; BMI is 24. There is no parotid gland hypertrophy and the teeth appear healthy. Abdominal examination discloses no tenderness or masses. Examination of the fingers and hands is normal.

Laboratory studies reveal a plasma glucose level of 317 mg/dL (17.6 mmol/L). Abdominal radiograph shows a normal small-bowel gas pattern.

Which of the following is the most likely diagnosis?

(A) Cannabinoid hyperemesis syndrome
(B) Cyclic vomiting syndrome
(C) Gastroparesis
(D) Rumination syndrome

Item 69

A 40-year-old woman is evaluated for a 5-year history of reflux symptoms. She experiences heartburn and regurgitation of gastric contents several times per week, and she notices worsening of symptoms in a recumbent position. Lifestyle modifications, such as elevation of the head of the bed, attempts at weight loss, and avoiding lying down after meals, have not been effective in controlling her symptoms. Over-the-counter antacids and H₂ blockers provide some relief, but the relief is not lasting. She has not had weight loss, dysphagia, gastrointestinal bleeding, or anemia. She does not smoke cigarettes.

On physical examination, vital signs are normal. BMI is 35. No mass or tenderness is noted on abdominal examination.

Which of the following is the most appropriate management?

(A) Ambulatory esophageal pH study
(B) Endoscopy
(C) Fundoplication
(D) Proton pump inhibitor

Item 70

An 18-year-old woman is admitted to the hospital for a 2-day history of fever, right upper quadrant abdominal pain, and jaundice. Her only medication is a daily oral contraceptive pill.

On physical examination, temperature is 37.9 °C (100.2 °F), blood pressure is 100/65 mm Hg, pulse rate is 100/min, and respiration rate is 18/min. BMI is 22. Scleral icterus is present. Abdominal examination discloses tenderness in the right upper quadrant.

Laboratory studies:
Hematocrit 38%
Leukocyte count 11,500/µL (11.5 × 10⁹/L)
Platelet count 450,000/µL (450 × 10⁹/L)
Alkaline phosphatase 180 units/L
Alanine aminotransferase 80 units/L
Aspartate aminotransferase 65 units/L
Total bilirubin 3.0 mg/dL (51.3 µmol/L)

Abdominal ultrasound discloses a dilated common bile duct with a diameter of 20 mm. The liver is otherwise normal. The spleen is normal. Endoscopic retrograde cholangiopancreatography reveals fusiform dilatation of the common bile duct with smooth tapering at the distal common bile duct. No stones are noted.

Which of the following is the most likely diagnosis?

(A) Biliary cyst
(B) Cholelithiasis
(C) Irritable bowel syndrome
(D) Primary biliary cirrhosis

Item 71

A 25-year-old man is evaluated in the emergency department for a 2-week history of progressive jaundice and the recent onset of confusion. His medical history is unremarkable.

On physical examination, he is confused. Temperature is 36.9 °C (98.4 °F), blood pressure is 96/60 mm Hg, pulse rate is 120/min, and respiration rate is 22/min. BMI is 21. He is deeply jaundiced and asterixis is noted. No organomegaly is present.

Laboratory studies:
Hematocrit 40%
Leukocyte count 12,400/µL (12.4 × 10⁹/L)
Platelet count 350,000/µL (350 × 10⁹/L)
INR 2.5 (normal range, 0.8-1.2)
Alanine aminotransferase 240 units/L
Aspartate aminotransferase 140 units/L
Total bilirubin 20.5 mg/dL (350.6 µmol/L)
Creatinine 2.5 mg/dL (221 µmol/L)

Abdominal ultrasonography discloses a normal liver and spleen size. There is minimal ascites but no organomegaly. The portal vein has a normal diameter. There is no bile duct dilatation.

Which of the following is the most appropriate management?

(A) Administer fresh frozen plasma
(B) Administer intravenous mannitol
(C) Perform endoscopic retrograde cholangiopancreatography
(D) Refer for liver transplantation

Item 72

A 65-year-old man is evaluated in the emergency department for painless bright red blood per rectum that began 6 hours ago. He has no other medical problems and takes no medications.

On physical examination, temperature is 36.6 °C (97.9 °F), blood pressure is 130/78 mm Hg, pulse rate is 96/min, and respiration rate is 18/min. Abdominal examination is normal. Rectal examination discloses no external hemorrhoids; bright red blood is noted in the rectal vault.

Laboratory studies reveal a hemoglobin level of 10.4 g/dL (104 g/L), a leukocyte count of 6000/µL (6 × 10⁹/L), and a platelet count of 380,000/µL (380 × 10⁹/L).

Which of the following is the most likely cause of this patient's bleeding?

(A) Colon cancer
(B) Diverticulosis
(C) Duodenal ulcer
(D) Ischemic colitis

Item 73

A 55-year-old man is evaluated for a 6-year history of typical gastroesophageal reflux symptoms treated on an as-needed basis with a proton pump inhibitor. However, the frequency of his reflux symptoms has recently increased and his episodes do not respond to treatment as completely as in the past. An upper endoscopy is scheduled to evaluate the cause of this change in his symptoms.

Endoscopy reveals a 4-cm segment of salmon-colored mucosa in the distal esophagus. Biopsy from the salmon-colored segment reveals intestinal metaplasia and goblet cells with no dysplasia.

In addition to starting a daily proton pump inhibitor, which of the following is the most appropriate management?

(A) Daily cyclooxygenase-2 (COX-2) inhibitor therapy
(B) Endoscopic ablation
(C) Fundoplication
(D) Repeat endoscopy in 1 year

Item 74

A 72-year-old man is evaluated for a 2-week history of painless jaundice. He also has pruritus, anorexia, and weight loss of 4.5 kg (10.0 lb) during the same time period. He takes no medications.

On physical examination, vital signs are normal. BMI is 22, and he appears thin. Scleral icterus and jaundice are present. There is no hepatosplenomegaly and no cutaneous signs of cirrhosis. The gallbladder is palpable.

Laboratory studies:

Complete blood count	Normal
Alkaline phosphatase	522 units/L
Alanine aminotransferase	354 units/L
Aspartate aminotransferase	215 units/L
Total bilirubin	12.1 mg/dL (206.9 µmol/L)
Direct bilirubin	10.7 mg/dL (183.0 µmol/L)

Contrast-enhanced CT scan demonstrates a dilated common bile duct with focal cutoff in the pancreas head. No focal mass is noted in the head. The pancreas duct is dilated. There is no evidence of mass lesions in the liver.

Which of the following is the most appropriate initial management?

(A) Obtain serum CA 19-9 concentration
(B) Perform abdominal MRI
(C) Perform endoscopic ultrasonography of the pancreas
(D) Refer for pancreaticoduodenectomy

Item 75

A 50-year-old man is evaluated in follow-up for a recent diagnosis of cirrhosis secondary to nonalcoholic steatohepatitis. He has a history of asthma, type 2 diabetes mellitus, hyperlipidemia, and obesity. His current medications are inhaled fluticasone, montelukast, insulin glargine, insulin lispro, simvastatin, and lisinopril.

On physical examination, temperature is 37.5 °C (99.5 °F), blood pressure is 120/70 mm Hg, pulse rate is 80/min, and respiration rate is 16/min; BMI is 31. Abdominal examination reveals a palpable spleen tip.

Laboratory studies disclose a platelet count of 100,000/µL (100 × 10⁹/L), an INR of 0.9 (normal range, 0.8-1.2), and a total bilirubin level of 1.2 mg/dL (20.5 µmol/L). Abdominal ultrasound discloses a nodular-appearing liver, splenomegaly, and intra-abdominal venous

collaterals consistent with portal hypertension. Upper endoscopy is notable for large (>5 mm) distal esophageal varices that persist despite air insufflation. There are no red wale signs.

Which of the following is the most appropriate treatment?

(A) Endoscopic ligation
(B) Endoscopic sclerotherapy
(C) Propranolol
(D) Transjugular intrahepatic portosystemic shunt

Item 76

A 29-year-old woman is evaluated for painful red spots on her shins and a recent increase in the frequency of loose stools with some bleeding. She has no other symptoms. She was diagnosed with ulcerative colitis 4 years ago. Her only medication is mesalamine.

On physical examination, she appears well. Vital signs are normal. Abdominal examination is normal. A few tender, erythematous subcutaneous nodules, each measuring about 1 to 3 cm in diameter, are noted on the anterior surfaces of the legs.

Laboratory studies reveal a leukocyte count of 9200/µL (9.2 × 10⁹/L).

Which of the following is the most appropriate therapy for the skin lesions?

(A) Broad-spectrum antibiotics
(B) Intensified therapy for ulcerative colitis
(C) NSAIDs
(D) Topical corticosteroid cream

Item 77

A 71-year-old woman is evaluated in follow-up for ascending colon cancer that was diagnosed at a recent screening colonoscopy. CT of the abdomen and pelvis showed no evidence of distant metastases. A right hemicolectomy was performed. The pathology review reports stage II cancer. No adjuvant chemotherapy is recommended. She is otherwise healthy.

Which of the following is the most appropriate management strategy for this patient?

(A) Colonoscopy in 2 to 6 months
(B) Colonoscopy in 1 year
(C) Colonoscopy in 3 years
(D) Colonoscopy in 5 years

Item 78

A 65-year-old woman is evaluated in the emergency department for transient right upper quadrant abdominal pain. It occurred midmorning, was unrelated to food, was crampy and gaslike, and resolved spontaneously after 90 minutes. She had never experienced this pain previously. She is otherwise healthy and takes no medications.

On physical examination, vital signs are normal. BMI is 28. Cardiac examination discloses a normal heart rate

CONT. with a regular rhythm. The lungs are clear. The abdomen is soft, nontender, and nondistended. Bowel sounds are normal, and no abdominal masses are palpable.

Abdominal ultrasound discloses a liver with normal echotexture. The spleen is normal. There is a 20-mm polyp in the gallbladder wall.

Which of the following is the most appropriate management?

(A) Cholecystectomy
(B) Endoscopic retrograde cholangiopancreatography
(C) Repeat ultrasound in 6 months
(D) Ursodeoxycholic acid

Item 79

A 65-year-old woman with a 6-month history of amyotrophic lateral sclerosis is evaluated for a 1-month history of difficulty swallowing. She experiences choking and coughing while attempting to swallow solids or liquids and has intermittent nasal regurgitation of liquids. Two weeks ago she was treated for pneumonia. Her only medication is riluzole.

On physical examination, vital signs are normal. Tongue fasciculations and jaw clonus are present, and there is definite weakness of the masseter and pterygoid muscles. There is weakness of the proximal arms and the intrinsic muscles of the hands, but deep tendon reflexes are preserved. The plantar response is extensor.

Which of the following is the most appropriate initial diagnostic test to evaluate this patient's swallowing disorder?

(A) Endoscopy
(B) Esophageal manometry
(C) Upper gastrointestinal series
(D) Videofluoroscopy

Item 80

A 65-year-old man is evaluated 48 hours after admission to the hospital for fever and a 9.1-kg (20.0-lb) weight loss due to poor oral intake and malnutrition. He has a B-cell lymphoproliferative disorder and has just finished a course of fludarabine and rituximab therapy.

On physical examination, temperature is 38.5 °C (101.3 °F), blood pressure is 120/70 mm Hg, pulse rate is 92/min, and respiration rate is 24. BMI is 21. Muscle wasting is noted. The general physical examination, including abdominal examination, is normal.

Laboratory studies:

Hemoglobin	8.5 g/dL (85 g/L)
Absolute neutrophil count	200/µL
Platelet count	90,000/µL (90 × 10⁹/L)
INR	0.9 (normal range, 0.8-1.2)
Albumin	2.1 g/dL (21 g/L)
Alkaline phosphatase	350 units/L
Alanine aminotransferase	120 units/L
Aspartate aminotransferase	90 units/L
Total bilirubin	1.2 mg/dL (20.5 µmol/L)
Creatinine	0.9 mg/dL (79.6 µmol/L)

Blood and urine cultures are pending, and empiric antibiotics are initiated. Abdominal CT discloses a distended gallbladder without cholelithiasis. The liver is normal. Periaortic lymphadenopathy is noted.

Which of the following is the most appropriate diagnostic test to perform next?

(A) Abdominal ultrasound
(B) Endoscopic ultrasound with lymph node fine-needle aspiration
(C) Liver biopsy
(D) MRI with magnetic resonance cholangiopancreatography

Item 81

A 67-year-old woman is evaluated for a 1-year history of loose stools. She reports approximately four episodes per day without abdominal pain. She has not had nausea, vomiting, weight loss, bright red blood per rectum, or melena.

On physical examination, temperature is 36.7 °C (98.1 °F), blood pressure is 115/85 mm Hg, pulse rate is 76/min, and respiration rate is 18/min; BMI is 25. No rashes are noted. Abdominal examination is normal. Rectal examination demonstrates normal resting anal tone.

Laboratory studies reveal a normal complete blood count, thyroid-stimulating hormone level, tissue transglutaminase IgA level, and total IgA level. Results of a routine screening colonoscopy for colon cancer done 1 year ago were normal.

Which of the following is the most appropriate next step in management?

(A) Begin dicyclomine
(B) Check antigliadin antibody
(C) Initiate loperamide
(D) Perform flexible sigmoidoscopy with colon biopsies

Item 82

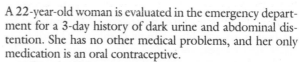

A 22-year-old woman is evaluated in the emergency department for a 3-day history of dark urine and abdominal distention. She has no other medical problems, and her only medication is an oral contraceptive.

On physical examination, temperature is 36.8 °C (98.2 °F), blood pressure is 100/62 mm Hg, pulse rate is 88/min, and respiration rate is 18/min. BMI is 24. Mental status is normal. Scleral icterus is noted. The lungs are clear, and the heart rate is normal and regular. The abdomen is distended, and bowel sounds are normal.

Laboratory studies:

Hematocrit	26%
Leukocyte count	7200/µL (7.2 × 10⁹/L)
Reticulocyte count	5%
Platelet count	138,000/µL (138 × 10⁹/L)
INR	3.1 (normal range, 0.8-1.2)
Alkaline phosphatase	32 units/L
Alanine aminotransferase	109 units/L
Aspartate aminotransferase	225 units/L
Total bilirubin	13 mg/dL (222.3 µmol/L)

Direct bilirubin	4.5 mg/dL (77.0 μmol/L)
Hepatitis A virus IgG	Positive
Hepatitis B surface antigen	Negative
Antibody to hepatitis B surface antigen	Positive
Hepatitis C virus antibody	Negative
Urine drug screen	Negative

Abdominal ultrasound discloses a nodular-appearing liver and an enlarged spleen. A small amount of ascites is noted.

Which of the following is the most likely diagnosis?

(A) Acetaminophen intoxication
(B) Acute viral hepatitis
(C) Primary biliary cirrhosis
(D) Wilson disease

Item 83

A 30-year-old man is evaluated for a 5-year history of solid-food dysphagia. He states that solid foods such as meats and breads tend to stick at the midesophagus. His symptoms are chronic but have been progressively increasing. He has occasional heartburn but no dysphagia to liquids, and he has not lost any weight. He went to the emergency department 2 weeks ago for an episode of food impaction and underwent disimpaction of a food bolus. He takes no medications.

Physical examination results are normal. Endoscopy reveals rings in the esophagus, and midesophageal biopsies show 30 eosinophils/hpf.

Which of the following is the most appropriate next step in management?

(A) Endoscopic dilation
(B) Food allergy testing
(C) Initiate omeprazole
(D) Initiate swallowed aerosolized fluticasone

Item 84

A 38-year-old woman is evaluated for a 12-month history of heartburn and intermittent dysphagia. There is no associated nausea, abdominal pain, or weight loss. Her medical history is unremarkable. Her only medication is esomeprazole.

On physical examination, vital signs are normal. BMI is 23. Abdominal examination is normal.

Endoscopy reveals a short, smooth-surfaced stricture in the distal esophagus, likely due to chronic gastroesophageal reflux, and hundreds of 2- to 4-mm gastric polyps. Biopsies reveal fundic gland polyps with no dysplasia.

Which of the following is the most appropriate management?

(A) Discontinue esomeprazole and repeat endoscopy in 3 months
(B) Order *APC* gene testing
(C) Perform colonoscopy
(D) Repeat endoscopy now for extensive polypectomy

Item 85

An 85-year-old man is evaluated in the emergency department for a 2-day history of confusion and poor appetite. His medical history is significant for type 2 diabetes mellitus. His medications are insulin glargine and metformin.

On physical examination, he is toxic appearing, cool, and clammy. Temperature is 36.5 °C (97.7 °F), blood pressure is 90/70 mm Hg, pulse rate is 110/min, and respiration rate is 32/min. BMI is 27. The cardiopulmonary examination is normal. The abdomen is unremarkable to palpation.

Laboratory studies:

Hemoglobin	13.5 g/dL (135 g/L)
Leukocyte count	7000/μL (7 × 10⁹/L)
Alkaline phosphatase	550 units/L
Alanine aminotransferase	120 units/L
Aspartate aminotransferase	190 units/L
Total bilirubin	3 mg/dL (51.3 μmol/L)

Abdominal ultrasound discloses a normal liver. There is no bile duct dilatation. Gallstones are present in the gallbladder. Ampicillin-sulbactam is begun.

Which of the following is the most appropriate next step in management?

(A) Cholecystectomy
(B) Endoscopic retrograde cholangiopancreatography
(C) Hepatobiliary iminodiacetic acid scan
(D) MRI with magnetic resonance cholangiopancreatography

Item 86

A 48-year-old man is evaluated in the emergency department for a 12-hour history of severe epigastric abdominal pain. He has a long-standing history of alcohol use. The pain developed gradually, radiates to his back, and is associated with nausea and diaphoresis.

On physical examination, temperature is 36.8 °C (98.2 °F), blood pressure is 118/62 mm Hg, pulse rate is 95/min, and respiration rate is 18/min. BMI is 35. The oral pharynx is dry. Absent breath sounds and dullness to percussion are noted in the left lower lung field. Abdominal examination discloses epigastric tenderness to palpation. There is no hepatosplenomegaly, cutaneous signs of cirrhosis, or peritoneal signs.

Laboratory studies:

Hematocrit	54%
Leukocyte count	14,100/μL (14.1 × 10⁹/L)
Alkaline phosphatase	105 units/L
Alanine aminotransferase	24 units/L
Aspartate aminotransferase	29 units/L
Amylase	2342 units/L
Bicarbonate	Normal
Total bilirubin	0.8 mg/dL (13.7 μmol/L)
Blood urea nitrogen	68 mg/dL (24.3 mmol/L)
Creatinine	1.9 mg/dL (168 μmol/L)
Lactate dehydrogenase	Normal
Lipase	1232 units/L

Contrast-enhanced CT scan demonstrates peripancreatic edema and hypoperfusion of the pancreatic body. A left pleural effusion is noted. There are no fluid collections or free air.

Which of the following is the most appropriate initial treatment?

(A) Aggressive hydration with intravenous fluids
(B) Broad-spectrum antibiotics
(C) Endoscopic retrograde cholangiopancreatography
(D) Nasogastric tube

Item 87

A 45-year-old woman is evaluated for a 2-year history of dysphagia to solids and liquids that is associated with intermittent nonexertional chest pain and regurgitation. Her weight has been stable and she has no other medical issues. She lives in a remote rural area.

Physical examination is normal, and BMI is 25.

Barium swallow reveals a dilated, smoothly tapering esophagus. Endoscopy reveals a dilated, aperistaltic esophagus with a tight gastroesophageal junction and no mass lesion. Manometry confirms esophageal aperistalsis.

Which of the following is the most appropriate management?

(A) Botulinum toxin injection into the lower esophageal sphincter
(B) Endoscopic pneumatic balloon dilatation
(C) Laparoscopic myotomy
(D) Medical therapy with nifedipine

Item 88

A 26-year-old man is evaluated for fatigue and has been newly diagnosed with iron-deficiency anemia. The patient has Down syndrome, and details of his clinical history are provided by his mother. There is no history of melena, hematochezia, or hematuria. His hemoglobin level was checked 2 years ago and was normal. His bowel movements are regular, and his weight is unchanged. He has no abdominal problems.

On physical examination, temperature is 36.3 °C (97.3 °F) and pulse rate is 88/min. Other vital signs are normal. BMI is 29. Mild skin pallor is noted. Abdominal and rectal examinations are normal.

Serum tissue transglutaminase IgA antibody testing is negative. Colonoscopy and upper endoscopy are unremarkable.

Which of the following is the most appropriate diagnostic test to perform next?

(A) Meckel scan
(B) Push enteroscopy
(C) Repeat upper endoscopy with small-bowel biopsies
(D) Small-bowel capsule endoscopy
(E) Stool guaiac examination

Item 89

A 49-year-old woman is evaluated for a 4-month history of watery diarrhea that occurs five to six times per day. The diarrhea is associated with cramping and urgency, but there is no bleeding. She has a history of gastroesophageal reflux disease. Her sister has celiac disease. Her only medication is lansoprazole.

On physical examination, vital signs are normal. Abdominal examination is normal. Colonoscopy reveals normal-appearing colonic mucosa, but colonic biopsies disclose an abnormally thickened subepithelial collagen band in the lamina propria.

Which of the following is the most appropriate next step for treatment of her diarrhea?

(A) Budesonide
(B) Gluten-free diet
(C) Mesalamine
(D) Prednisone
(E) Stop lansoprazole

Item 90

A 67-year-old man is admitted to the hospital for pain control in the setting of metastatic pancreatic adenocarcinoma that was diagnosed 3 months ago. Although the cancer was found incidentally, the patient has had progressive abdominal pain over the last few weeks that has not been responsive to outpatient escalation of his oral analgesics. Over the last few days in the hospital, pain control was achieved with intravenous morphine (both short-acting and time-released), with transition to equivalent oral dosing planned. He has reported constipation due to his pain medications, and he has not had relief of constipation despite the use of docusate sodium and senna. He did not tolerate polyethylene glycol, and fiber caused excessive bloating. He is still passing gas and infrequent, small bowel movements.

On physical examination, he appears thin and cachectic. Blood pressure is 115/80 mm Hg, pulse rate is 76/min, and respiration rate is 14/min. BMI is 20. Abdominal examination discloses mild tenderness in the upper abdomen without significant distention. There is no guarding or rebound. Rectal examination is normal with firm stool in the rectal vault.

Laboratory studies, including a complete blood count and glucose, calcium, and thyroid-stimulating hormone levels, are normal. Abdominal radiograph reveals stool throughout the colon with no air-fluid levels.

Which of the following is the most appropriate management?

(A) Add methylnaltrexone
(B) Add naloxone
(C) Administer a diatrizoate sodium enema
(D) Decrease the morphine dose

Item 91

A 65-year-old woman is evaluated in follow-up after recent discharge from her third hospitalization for an acute exacerbation of hepatic encephalopathy. No specific trigger was identified for the worsening encephalopathy. Her medical history is significant for cirrhosis due to primary biliary cirrhosis, as well as esophageal varices and ascites. Her medications are lactulose, nadolol, furosemide, spironolactone, and zinc sulfate; she is adherent to her lactulose therapy.

On physical examination, temperature is 37.5 °C (99.5 °F), blood pressure is 105/65 mm Hg, pulse rate is 68/min, and respiration rate is 16/min. BMI is 33. There are no gross or focal neurologic deficits. The spleen tip is palpable.

Which of the following is the most appropriate additional treatment?

(A) Ciprofloxacin
(B) Metronidazole
(C) Protein restriction
(D) Rifaximin

Item 92

A 50-year-old man is evaluated for a 6-month history of dysphagia. He describes a sensation of both solids and liquids sticking in the midesophageal area. This sensation has slowly worsened over time. He also describes intermittent midsternal discomfort that is nonexertional and is usually precipitated by swallowing food. He has lost 4.5 kg (10.0 lb). He has had no history of heartburn or acid regurgitation.

Physical examination is normal.

A barium swallow is shown. Esophageal manometry shows aperistalsis with swallowing of liquids.

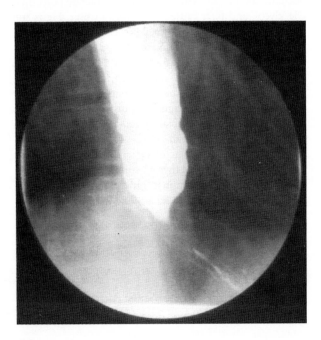

Which of the following is the most appropriate management?

(A) CT of the chest and abdomen
(B) Endoscopy
(C) Myotomy
(D) Trial of swallowed aerosolized corticosteroids

Item 93

A 60-year-old woman is evaluated for elevated serum liver chemistry tests for the past 6 months that were originally discovered at a health screening fair sponsored by her church. She is asymptomatic. Her medical history is significant for hyperlipidemia, hypothyroidism, and osteopenia. Her medications are levothyroxine, atorvastatin, calcium, and vitamin D.

The physical examination is unremarkable.

Laboratory studies:

Platelet count	200,000/µL (200 × 10⁹/L)
INR	0.9 (normal range, 0.8-1.2)
Alkaline phosphatase	450 units/L
Alanine aminotransferase	80 units/L
Aspartate aminotransferase	70 units/L
Total bilirubin	0.9 mg/dL (15.4 µmol/L)
Creatinine	0.9 mg/dL (79.6 µmol/L)
Serum antimitochondrial antibody	1:256

Abdominal ultrasound discloses a coarsened hepatic echotexture. No splenomegaly or ascites is noted.

Which of the following is the most appropriate treatment?

(A) Azathioprine
(B) Colchicine
(C) Methotrexate
(D) Ursodeoxycholic acid

Item 94

A 73-year-old woman is evaluated for a 6-month history of abdominal pain that occurs about 30 minutes after eating. She has lost 9.1 kg (20.0 lb) since the onset of symptoms. She has a history of hypertension and hypercholesterolemia. Her medications are lisinopril, simvastatin, and aspirin. She has a 50-pack-year history of smoking and is a lifelong nondrinker.

On physical examination, temperature is 37.2 °C (99.0 °F), blood pressure is 155/92 mm Hg, pulse rate is 88/min, and respiration rate is 22/min. BMI is 34. Oxygen saturation is 92% with the patient breathing ambient air. Abdominal examination is normal.

Laboratory studies reveal a leukocyte count of 8700/µL (8.7 × 10⁹/L) and a bicarbonate level of 24 meq/L (24 mmol/L).

Which of the following is the most likely diagnosis?

(A) Chronic mesenteric ischemia
(B) Chronic pancreatitis
(C) Colonic ischemia
(D) Gastroparesis

Item 95

A 53-year-old man is evaluated in follow-up 1 week after his first screening colonoscopy. He has no history of colorectal neoplasia in first- or second-degree relatives.

Physical examination is normal. A colonoscopy to the cecum was performed. The preparation was described as poor, with collections of semisolid debris that could not be effectively cleared from several colonic segments. According to the colonoscopy report, mass lesions 1 cm or larger are unlikely to have been obscured by the debris. Three diminutive (<3 mm) hyperplastic polyps were removed from the rectum.

Which of the following is the most appropriate management for this patient?

(A) Repeat colonoscopy now following adequate preparation
(B) Repeat colonoscopy in 3 years
(C) Repeat colonoscopy in 5 years
(D) Repeat colonoscopy in 10 years

Item 96

A 35-year-old man is evaluated in follow-up 8 weeks after the diagnosis of a *Helicobacter pylori*–positive duodenal ulcer. He has had persistent epigastric pain despite adhering to a 2-week course of treatment with amoxicillin, clarithromycin, and omeprazole.

On physical examination, vital signs are normal. There is tenderness to palpation in the epigastrium without guarding. Stool examination is negative for occult blood. The remainder of the physical examination is normal. A repeat *H. pylori* stool antigen test is positive.

Which of the following is the most appropriate treatment?

(A) Amoxicillin, clarithromycin, and omeprazole
(B) Bismuth, metronidazole, tetracycline, and omeprazole
(C) Pantoprazole
(D) Observation

Answers and Critiques

Item 1   Answer: A

Educational Objective: Manage colorectal cancer surveillance in a patient with hereditary nonpolyposis colorectal cancer syndrome (Lynch syndrome).

The most appropriate management strategy is a colonoscopy now. This patient's family history meets the Amsterdam criteria II, supporting a possible hereditary nonpolyposis colorectal cancer (HNPCC) kindred. The Amsterdam criteria II can be remembered by the "3-2-1 rule" (3 affected members, 2 generations, 1 under age 50 years). HNPCC (or Lynch syndrome) is an autosomal dominant syndrome that carries an 80% lifetime risk for colon cancer. HNPCC is the most common of the hereditary colon cancer syndromes, accounting for 2% to 3% of all colorectal adenocarcinomas. Colorectal adenomas develop at a relatively young age (by age 20 to 30 years) and are thought to progress to colorectal cancer more quickly than sporadic adenomas. HNPCC-associated extracolonic cancers include uterine cancer (40% to 60% lifetime risk) and ovarian cancer (10% to 12% lifetime risk). Colorectal evaluation should be initiated by age 20 to 25 years or 10 years prior to the earliest age of colorectal cancer diagnosis in the family, whichever comes first. Colonoscopy is the test of choice. In addition, gynecologic (transvaginal ultrasound or endometrial aspirate) and genitourinary (urine cytology) cancer screening should be performed.

Colonoscopy at age 40 years would be an acceptable option for a patient with a nonsyndromic family history of colorectal cancer in a first-degree relative but not in a patient with a possible hereditary nonpolyposis colorectal cancer syndrome.

Colonoscopy at age 50 years is one of several endorsed options for average-risk colorectal cancer screening, but it is not appropriate for this patient who is in a high-risk category.

Neither stool DNA testing nor CT colonography is currently endorsed for colorectal cancer screening/surveillance among patients at increased risk because of family history.

KEY POINT

- In patients with hereditary nonpolyposis colorectal cancer syndrome (Lynch syndrome), colonoscopy should be initiated by age 20 to 25 years or 10 years prior to the earliest age of colorectal cancer diagnosis in the family, whichever comes first.

Bibliography

Goodenberger M, Lindor NM. Lynch syndrome and MYH-associated polyposis: review and testing strategy. J Clin Gastroenterol. 2011;45(6):488-500. [PMID: 21325953]

Item 2   Answer: D

Educational Objective: Manage nonalcoholic steatohepatitis.

The most appropriate management is serial monitoring of aminotransferases, in addition to weight loss through dietary and lifestyle changes. There is no definitive treatment for nonalcoholic fatty liver disease. The reduction of underlying risk factors is essential. Weight loss, exercise, and aggressive control of plasma glucose, lipids, and blood pressure are the mainstays of treatment. Nonalcoholic fatty liver disease has become a leading cause of liver disease in the Western world, along with hepatitis C and alcoholic liver disease. When hepatic steatosis is associated with liver inflammation, as is seen in this patient with elevated hepatic aminotransferases, nonalcoholic steatohepatitis (NASH) is diagnosed. The association of NASH with the metabolic syndrome (obesity, dyslipidemia, hypertension, insulin resistance) is well established. Although most cases of nonalcoholic fatty liver disease are seen in patients who are overweight, the condition has also been described in patients who have a normal BMI. The cornerstone of management of NASH is typically weight loss through diet and lifestyle modification. Monitoring of hepatic aminotransferases is appropriate to confirm that weight loss results in improved markers of liver inflammation. Associated medical conditions such as dyslipidemia should be treated, and statins such as simvastatin should not be discontinued in this setting. The risks of hepatoxicity due to the use of medications such as simvastatin are usually outweighed by the benefits derived from these medications in regard to cardiovascular risk reduction.

This patient's hepatitis B serologies indicate immunity to hepatitis B virus; therefore, an antiviral medication such as entecavir is not appropriate.

This patient's iron stores are not elevated, with a transferrin saturation (iron/total iron binding capacity) of less than 45%; therefore, phlebotomy is not warranted as a treatment in this setting.

KEY POINT

- Weight loss, exercise, and aggressive control of plasma glucose, lipids, and blood pressure are the mainstays of treatment for nonalcoholic steatohepatitis; monitoring of hepatic aminotransferases is appropriate to confirm that weight loss results in improved markers of liver inflammation.

Bibliography

Perlemuter G, Bigorgne A, Cassard-Doulcier AM, Naveau S. Nonalcoholic fatty liver disease: from pathogenesis to patient care. Nat Clin Pract Endocrinol Metab. 2007;3(6):458-469. [PMID: 17515890]

Item 3   Answer: B

Educational Objective: Treat spontaneous bacterial peritonitis in a patient with significant hepatic and kidney dysfunction.

The most appropriate treatment is cefotaxime and albumin. The diagnosis of spontaneous bacterial peritonitis (SBP) is made in the setting of a positive ascitic fluid bacterial culture and/or an elevated ascitic fluid absolute polymorphonuclear (PMN) cell count (≥250/microliter) without evidence of secondary causes of peritonitis. Patients with negative cultures have the same clinical presentation and outcomes compared with those with positive cultures. Intravenous cefotaxime or a similar third-generation cephalosporin is the treatment of choice for SBP. Three of the most common isolates are *Escherichia coli*, *Klebsiella pneumoniae*, and pneumococci. Oral fluoroquinolone treatment may be indicated in ambulatory patients with stable hepatic and kidney function and ascitic fluid absolute PMN cell count of 250/microliter or greater. While a significant number of hospitalized patients with SBP recover, it has been shown that kidney failure associated with SBP increases the risk for mortality. The use of cefotaxime plus intravenous albumin at 1.5 g/kg on admission and 1 g/kg on day 3 has been shown to decrease in-hospital mortality by 20% in patients with serum creatinine values of 1.5 mg/dL (133 micromoles/L) or greater, as in this patient. Patients with advanced liver disease, including those with a serum total bilirubin of 4 mg/dL (68.4 micromoles/L) or greater, as seen in this patient, also benefit from intravenous albumin to prevent kidney failure associated with SBP.

The use of cefotaxime alone in this patient is not appropriate, because the risk for progressive kidney dysfunction could still exist in the absence of intravenous albumin.

Oral diuretics such as furosemide and spironolactone should be withheld in patients with ascites and SBP to minimize the risk of worsening kidney function.

There is no evidence that large-volume paracentesis improves outcomes in patients with SBP; in fact, it may worsen kidney function owing to excessive fluid shifts.

KEY POINT

- In patients with spontaneous bacterial peritonitis, the concomitant use of intravenous albumin with antibiotic therapy is associated with a survival benefit compared with antibiotic therapy alone.

Bibliography

Runyon BA; AASLD Practice Guidelines Committee. Management of adult patients with ascites due to cirrhosis: an update. Hepatology. 2009;49(6):2087-2107. [PMID: 19475696]

Item 4   Answer: E

Educational Objective: Manage acute diarrhea.

This patient needs no additional studies at this time. She has had acute diarrhea for only 1 day; for most patients this represents a self-limited gastroenteritis. This is supported by the fact that this patient's work colleagues have recently been sick with similar symptoms. Features or clinical characteristics that require additional evaluation for acute diarrhea include fever, bloody stools, pregnancy, elderly or immunocompromised state, hospitalization, employment as a food handler, recent antibiotic use, volume depletion, or significant abdominal pain. This patient has none of these features requiring additional evaluation, so she should be encouraged to stay well hydrated, use antidiarrheal agents as needed, and follow up if symptoms change or persist.

Stool cultures and *Clostridium difficile* evaluation should be considered in patients with any features that require additional evaluation, as described previously. Additional studies may be necessary for acute diarrhea in patients with unique clinical situations or exposures.

The presence of fecal leukocytes is nonspecific and may represent infection, ischemia, or idiopathic inflammation; evaluation for fecal leukocytes rarely adds much information in the evaluation of acute diarrhea.

A flexible sigmoidoscopy with random biopsies can be used in the evaluation of chronic watery diarrhea to assess for microscopic colitis, but this would not be indicated in the acute setting unless the patient had clinical features that suggest ischemic colitis (sudden onset of mild crampy abdominal pain and bloody diarrhea). These features are not present in this patient.

KEY POINT

- Most patients with acute diarrhea have a self-limited gastroenteritis that requires no further evaluation.

Bibliography

Baldi F, Bianco MA, Nardone G, Pilotto A, Zamparo E. Focus on acute diarrhoeal disease. World J Gastroenterol. 2009;15(27):3341-3348. [PMID: 19610134]

Item 5   Answer: A

Educational Objective: Diagnose acute viral hepatitis in a patient with new-onset jaundice.

The most likely diagnosis is acute viral hepatitis. This patient has marked hepatitis with jaundice and significant elevations of hepatic aminotransferases (greater than 15 times the upper limit of normal). In addition, the short duration of her symptoms suggests an acute onset. Elevation of aspartate aminotransferase and alanine aminotransferase to this severe degree is seen in acute viral hepatitis. Typically, the only other causes of this degree of liver chemistry test elevation are medication reactions/toxicity, autoimmune liver disease, ischemic hepatitis (referred to as "shock liver"), or acute bile duct obstruction.

Fulminant liver failure should always be a consideration in patients with acute hepatitis. However, fulminant liver failure is manifested by hepatic encephalopathy that occurs within 8 weeks of the onset of jaundice; this patient has normal mental status. In addition, laboratory studies demonstrate a normal INR and normal albumin level, confirming that this patient's liver function remains intact despite her liver inflammation.

Hemochromatosis is a chronic metabolic cause of chronic liver disease and is associated with much lower elevations of liver inflammation markers than are seen in this patient.

Primary biliary cirrhosis is an immune-mediated cause of chronic liver inflammation. This is not the correct diagnosis because the degree of elevation of aminotransferases vastly exceeds the levels seen in patients with primary biliary cirrhosis, who have elevated alkaline phosphatase and bilirubin levels disproportionately higher than the aminotransferase elevation.

KEY POINT

- Acute viral hepatitis is characterized by jaundice and significant elevations of hepatic aminotransferases (greater than 15 times the upper limit of normal).

Bibliography

Green RM, Flamm S. AGA technical review on the evaluation of liver chemistry tests. Gastroenterology. 2002;123(4):1367-1384. [PMID: 12360498]

Item 6 Answer: D

Educational Objective: Manage colorectal cancer risk reduction.

There are no specific medications that should be recommended strictly to reduce colorectal cancer risk. Based on existing data, there does not appear to be a sufficient risk-to-benefit ratio for routine use of any colorectal chemoprevention agents outside of high-risk patient populations. Although many observational studies and clinical trials have reported that regular use of aspirin or other NSAIDs can reduce colorectal cancer risk, these medications may also induce serious toxicities such as gastrointestinal bleeding, hemorrhagic stroke, hypertension, or kidney impairment. Based on a comprehensive systematic review, the U.S. Preventive Services Task Force concluded that the potential harms outweigh the anticipated benefits of using aspirin or NSAIDs solely to prevent colorectal cancer in asymptomatic adults, including patients with a family history of colorectal cancer (but excluding patients with hereditary cancer syndromes).

Celecoxib is a selective cyclooxygenase-2 inhibitor (a class of NSAIDs) with potential polyp prevention effects, but it has not been approved by the FDA for use as a colorectal cancer chemoprevention agent in patients with a nonsyndromic family history.

In epidemiologic studies, systematic reviews, and secondary analyses from some clinical trials, postmenopausal hormone therapy using estrogen (with or without progesterone) has been inconsistently associated with a reduced risk of colorectal cancer. Postmenopausal hormone replacement therapy is not currently recommended for colorectal cancer chemoprevention because of the associated risks for significant adverse events, including breast and endometrial cancer.

KEY POINT

- Based on current data, the risks outweigh the benefits of using NSAIDs or estrogen replacement therapy for colorectal cancer chemoprevention.

Bibliography

Dubé C, Rostom A, Lewin G, et al; U.S. Preventive Services Task Force. The use of aspirin for primary prevention of colorectal cancer: a systematic review prepared for the U.S. Preventive Services Task Force. Ann Intern Med. 2007;146(5):365-375. [PMID: 17339622]

Item 7 Answer: A

Educational Objective: Diagnose acute mesenteric ischemia.

This patient most likely has acute mesenteric ischemia based on the suggestive CT scan findings, the presence of metabolic acidosis with an elevated serum lactate level, and the finding of pain out of proportion to the examination. CT scan of the abdomen may show bowel-wall thickening or intestinal pneumatosis (air within the wall of the bowel). The most common cause of acute mesenteric ischemia is an embolus to the superior mesenteric artery originating from the left atrium or a ventricular mural thrombus. The next most common cause is nonocclusive mesenteric ischemia subsequent to a cardiovascular event, such as hypotension following a myocardial infarction. These two causes account for 75% of cases of acute mesenteric ischemia. Traditional angiography has been the diagnostic gold standard and can be used for administration of therapeutic vasodilators and stenting. CT angiography is becoming increasingly recognized as a highly sensitive and specific modality to diagnose acute mesenteric ischemia. The procedure is more readily available than traditional angiography and also permits the evaluation of the abdomen in addition to the vasculature.

Crohn disease could cause thickening of the small bowel on imaging, but it would not be consistent with this patient's acute onset of severe abdominal pain, hemodynamic instability, and metabolic acidosis.

An intussusception causes bowel obstruction rather than intestinal ischemia.

Acute pancreatitis is unlikely to lead to shock within 1 hour of onset. In addition, the CT scan does not support

CONT.

a diagnosis of acute pancreatitis, which would be characterized by pancreatic edema.

- Acute mesenteric ischemia should be suspected in patients with the acute onset of severe abdominal pain and an abdominal examination that discloses less tenderness than expected based on the patient's symptoms (pain out of proportion to the examination).

Bibliography

Brandt LJ, Boley SJ. AGA technical review on intestinal ischemia. American Gastrointestinal Association. Gastroenterology. 2000;118(5):954-968. [PMID: 10784596]

Item 8   Answer: D

Educational Objective: Manage decompensated cirrhosis by referring for liver transplantation.

The most appropriate management is referral for consideration of liver transplantation. The major indications for liver transplantation are acute liver failure, hepatic decompensation due to chronic liver disease, primary liver cancer, and inborn errors of metabolism. The most common chronic liver diseases that prompt referral for liver transplantation are hepatitis C, cirrhosis due to nonalcoholic steatohepatitis, and alcoholic liver disease. This patient has end-stage liver disease due to alcoholic cirrhosis with manifestations of liver failure (ascites and hepatic encephalopathy). Patients who develop manifestations of decompensated liver disease such as ascites, hepatic encephalopathy, or gastroesophageal variceal hemorrhage have an estimated 50% mortality rate at 2 years and should be considered for eventual liver transplantation. Liver transplant centers typically require that a patient abstain from alcohol, usually for a period of 6 months, prior to consideration of liver transplantation.

A nonselective β-blocker such as nadolol or propranolol is indicated for primary prevention of variceal bleeding in patients with medium or large varices or varices otherwise defined as high risk for bleeding. Patients without varices should be periodically screened with upper endoscopy, but initiating β-blocker therapy in the absence of varices, as in this patient, is not indicated.

The prevalence of protein-calorie malnutrition ranges from 35% to 80% in both alcoholic and nonalcoholic cirrhosis. Protein-calorie malnutrition is an independent predictor of mortality in patients with cirrhosis. Protein restriction is not necessary for most patients with cirrhosis and hepatic encephalopathy; protein-intake modification is usually reserved for patients whose symptoms cannot be managed with lactulose alone.

Liver transplantation rather than ongoing medical management offers this patient the best chance of longer-term survival.

- Patients who develop decompensated cirrhosis (manifested by the complications of ascites, hepatic encephalopathy, jaundice, or portal-hypertension–related bleeding) should be considered for liver transplantation.

Bibliography

Ahmed A, Keeffe EB. Current indications and contraindications for liver transplantation. Clin Liver Dis. 2007;11(2):227-247. [PMID: 17606204]

Item 9   Answer: A

Educational Objective: Manage colorectal cancer screening in a patient with ulcerative colitis.

The most appropriate management for this patient is colonoscopy now and every 1 to 2 years. Patients with ulcerative colitis with disease extending beyond the rectum are at an increased risk of colorectal cancer. Cancer risk has been widely reported to be between 0.5% and 1% per year after having extensive disease for 10 years or more. The exact risk for an individual patient is uncertain and is probably based on the duration and extent of disease, severity of inflammation, and other personal factors. Based on this increased cancer risk, routine surveillance colonoscopy with biopsies every 1 to 2 years is warranted beginning 8 to 10 years after diagnosis. Because cancers associated with ulcerative colitis tend to arise from the mucosa as opposed to the usual adenoma-cancer sequence, biopsies are taken from flat mucosa throughout the colon and are evaluated for dysplastic changes. A finding of flat, high-grade dysplasia is grounds for recommending colectomy owing to the high rate of concomitant undetected cancer. A finding of flat, low-grade dysplasia warrants colectomy or continued surveillance colonoscopy at more frequent intervals.

Colonoscopy now for this patient is appropriate, but the interval should be every 1 to 2 years rather than every 5 years. For persons without ulcerative colitis but with a family history of colorectal cancer in a first-degree relative, screening is initiated either at age 40 years or beginning 10 years earlier than the diagnosis of the youngest affected family member. Colonoscopy every 10 years starting at age 40 is not appropriate for this patient.

- Patients with ulcerative colitis with disease extending beyond the rectum should undergo routine surveillance colonoscopy with biopsies every 1 to 2 years beginning 8 to 10 years after diagnosis.

Bibliography

Kornbluth A, Sachar DB; Practice Parameters Committee of the American College of Gastroenterology. Ulcerative colitis practice guidelines in adults: American College Of Gastroenterology, Practice Parameters Committee [erratum in Am J Gastroenterol.

2010;105(3):500.]. Am J Gastroenterol. 2010;105(3):501-523. [PMID: 20068560]

Item 10   Answer: D

Educational Objective: Evaluate for celiac disease in a patient with diarrhea-predominant irritable bowel syndrome.

This patient should undergo tissue transglutaminase antibody testing. The American College of Gastroenterology recommends routine serologic testing for celiac disease in patients who present with symptoms of diarrhea-predominant or mixed irritable bowel syndrome (IBS). Additionally, there is a well-established association between comorbid autoimmune disorders and celiac disease, especially type 1 diabetes mellitus and autoimmune thyroid disease.

Although some evidence suggests a role of small-bowel bacterial overgrowth in the pathogenesis of IBS, evidence is insufficient to warrant testing for this condition with a breath test.

Approximately 2% of patients with features of diarrhea-predominant IBS are found to have microscopic colitis. A history of nocturnal or large-volume diarrhea or a stool osmotic gap less than 50 mOsm/kg (50 mmol/kg) would make a compelling case for microscopic colitis. In the absence of these features, a colonoscopy and random biopsies might be indicated, but the yield is low.

In patients who meet clinical criteria for IBS without alarm features, routine testing with stool culture is unlikely to result in an alternative diagnosis. Similarly, other laboratory tests such as the erythrocyte sedimentation rate and thyroid-stimulating hormone have a low yield. Patients who should be considered for colonoscopy and additional evaluation with blood and urine studies include those older than 50 years or those with a short history of symptoms, documented weight loss, nocturnal symptoms, family history of colon cancer or rectal bleeding, and recent antibiotic use.

KEY POINT

- The American College of Gastroenterology recommends routine serologic testing for celiac disease in patients with symptoms of diarrhea-predominant or mixed irritable bowel syndrome.

Bibliography
Ford AC, Chey WD, Talley NJ, Malhotra A, Spiegel BM, Moayyedi P. Yield of diagnostic tests for celiac disease in individuals with symptoms suggestive of irritable bowel syndrome: systematic review and meta-analysis. Arch Intern Med. 2009;169(7):651-658. [PMID: 19364994]

Item 11   Answer: D

Educational Objective: Diagnose intrahepatic cholestasis of pregnancy.

The most likely diagnosis is intrahepatic cholestasis of pregnancy (ICP), which occurs during the second or third trimester of pregnancy and resolves after delivery. ICP is more common in women of South Asian, South American, and Scandinavian ancestry. ICP is characterized by generalized pruritus and can result in excoriations. The most common laboratory findings are mildly elevated bilirubin and alkaline phosphatase levels; mildly elevated hepatic aminotransferases can also be noted. The most consistently abnormal laboratory test is an elevated serum bile acid concentration, which may be the only laboratory abnormality in some patients. ICP is believed to result from sex hormone–induced inhibition of bile salt export from hepatocytes. ICP is treated with ursodeoxycholic acid, which can result in improvement of symptoms. While maternal effects of ICP are mild, ICP can cause fetal distress and premature labor that are not necessarily improved by the use of ursodeoxycholic acid. High maternal bile acid levels are an indication for early delivery.

Acute fatty liver of pregnancy and HELLP (Hemolysis, Elevated Liver enzymes, and Low Platelets) syndrome are life-threatening complications of pregnancy. Both of these typically occur during the third trimester of pregnancy and are treated with urgent delivery. HELLP syndrome is characterized by microangiopathic hemolytic anemia, elevated liver chemistry tests, and low platelets. This patient's normal complete blood count excludes HELLP syndrome. Acute fatty liver of pregnancy is always defined by liver failure and coagulopathy; however, this patient has normal liver function and no evidence of coagulopathy.

Hyperemesis gravidarum occurs in the first trimester of pregnancy and resolves by week 16. It is characterized by unrelenting nausea and vomiting. Elevated hepatic aminotransferases are seen in up to 50% of cases and typically normalize when symptoms abate. Cholestasis and pruritus are not part of this syndrome.

KEY POINT

- Intrahepatic cholestasis of pregnancy is characterized by generalized pruritus, elevated serum bile acid concentration, and variable elevations of serum bilirubin, alkaline phosphatase, and aminotransferase levels.

Bibliography
Pan C, Perumalswami PV. Pregnancy-related liver diseases. Clin Liver Dis. 2011;15(1):199-208. [PMID: 21112001]

Item 12   Answer: D

Educational Objective: Manage gastrointestinal bleeding in a patient taking warfarin.

The most appropriate management is to proceed with upper endoscopy without attempting to correct the INR with fresh frozen plasma or vitamin K. The characteristic gnawing epigastric pain with coffee-ground emesis in an older patient points to the diagnosis of bleeding peptic

CONT.

ulcer disease. After initial resuscitation, patients with non-variceal upper gastrointestinal bleeding should undergo an upper endoscopic evaluation within 24 hours of presentation. Clinical guidelines state that the risk of continued bleeding on warfarin therapy must be weighed against the risk of stopping anticoagulation. In this hemodynamically stable patient with a prosthetic mitral valve, atrial fibrillation, and previous history of a transient ischemic attack, the risk of thrombosis following discontinuation of warfarin is high, and withholding reversal of anticoagulation is a reasonable option. The guidelines further state that endoscopy should not be delayed for anticoagulation reversal unless the INR is supratherapeutic (INR >3.0). This patient's INR is not supratherapeutic; therefore, he can undergo upper endoscopy promptly.

Of the remaining options, fresh frozen plasma would be the best option for immediate reversal of INR. Intravenous and oral vitamin K have a delayed effect in reversal of coagulopathy. However, no reversal agent is necessary in this patient who is able to undergo immediate endoscopy.

KEY POINT

- Upper endoscopy can be performed without delay in patients with upper gastrointestinal bleeding and an INR less than 3.0.

Bibliography

Barkun AN, Bardou M, Kuipers EJ, et al; International Consensus Upper Gastrointestinal Bleeding Conference Group. International consensus recommendations on the management of patients with nonvariceal upper gastrointestinal bleeding. Ann Intern Med. 2010;152(2):101-113. [PMID: 20083829]

Item 13   Answer: A
Educational Objective: Manage recently resolved acute diverticulitis.

The most appropriate management strategy is colonoscopy. Uncomplicated, acute diverticulitis should be treated for 7 to 10 days using relatively broad-spectrum antibiotics with activity against both anaerobes and gram-negative rods. Hospitalization with intravenous antibiotic therapy is necessary for patients who cannot tolerate oral intake. After the presenting symptoms have improved and oral diet can be resumed, transition to oral antibiotic therapy is appropriate. Following resolution of acute diverticulitis, the entire colorectum should be evaluated to rule out other disorders that may mimic diverticulitis, such as adenocarcinoma or Crohn disease.

Elective segmental colon resection can be considered to reduce the risk of recurrent diverticulitis, but the timing of prophylactic operative intervention remains somewhat controversial. On average, only about one third of patients who respond to medical management for their first attack of acute diverticulitis will experience a second attack. Therefore, in the absence of other high risk factors such as

young age at onset (<50 years), immunocompromised state, or multiple comorbid conditions, elective surgery is generally not advised for a single episode of uncomplicated, acute diverticulitis.

Alterations in the peridiverticular microflora may play a role in the pathogenesis of acute or chronic diverticular inflammation, but existing data are insufficient to support probiotic therapy as a routine clinical intervention after antibiotic therapy is completed.

KEY POINT

- Following resolution of acute diverticulitis, the entire colorectum should be evaluated with colonoscopy to rule out other disorders that may mimic diverticulitis, such as adenocarcinoma or Crohn disease.

Bibliography

Hemming J, Floch M. Features and management of colonic diverticular disease. Curr Gastroenterol Rep. 2010;12(5):399-407. [PMID: 20694839]

Item 14   Answer: B
Educational Objective: Diagnose diffuse esophageal spasm.

This patient has diffuse esophageal spasm. His symptoms (dysphagia to both solids and liquids) are suggestive of an esophageal dysmotility disorder. The differential diagnosis includes disorders like achalasia and diffuse esophageal spasm. Both may be associated with chest pain. Findings of a "corkscrew esophagus" (caused by multiple simultaneous contractions) on barium swallow are typical of diffuse esophageal spasm. Multiple simultaneous contractions are also seen on manometry. Treatment is usually initiated with calcium channel blockers.

On barium radiography, achalasia is characterized by esophageal dilatation with the classic "bird's beak" appearance distally and the to-and-fro movement of barium (loss of peristalsis).

The diagnosis of eosinophilic esophagitis is made endoscopically and is characterized by multiple rings or esophageal strictures and increased mucosal friability, none of which are present in this patient.

A Schatzki ring is characterized by an isolated ring at the gastroesophageal junction that causes intermittent dysphagia. It is usually not associated with chest pain.

KEY POINT

- Findings of a "corkscrew esophagus" (caused by multiple simultaneous contractions) on barium swallow are typical of diffuse esophageal spasm.

Bibliography

Lacy BE, Weiser K. Esophageal motility disorders: medical therapy. J Clin Gastroenterol. 2008;42(5):652-658. [PMID: 18364589]

Item 15   Answer: A

Educational Objective: Manage dyspepsia and heartburn with proton pump inhibitor therapy.

The best first-line treatment for this patient is acid suppression with a proton pump inhibitor (PPI). This patient is considered to have gastroesophageal reflux disease (GERD) with dyspeptic features. Community studies have shown that the majority of patients with dyspepsia who undergo upper endoscopy have normal findings. However, the most common finding in patients with abnormalities is esophagitis. Thus, there are likely a minority of patients with dyspepsia who actually have atypical symptoms of GERD. PPI therapy is thought to be superior to H$_2$ blockers for both dyspepsia and heartburn.

Sucralfate does not have a role in the treatment of GERD and has no advantage when compared with placebo for treatment of functional dyspepsia.

A test-and-treat strategy for *Helicobacter pylori* would be appropriate for patients with dyspeptic symptoms without heartburn or alarm symptoms, and who are from an area with a high prevalence of *H. pylori* infection (>20%). Because this patient also has heartburn, this approach is incorrect. There has recently been some controversy as to whether eradication of *H. pylori* in patients with dyspepsia may increase the risk of posteradication GERD, but a recent meta-analysis has not shown this to be true.

An upper endoscopy is incorrect, because this patient does not have any alarm features (onset after age 50 years; anemia; dysphagia; odynophagia; vomiting; weight loss; family history of upper gastrointestinal malignancy; personal history of peptic ulcer disease, gastric surgery, or gastrointestinal malignancy; and abdominal mass or lymphadenopathy on examination). The diagnostic yield of endoscopy in the absence of these findings is very low.

KEY POINT

- Patients with gastroesophageal reflux disease with dyspeptic features should be treated with proton pump inhibitor therapy.

Bibliography

Tack J, Talley NJ. Gastroduodenal disorders. Am J Gastroenterol. 2010;105(4):757-763. [PMID: 20372127]

Item 16   Answer: C

Educational Objective: Evaluate the source of gastrointestinal bleeding with upper endoscopy.

The most appropriate diagnostic test is upper endoscopy. In a patient with suspected upper gastrointestinal bleeding, the presenting symptoms can suggest the degree and volume of blood loss. The presence of melena (black, tarry stools) suggests an upper gastrointestinal tract source but

can be associated with loss of as little as 150 to 200 mL of blood. Hematemesis of bright red blood is associated with ongoing upper gastrointestinal bleeding, whereas hematochezia secondary to an upper source is suggestive of brisk ongoing bleeding of at least 1000 mL of blood. Presyncope and syncope may occur with hypovolemia secondary to bleeding. This patient has hematochezia, significant anemia, and hemodynamic instability. His regular use of ibuprofen for his arthritis increases the chance of an upper gastrointestinal source of bleeding. The absence of blood or coffee-ground material in the nasogastric tube aspirate does not rule out an upper gastrointestinal bleeding source; nasogastric tube placement can miss up to 15% of actively bleeding lesions, especially if no bile is noted on the aspirate. Therefore, placement of a nasogastric tube when there is a high suspicion of upper gastrointestinal bleeding is not very helpful and should not guide a decision on whether or not to perform upper endoscopy. A brisk upper gastrointestinal source of bleeding can cause hematochezia and can be life threatening if not acted upon early. If an upper gastrointestinal source is suspected, urgent upper endoscopy should be performed. If the upper endoscopy is unrevealing, a rapid lavage and colonoscopy is the next step, followed by a tagged red blood cell scan if no source is found.

Video capsule endoscopy is reserved for persistent occult (or overt) gastrointestinal bleeding without an identified upper or lower gastrointestinal source.

KEY POINT

- If an upper gastrointestinal source of bleeding is suspected in a patient with hematochezia, upper endoscopy is the most appropriate diagnostic procedure.

Bibliography

Davila RE, Rajan E, Adler DG, et al; Standards of Practice Committee. ASGE Guideline: the role of endoscopy in the patient with lower-GI bleeding. Gastrointest Endosc. 2005;62(5):656-660. [PMID: 16246674]

Item 17   Answer: B

Educational Objective: Treat new-onset Crohn disease.

The most appropriate treatment is an anti–tumor necrosis factor (anti-TNF) agent such as infliximab. This patient has moderately to severely active Crohn ileitis associated with weight loss and significant symptoms. The SONIC study showed better clinical outcomes when patients with recently diagnosed moderate to severe Crohn disease were treated aggressively with anti-TNF therapy with or without an immunomodulator such as azathioprine or 6-mercaptopurine. Anti-TNF therapy alone was superior to azathioprine monotherapy, and the combination of these two agents resulted in the highest rates of remission and mucosal healing. The decision to use thiopurine or anti-TNF monotherapy versus combination therapy is based on an individual patient's severity of symptoms and risk factors for developing complications of their disease balanced against the potential side effects of these treatments. An alternative to the immediate use of anti-TNF therapy is the simultaneous initiation of an immunomodulator and corticosteroids with a goal to taper off of corticosteroids within 3 months. If symptoms are not completely controlled after stopping the corticosteroids, then an anti-TNF agent could be added at that time.

Antibiotics are effective in the treatment of abscess and wound infections associated with inflammatory bowel diseases, but their efficacy as primary treatment for Crohn disease and ulcerative colitis is not well established.

Because Crohn disease is a transmural disease, the 5-aminosalicylic acid agents have not proved to be as efficacious as they are in ulcerative colitis. They are often used in the treatment of mild disease but are ineffective in moderate to severe disease.

Corticosteroid therapy on its own may help improve initial symptoms, but the majority of patients will also require maintenance therapy with an immunosuppressant medication to avoid becoming corticosteroid dependent. More aggressive use of anti-TNF agents with an immunomodulator results in higher rates of remission and mucosal healing compared with initial treatment with corticosteroids.

Surgical evaluation would be important if there was concern for perforation, abscess, obstruction, or medically refractory disease, but it would not be the appropriate next step in this patient's management.

> **KEY POINT**
> - The most effective treatment for patients with recently diagnosed moderately to severely active Crohn disease is anti–tumor necrosis factor therapy with or without an immunomodulator such as azathioprine or 6-mercaptopurine.

Bibliography
Colombel JF, Sandborn WJ, Reinisch W, et al; SONIC Study Group. Infliximab, azathioprine, or combination therapy for Crohn's disease. N Engl J Med. 2010;362(15):1383-1395. [PMID: 20393175]

Item 18   Answer: C
Educational Objective: Treat severe alcoholic hepatitis.

The most appropriate additional treatment is pentoxifylline. Assessment of the severity of acute alcoholic hepatitis is important because, in addition to abstinence from alcohol and nutritional therapy, pharmacologic therapy may be beneficial. Severe alcoholic hepatitis is defined by a Maddrey discriminant function (MDF) score of 32 or greater. For these patients, a significant increase in short-term survival has been demonstrated with systemic corticosteroids compared with placebo or supportive care (85% versus 65%). However, systemic corticosteroids such as prednisolone are contraindicated in the presence of gastrointestinal bleeding, kidney failure, or active infection such as spontaneous bacterial peritonitis, which is present in this patient. In addition to abstinence from alcohol and efforts to improve nutrition, patients with severe alcoholic hepatitis may benefit from pentoxifylline if corticosteroid therapy is contraindicated.

Drugs such as infliximab and etanercept have been studied for use in patients with moderate to severe alcoholic hepatitis, but both agents have been associated with increased mortality compared with systemic corticosteroid therapy or supportive care. Therefore, they are not currently recommended for use in clinical practice.

> **KEY POINT**
> - In addition to abstinence from alcohol and efforts to improve nutrition, patients with severe alcoholic hepatitis (Maddrey discriminant function score ≥32) may benefit from pentoxifylline if corticosteroid therapy is contraindicated.

Bibliography
O'Shea RS, Dasarathy S, McCullough AJ; Practice Guideline Committee of the American Association for the Study of Liver Diseases; Practice Parameters Committee of the American College of Gastroenterology. Alcoholic liver disease. Hepatology. 2010;51(1):307-328. [PMID: 20034030]

Item 19   Answer: D
Educational Objective: Manage a high-risk peptic ulcer after endoscopic treatment.

For this patient with a high-risk lesion on upper endoscopy, it is appropriate to observe him in the hospital for at least 72 hours. Peptic ulcer disease is graded based upon the endoscopic appearance according to the Forrest classification, which ranges from grade IA to III. High-risk lesions or stigmata are peptic ulcers with pulsatile bleeding (IA); oozing blood (IB); a nonbleeding visible vessel (IIA), also called a pigmented protuberance; or an adherent clot (IIB). High-risk stigmata constitute approximately one third to one half of bleeding peptic ulcers seen on upper endoscopy. The risk of rebleeding is highest for Forrest grade I and II lesions (20% to 50% without endoscopic treatment). The risk of rebleeding is lowest for peptic ulcers with a flat pigmented spot (IIC) or a clean ulcer base (III). This patient has a high-risk lesion that was treated endoscopically. The risk of rebleeding is highest in the first 72 hours following treatment. Furthermore, it takes about 72 hours for an endoscopically treated high-risk peptic ulcer to become a low-risk peptic ulcer. Therefore, hospitalization for at least 72 hours is the correct answer, and shorter intervals of 12, 24, and 48 hours are incorrect.

KEY POINT

- Patients with high-risk peptic ulcers (active bleeding or a visible vessel in an ulcer base) require hospitalization for at least 72 hours after endoscopic therapy.

Bibliography

Gralnek IM, Barkun AN, Bardou M. Management of acute bleeding from a peptic ulcer. N Engl J Med. 2008;359(9):928-937. [PMID: 18753649]

Item 20   Answer: A

Educational Objective: Manage obscure gastrointestinal bleeding associated with aortic stenosis.

The most appropriate treatment is aortic valve replacement. Heyde syndrome is the combination of bleeding angioectasias in patients with aortic stenosis. This association is attributed to mechanical disruption of von Willebrand multimers during nonlaminar flow through a critically narrowed aortic valve. The deficiency of von Willebrand factor is directly related to the severity of the aortic stenosis, as measured by the mean transvalvular gradient. The destruction of the von Willebrand multimers can lead to anemia and bleeding from mucosal angioectasias. The best treatment for this condition is operative aortic valve replacement. In most patients with aortic stenosis and angioectasias, bleeding improves after aortic valve replacement.

Localized endoscopic treatment of angioectasias would not be optimal because it is very difficult to control bleeding from multiple angioectasias endoscopically. In addition, the underlying cause of disease would not be addressed.

Gastric acidity has no impact on bleeding from mucosal angioectasias, and a proton pump inhibitor would do nothing to reduce the destruction of von Willebrand factor by a stenotic aortic valve. Therefore, therapy with a proton pump inhibitor would not be an effective therapy for this problem.

Although conjugated estrogens have been used for systemic treatment of refractory angioectasias and as treatment for congenital von Willebrand disease, they would not be first-line therapy in this situation. The best approach would be to improve this patient's cardiac status and reduce the risk of gastrointestinal bleeding with aortic valve replacement.

KEY POINT

- In patients with angioectasias associated with aortic stenosis (Heyde syndrome), operative aortic valve replacement is usually successful in preventing further gastrointestinal bleeding.

Bibliography

Gola W, Lelonek M. Clinical implication of gastrointestinal bleeding in degenerative aortic stenosis: an update. Cardiol J. 2010;17(4):330-334. [PMID: 20690087]

Item 21   Answer: C

Educational Objective: Manage endoscopic surveillance for ampullary adenocarcinoma in a patient with familial adenomatous polyposis.

The most appropriate surveillance procedure is upper endoscopy. Familial adenomatous polyposis (FAP) syndrome not only is associated with a very high risk of colon cancer, but there is a significantly increased risk for malignancy of the biliary ampulla. Therefore, in patients with a history of FAP, a strict long-term endoscopic surveillance protocol of the duodenum is indicated. Patients with ampullary cancer typically have a 5-year survival rate of 45%, which is a better prognosis than cancer of the common bile duct (cholangiocarcinoma). Treatment of ampullary cancer typically is with pancreaticoduodenectomy.

Although ampullary adenocarcinoma can result in biliary obstruction and bile duct dilatation, ultrasound is not indicated as a screening strategy for ampullary cancer because it lacks sufficient sensitivity. Centers that offer endoscopic ultrasound sometimes employ this procedure to diagnose and stage ampullary adenomas and adenocarcinomas.

The development of ampullary carcinoma can result in obstructive jaundice and elevated hepatic aminotransferases, but the goal of surveillance for ampullary adenocarcinoma is to diagnose impending adenocarcinoma before it results in abnormal liver chemistry tests; therefore, serial monitoring of aminotransferases for the purpose of surveillance is not indicated.

KEY POINT

- Ampullary adenocarcinoma is a rare cancer that occurs most often in hereditary polyposis syndromes such as familial adenomatous polyposis or Peutz-Jeghers syndrome; patients with these syndromes should undergo regular surveillance endoscopy.

Bibliography

Heinrich S, Clavien PA. Ampullary cancer. Curr Opin Gastroenterol. 2010;26(3):280-285. [PMID: 20168227]

Item 22   Answer: E

Educational Objective: Manage an asymptomatic pancreatic pseudocyst following acute pancreatitis.

This patient requires no further diagnostic testing or therapy. She has an asymptomatic pancreatic pseudocyst that developed as a result of her acute pancreatitis 8 weeks earlier. Pancreatic pseudocysts (cysts of pancreatic juice that have a fibrous, nonepithelial lining that occurs around the gland) are the most common complication of acute pancreatitis. The cysts generally take at least 4 weeks to form, often resolve spontaneously, and are asymptomatic; they may, however, cause pain or obstruction by pressing against other organs. Because this patient did not have a fluid collection at the time of initial presentation, the collection is a result of the pancreatitis and not a cause. She requires no further testing or therapy because she is currently asymptomatic, and it is very likely that the pseudocyst will resolve spontaneously.

Endoscopic ultrasonography (EUS) is used to evaluate cystic lesions of the pancreas. Several criteria can be used to identify a mucinous cystic lesion that requires removal, including the presence of septation, echogenic mucin, or a mass. In this patient, EUS is not necessary because there is no concern about a mucinous cystic lesion.

Magnetic resonance cholangiopancreatography (MRCP) is a noninvasive technique for imaging the bile ducts and the pancreatic duct. In a patient with a pancreatic pseudocyst, MRCP might be useful to determine if the cyst is connected to the biliary tree. However, in this patient, MRCP is not necessary because the CT scan does not document a connection between the lesion and the main pancreatic duct.

Percutaneous or surgical drainage is not indicated at this time because the patient is asymptomatic. Drainage would be advised only if the patient developed symptoms such as pain, fever, or anorexia.

KEY POINT

- Asymptomatic pancreatic pseudocysts following acute pancreatitis typically resolve spontaneously and do not require treatment.

Bibliography

Gumaste VV, Aron J. Pseudocyst management: endoscopic drainage and other emerging techniques. J Clin Gastroenterol. 2010;44(5):326-331. [PMID: 20142757]

Item 23 Answer: A

Educational Objective: Diagnose new-onset ascites.

The most appropriate diagnostic test to perform next is echocardiography. Clinical practice guidelines recommend that all patients with new-onset ascites undergo diagnostic paracentesis. The serum-ascites albumin gradient (SAAG) is an efficient and highly accurate test to categorize the cause of ascites. The SAAG is calculated by subtracting the ascitic fluid albumin concentration from the serum albumin concentration. If the SAAG is 1.1 g/dL (11 g/L) or greater, then portal hypertension is the cause of ascites in up to 97% of suspected cases. When the SAAG is less than 1.1 g/dL (11 g/L), the cause of ascites is very likely to be unrelated to portal hypertension. A SAAG value of 1.1 g/dL (11 g/L) or greater with a total protein level greater than 2.5 g/dL (25 g/L) indicates cardiac disease, such as right ventricular failure or constrictive pericarditis. This patient has an ascites fluid total protein greater than 2.5 g/dL (25 g/L) and a SAAG

value of 1.3 g/dL (13 g/L) without evidence of cirrhosis by laboratory and imaging studies. The next best test to order is an echocardiogram.

Hepatic venous pressure gradient measurement and transjugular liver biopsy would be indicated if the echocardiogram was negative. In up to 10% of patients, ascites may be caused by noncirrhotic or idiopathic portal hypertension, and a liver biopsy is usually required to confirm or exclude this diagnosis.

Serum CA-125 levels can be elevated in patients with ascites from any cause. However, regular testing is not recommended unless there is suspicion for an underlying gynecologic malignancy in female patients.

Nephrotic syndrome is uncommon in a patient with a SAAG of 1.1 g/dL (11 g/L) or greater; therefore, a 24-hour urine collection for total protein is not recommended. Additionally, a normal urinalysis would argue against nephrotic syndrome.

KEY POINTS

- A serum-ascites albumin gradient value of 1.1 g/dL (11 g/L) or greater with total ascites protein greater than 2.5 g/dL (25 g/L) is indicative of cardiac disease, such as heart failure or constrictive pericarditis.

Bibliography

Runyon BA; AASLD Practice Guidelines Committee. Management of adult patients with ascites due to cirrhosis: an update. Hepatology. 2009;49(6):2087-2107. [PMID: 19475696]

Item 24 Answer: A

Educational Objective: Diagnose hepatocellular carcinoma.

The most appropriate next diagnostic test is a contrast-enhanced abdominal CT. Hepatocellular carcinoma (HCC) usually develops in patients with advanced chronic liver disease; however, patients with hepatitis B may develop HCC in the absence of advanced liver disease. HCCs derive their blood supply through neovascularization, whereby the cancer develops a new blood supply fed through small branches of the hepatic artery. It is this characteristic vascular supply that helps identify potential cancers on contrast-enhanced imaging, such as triple-phase CT and gadolinium MRI. Although these modalities tend to be better at identifying HCC than ultrasonography, the current screening guidelines for HCC recommend ultrasonography every 6 to 12 months.

The diagnosis of HCC can be made using noninvasive radiologic criteria in patients with cirrhosis. Multiple studies have documented the high sensitivity and specificity of CT and MRI for HCC in patients with cirrhosis with lesions 2 cm or larger in diameter. If CT and MRI radiologic criteria are typical of HCC, a biopsy is not necessary and the lesion should be treated as HCC.

Repeat ultrasound at 6 months is within the recommended surveillance interval of 6 to 12 months for patients with no liver masses on a previous ultrasound; it is not the correct diagnostic test in a patient with a liver lesion that is between 1 and 2 cm.

Serum carcinoembryonic antigen (CEA) levels are not clinically useful in the diagnosis of HCC.

> **KEY POINT**
> - In patients with chronic hepatitis B infection or cirrhosis and a positive screening abdominal ultrasound for hepatocellular carcinoma, triple-phase CT or gadolinium MRI is the most appropriate next diagnostic test.

Bibliography

Forner A, Vilana R, Ayuso C, et al. Diagnosis of hepatic nodules 20 mm or smaller in cirrhosis: prospective validation of the noninvasive diagnostic criteria for hepatocellular carcinoma [erratum in Hepatology. 2008;47(2):769.]. Hepatology. 2008;47(1):97-104. [PMID: 18069697]

Item 25   Answer: C

Educational Objective: Manage gastroesophageal reflux disease that does not respond to an empiric trial of proton pump inhibitor therapy.

This patient should undergo endoscopy. Her symptoms suggest gastroesophageal reflux disease (GERD) and there has been no response to empiric trials of high-dose proton pump inhibitors (PPIs) for an adequate period of time (8-12 weeks). Further evaluation with endoscopy is required in patients with symptoms of weight loss, dysphagia, odynophagia, bleeding, or anemia and in men with long-standing symptoms (>5 years) or symptoms that are refractory to acid-suppression therapy. This patient has intermittent dysphagia for solid food, and her symptoms appear to be refractory to PPI therapy; she should therefore undergo endoscopy to explore complications and alternative diagnoses such as eosinophilic esophagitis, stricture, malignancy, and achalasia.

PPIs are much more effective in healing esophagitis (particularly severe esophagitis) compared with H_2 blockers. Adding H_2 blockers to maximal PPI therapy does not result in a meaningful increase in acid blockade. Therefore, an additional dose of an H_2 blocker is unlikely to produce relief for patients who continue to have heartburn after 6 weeks of treatment with a PPI.

Ambulatory esophageal pH monitoring is most commonly used to confirm GERD in patients with persistent symptoms despite maximal medical therapy and an unrevealing endoscopy study (no evidence of reflux-induced esophagitis or Barrett esophagus). However, in this patient with persistent symptoms and intermittent dysphagia, endoscopy is the most appropriate next diagnostic test to assess for evidence of reflux-induced complications. If endoscopy is unrevealing, ambulatory pH monitoring should be considered.

Persistent or recurrent symptoms despite maximal medical therapy for GERD are indications for antireflux surgery such as fundoplication. However, before consideration of antireflux surgery, this patient should undergo endoscopy (to confirm the presence of esophagitis and to eliminate the possibility of an alternative diagnosis) and possibly ambulatory pH recording (to document continued acid reflux while taking maximal doses of a PPI).

> **KEY POINT**
> - Patients with suspected gastroesophageal reflux disease whose symptoms do not respond to an empiric trial of proton pump inhibitor therapy should undergo endoscopy to assess for alternative diagnoses.

Bibliography

Kahrilas PJ, Shaheen NJ, Vaezi MF, et al; American Gastroenterological Association. American Gastroenterological Association Medical Position Statement on the management of gastroesophageal reflux disease. Gastroenterology. 2008;135(4):1383-1391. [PMID: 18789939]

Item 26   Answer: D

Educational Objective: Manage acute uncomplicated diverticulitis.

The most appropriate management strategy for this patient with acute diverticulitis is oral antibiotic therapy with metronidazole and ciprofloxacin. Diverticulitis results from obstruction at the diverticulum neck by fecal matter, leading to mucus and bacterial overgrowth. Left lower quadrant pain is the most common clinical manifestation, often accompanied by fever. Other symptoms may include nausea, vomiting, and anorexia. More than half of patients with diverticulitis have leukocytosis. Diverticulitis is diagnosed based on history and physical examination, but imaging is often helpful when the diagnosis is unclear or when complications are suspected. Oral antibiotic therapy with agents that are effective against anaerobes and gram-negative rods is a reasonable option for immunocompetent patients with isolated, uncomplicated acute diverticulitis who are able to tolerate oral intake.

Lower endoscopy should be avoided in the acute setting because air insufflation may increase the risk for perforation. After resolution, however, patients who have not had a recent colonoscopy should undergo the procedure to rule out malignancy.

CT-guided percutaneous drainage can be considered for patients who have a large (≥4 cm) peridiverticular abscess to hasten recovery and convert surgical intervention from emergent to elective, thereby increasing the likelihood of a one-stage procedure.

Hospitalization and intravenous antibiotics are generally reserved for patients with evidence of peritonitis, those with significant comorbidities, or those who cannot tolerate oral intake.

Surgical consultation can be considered for acute diverticulitis that is unresponsive to antibiotic therapy, complicated diverticulitis (associated with abscess, fistula, obstruction, peritonitis, or stricture), recurrent diverticulitis, or smoldering diverticulitis.

KEY POINT

- Oral antibiotic therapy with agents that are effective against anaerobes and gram-negative rods is a reasonable option for immunocompetent patients with isolated, uncomplicated acute diverticulitis who are able to tolerate oral intake.

Bibliography

Jacobs DO. Clinical practice. Diverticulitis. N Engl J Med. 2007;357(20):2057-2066. [PMID: 18003962]

Item 27   Answer: B
Educational Objective: Diagnose hepatopulmonary syndrome.

The most likely diagnosis is hepatopulmonary syndrome (HPS). HPS is characterized by arterial hypoxemia from pulmonary vascular dilatation in the setting of portal hypertension. Most cases of HPS are associated with cirrhosis, but noncirrhotic causes of portal hypertension can also exist. Dyspnea on exertion or rest is the hallmark symptom of HPS, and some patients have platypnea (worsening dyspnea when moving from the supine to upright position). Chest radiograph is frequently nonspecific, but hypoxemia on arterial blood gas testing is common, with a PO_2 of less than 70 mm Hg (9.3 kPa) (breathing ambient air) in symptomatic patients. Contrast-enhanced transthoracic echocardiography with agitated saline is the most efficient method to detect HPS. Microbubbles in the left atrium within three to six cardiac cycles indicate the presence of an abnormally dilated vascular bed. Currently, liver transplantation is the only successful treatment.

Although patients with cirrhosis commonly have reduced physical strength and function, deconditioning is not associated with hypoxemia.

This patient's symptoms, physical examination findings, electrocardiogram, and echocardiogram do not suggest ischemic heart disease, and myocardial blood flow is unaffected by HPS.

Portopulmonary hypertension (POPH) refers to the development of pulmonary arterial hypertension in patients with portal hypertension. Right heart catheterization is required to make a diagnosis of POPH. However, POPH is rarely associated with moderate to severe arterial hypoxemia, and this patient's estimated normal right ventricular systolic pressure on echocardiography makes this diagnosis unlikely.

KEY POINT

- Hepatopulmonary syndrome should be suspected in patients with dyspnea, cirrhosis, and a PO_2 less than 70 mm Hg (9.3 kPa).

Bibliography

Rodríguez-Roisin R, Krowka MJ. Hepatopulmonary syndrome—a liver-induced lung vascular disorder. N Engl J Med. 2008;358(22):2378-2387. [PMID: 18509123]

Item 28   Answer: C
Educational Objective: Manage a type I gastric carcinoid tumor.

The most appropriate management strategy is to repeat endoscopy in 6 months. Gastric carcinoid tumors are often identified as incidental findings during evaluation for nonspecific gastrointestinal symptoms and signs. Three gastric carcinoid subtypes are recognized. Type I gastric carcinoid tumors, which occur in the setting of chronic atrophic gastritis (as described in this patient), are the most common subtype and account for approximately 65% of these lesions. Type I gastric carcinoids can be single or multifocal tumors. Lesions less than or equal to 2 cm in diameter typically have an indolent natural history; metastases occur rarely and the 5-year survival rate exceeds 95%. For this patient, endoscopic removal of the nodules followed by regular endoscopic surveillance (every 6 to 12 months for at least 3 years) is the preferred management strategy.

Antrectomy can be performed to reduce G-cell mass and lower serum gastrin concentration, which is thought to stimulate the growth of type I gastric carcinoid tumors. However, this procedure is generally recommended for numerous (≥5) and/or larger tumors than those described in this patient.

Octreotide therapy is most often used for symptom control of flushing and diarrhea in patients with carcinoid syndrome, particularly for type II tumors that arise in the setting of Zollinger-Ellison syndrome or multiple endocrine neoplasia type 1. Octreotide inhibits the hormone secretion of a variety of tumors, including carcinoid, insulinomas, and gastrinomas, by binding to somatostatin receptors.

Total gastrectomy is usually reserved for patients with type III, or sporadic, gastric carcinoid tumors. Type III lesions (which account for approximately 20% of gastric carcinoids) are associated with normal serum gastrin levels and have a relatively unfavorable prognosis, justifying aggressive surgical intervention.

KEY POINT

- Patients with small (≤2 cm) type I gastric carcinoid tumors should be followed with endoscopic surveillance every 6 to 12 months for at least 3 years after initial endoscopic removal.

Bibliography
Hwang JH, Rulyak SD, Kimmey MB; American Gastroenterological Association Institute. American Gastroenterological Association Institute technical review on the management of gastric subepithelial masses. Gastroenterology. 2006;130(7):2217-2228. [PMID: 16762644]

Item 29   Answer: D

Educational Objective: Manage a flare of ulcerative colitis with testing for *Clostridium difficile.*

The most appropriate diagnostic test is stool studies for *Clostridium difficile. C. difficile* has become a common problem in patients with inflammatory bowel disease, and it has a high associated morbidity and mortality. Although the typical clinical scenario for *C. difficile* colitis is an older hospitalized or institutionalized patient with recent antibiotic use, outpatient *C. difficile* infection in young people without recent antibiotic use is being described more frequently. Rapid identification is essential to initiate proper antibiotic therapy and to minimize immune suppression during treatment. A classic associated finding is leukocytosis, which can be quite marked. The most serious associated complication is toxic megacolon, which can be assessed with plain abdominal films. Standard treatment is with oral metronidazole; however, oral vancomycin is becoming more frequently recommended for patients with inflammatory bowel disease owing to better clinical response and the patient's already compromised colon. Intravenous metronidazole or vancomycin retention enemas can also be effective if oral intake is not possible. Stool should also be tested for routine enteric pathogens and parasitic infections, because these can mimic or exacerbate a flare of ulcerative colitis and should be appropriately treated.

CT would be recommended in a patient with increasing abdominal pain and distention, rebound tenderness, and hypoactive bowel sounds to evaluate for toxic megacolon or perforation. However, these symptoms are not present in this patient.

Colonoscopy is an appropriate second-line evaluation if the patient does not respond to appropriate therapy for *C. difficile*, another infection, or a flare of ulcerative colitis. It is not a very good first-line evaluation owing to its invasive nature, the time required to receive biopsy results, and the frequent lack of pseudomembranes during a *C. difficile* infection in the setting of inflammatory bowel disease. Superimposed cytomegalovirus infection should be considered in patients on long-standing corticosteroid therapy, and in this case colonoscopy could be beneficial to obtain biopsy specimens.

Patients with inflammatory bowel disease have an increased rate of cholelithiasis, but this patient's symptoms are not consistent with gallstone disease and a right upper quadrant ultrasound would not be helpful.

> **KEY POINT**
> - *Clostridium difficile* has become a common problem in patients with inflammatory bowel disease; patients with disease flares should undergo stool studies for routine enteric pathogens, ova and parasites, and *C. difficile.*

Bibliography
Ananthakrishnan AN, Issa M, Binion DG. Clostridium difficile and inflammatory bowel disease. Gastroenterol Clin North Am. 2009;38(4):711-728. [PMID: 19913210]

Item 30   Answer: E

Educational Objective: Manage vaccination in an immunosuppressed patient with inflammatory bowel disease.

Varicella vaccination is contraindicated in this patient. Varicella vaccine is a live-virus vaccine; live-virus vaccines are generally contraindicated for immunocompromised patients. Other live vaccines include yellow fever, intranasal influenza, measles-mumps-rubella, bacillus Calmette-Guérin, and oral typhoid. Patients with inflammatory bowel disease (IBD) are considered immunosuppressed if they have significant protein-calorie malnutrition or are receiving corticosteroids (equivalent of prednisone 20 mg/d or higher); effective doses of 6-mercaptopurine, azathioprine, or methotrexate; anti–tumor necrosis factor (anti-TNF) therapy; or natalizumab. If patients have not had varicella infection or vaccination, they should ideally be vaccinated before initiating immunosuppression.

Reactivation of hepatitis B has been reported during treatment with anti-TNF therapy, so patients should be offered hepatitis B vaccination if they are not already immune. Women with IBD between the ages of 9 and 26 years should be offered vaccination for human papillomavirus (HPV), because immunosuppressed patients appear to be at higher risk for HPV infection and abnormal Pap smears. Pneumococcal vaccination is recommended for all immunosuppressed patients with a single revaccination if 5 or more years have passed since the first dose. Trivalent inactivated influenza vaccination is recommended annually. Pneumococcal, inactivated influenza, HPV, and hepatitis B vaccinations have been shown to be safe and effective in immunosuppressed patients with IBD.

> **KEY POINT**
> - Live-virus vaccines such as varicella are generally contraindicated for immunocompromised patients with inflammatory bowel disease.

Bibliography
Melmed GY. Vaccination strategies for patients with inflammatory bowel disease on immunomodulators and biologics. Inflamm Bowel Dis. 2009;15(9):1410-1416. [PMID: 19462435]

Item 31   Answer: A

Educational Objective: Manage colorectal cancer screening in a patient with a positive fecal occult blood test.

The most appropriate management strategy is colonoscopy now. When performed correctly, guaiac fecal occult blood testing (gFOBT) is an effective screening test for colorectal cancer; proper performance requires a dedicated clinician and a motivated patient. The test is inexpensive, noninvasive, generally acceptable to patients, and can detect bleeding anywhere in the colon. Occult blood is detected by either gFOBT or fecal immunochemical test (FIT). If performed correctly, gFOBT has been shown to reduce colorectal cancer–related mortality by up to 33%. This patient meets criteria for average-risk colorectal cancer screening, so high-sensitivity gFOBT is an acceptable choice for the initial assessment. Single-sample gFOBT of a stool specimen collected following digital rectal examination is not adequate for colorectal cancer screening, but this practice was reported by nearly 25% of internists in a recent national survey. For any positive screening gFOBT result, colonoscopy is the indicated diagnostic test.

Immediate retesting with gFOBT does not provide useful diagnostic information, because a negative result is insufficient to exclude clinically relevant pathology. Repeat fecal occult blood testing in 1 year, by either gFOBT or FIT, is a similarly insensitive follow-up strategy.

Flexible sigmoidoscopy permits structural evaluation of the distal colorectum but would miss a bleeding source located proximal to the splenic flexure. It is therefore not the most appropriate test for this patient.

> **KEY POINT**
> - Colonoscopy should be performed in any patient with a single positive screening guaiac fecal occult blood test.

Bibliography

Levin B, Lieberman DA, McFarland B, et al; American Cancer Society Colorectal Cancer Advisory Group; US Multi-Society Task Force; American College of Radiology Colon Cancer Committee. Screening and surveillance for the early detection of colorectal cancer and adenomatous polyps, 2008: a joint guideline from the American Cancer Society, the US Multi-Society Task Force on Colorectal Cancer, and the American College of Radiology. CA Cancer J Clin. 2008;58(3):130-160. [PMID: 18322143]

Item 32   Answer: B

Educational Objective: Treat chronic hepatitis C infection.

In this patient with chronic hepatitis C virus (HCV) infection and advanced fibrosis, antiviral therapy with peginterferon and ribavirin is indicated. Chronic HCV infection is often progressive and may result in cirrhosis and hepatocellular carcinoma. Effective therapy for active HCV infection can delay or prevent these complications. The best available therapy for chronic hepatitis C is the combination of peginterferon and ribavirin, as well as an NS3/4A protease inhibitor if the patient has genotype 1 hepatitis C. The ideal candidate for therapy is the patient with detectable virus, some indication of hepatic inflammation (elevated liver chemistry tests or inflammation on the biopsy), and no contraindication to therapy (decompensated liver disease [ascites, hepatic encephalopathy, jaundice], pregnancy, severe psychiatric disease, or severe preexisting cytopenias). The goal of therapy is to achieve a sustained virologic response, which is defined as undetectable HCV beyond 6 months after the end of treatment. Antiviral therapy for hepatitis C is associated with significant morbidity; therefore, careful consideration should be made regarding which patients are candidates for antiviral therapy.

Extrahepatic manifestations of chronic HCV infection include hematologic conditions (mixed cryoglobulinemia, lymphoma), skin diseases, autoimmune diseases (thyroiditis), and kidney disease. Some of these conditions may benefit from corticosteroid and antiviral therapy, but this patient has no indication for corticosteroid therapy. Corticosteroid therapy results in increased viral replication and should not be given to patients with hepatitis C unless there is a defined indication for corticosteroids.

Liver transplantation is performed when patients with hepatitis C develop decompensated cirrhosis. This patient has good liver function without signs or symptoms of liver decompensation; therefore, referral for liver transplantation is not warranted at this time.

Repeating the liver biopsy in 6 months will provide no additional information that will be helpful in this patient's management.

Serial monitoring of aminotransferases without consideration of antiviral therapy is not appropriate because this patient has advanced fibrosis. Although the overall risk of developing cirrhosis from hepatitis C is up to 25%, one of the risk factors for progression to cirrhosis is advanced fibrosis. Therefore, this patient's lack of established cirrhosis should not be reassuring that cirrhosis will not develop.

> **KEY POINT**
> - The best available therapy for chronic hepatitis C is the combination of peginterferon and ribavirin, with the addition of an NS3/4A protease inhibitor for genotype 1 hepatitis C virus.

Bibliography

Ghany MG, Strader DB, Thomas DL, Seeff LB; American Association for the Study of Liver Diseases. Diagnosis, management, and treatment of hepatitis C: an update. Hepatology. 2009;49(4):1335-1374. [PMID: 19330875]

Item 33   Answer: C

Educational Objective: Treat infectious esophagitis caused by cytomegalovirus.

This patient's findings are consistent with cytomegalovirus (CMV) infectious esophagitis, which should be treated

CONT.

with intravenous ganciclovir. The differential diagnosis of odynophagia (painful swallowing) includes infectious esophagitis (caused by CMV or herpes simplex virus [HSV]) or pill-induced esophagitis (associated with tetracycline, iron sulfate, bisphosphonates, potassium, NSAIDs, and quinidine). Infectious esophagitis caused by CMV is diagnosed by the finding of isolated, deep ulcers on endoscopy and typical CMV inclusion bodies on biopsy.

Acyclovir is used for treatment of HSV infection. Infectious esophagitis caused by HSV is characterized by multiple superficial ulcers on endoscopy and ground-glass nuclei with multinucleated giant cells on histology, with biopsies positive for HSV by polymerase chain reaction or viral culture. Because this patient has CMV infection, acyclovir is not appropriate.

Fluconazole is used in the treatment of *Candida* esophagitis, which usually presents with dysphagia and is characterized on endoscopy by curdy white deposits that adhere to the mucosa. These findings are not present in this patient.

Swallowed aerosolized fluticasone would not be used for the treatment of infectious esophagitis and would be more appropriate in patients with eosinophilic esophagitis.

> **KEY POINT**
> * Intravenous ganciclovir is the appropriate treatment for infectious esophagitis caused by cytomegalovirus.

Bibliography
Pace F, Pallotta S, Antinori S. Nongastroesophageal reflux disease-related infectious, inflammatory and injurious disorders of the esophagus. Curr Opin Gastroenterol. 2007;23(4):446-451. [PMID: 17545784]

Item 34   Answer: B
Educational Objective: Manage toxic megacolon in a patient with ulcerative colitis.

The most appropriate management is immediate surgery. Most patients with toxic megacolon related to ulcerative colitis have at least 1 week of bloody diarrhea symptoms that are unresponsive to medical therapy. On examination, patients have tachycardia, fever, hypotension, decreased or absent bowel sounds, and lower abdominal distention and tenderness, often with peritoneal signs. On plain film radiography, the transverse colon is most affected, with dilatation exceeding 6 cm. This patient has toxic megacolon based on the clinical history, examination findings, and imaging studies. Toxic megacolon is the most severe complication associated with ulcerative colitis; it is associated with a 40% mortality rate in patients undergoing emergency colectomy after a perforation has occurred (compared with 2% without a perforation). About 50% of patients with toxic megacolon may improve with medical therapy (bowel rest, intravenous corticosteroids, antibiotics, and fluids); however, progressive abdominal distention and tenderness with

hemodynamic instability are indications for immediate surgery.

A CT scan could further identify the extent of colonic dilatation and wall thickening as well as possible abscess formation or microperforation, but this would not change the required management of this patient.

Infliximab is a good treatment for flares of ulcerative colitis, but it is not an effective therapy for toxic megacolon and would not be indicated in this patient.

Intravenous hydrocortisone would be a good choice for an ulcerative colitis flare or possibly toxic megacolon, but only if the patient was clinically stable.

> **KEY POINT**
> * Toxic megacolon is the most severe complication associated with ulcerative colitis; progressive abdominal distention and tenderness with hemodynamic instability are indications for immediate surgery.

Bibliography
Gan SI, Beck PL. A new look at toxic megacolon: an update and review of incidence, etiology, pathogenesis, and management. Am J Gastroenterol. 2003;98(11):2363-2371. [PMID: 14638335]

Item 35   Answer: B
Educational Objective: Treat autoimmune pancreatitis.

This patient has autoimmune pancreatitis (AIP) and should receive corticosteroids. Painless jaundice in the context of a diffusely enlarged pancreas with a narrowed pancreatic duct is the hallmark of this condition. Endoscopic ultrasound and CT scan have ruled out a pancreatic mass and he has a normal CA 19-9 level, both of which help exclude pancreatic cancer as the cause of this patient's findings. Elevated serum concentrations of IgG4 are highly suggestive of AIP but may also occur in association with pancreatic cancer. A trial of corticosteroids is indicated to treat AIP. A biopsy typically would not be performed because it would put the patient at risk for complications such as pancreatitis and ductal injury. Patients typically are given a 3- to 4-month course of treatment and then undergo cross-sectional imaging to determine resolution of pancreatic inflammation. Failure to identify improvement on follow-up imaging is cause to consider an alternative diagnosis. For patients who do not respond to corticosteroids or who relapse when corticosteroids are withdrawn, a trial of immunomodulatory therapy (for example, azathioprine) is indicated.

Broad-spectrum antibiotics may be indicated in patients with ascending cholangitis or infected pancreatic necrosis, but the patient is not sufficiently ill or febrile to consider these diagnoses. Antibiotics are not effective in treating AIP.

Many but not all biliary strictures associated with AIP respond to corticosteroid therapy. For those that do respond, an invasive procedure like endoscopic retrograde biliary cholangiopancreatography with biliary stent placement can be avoided. The best course of action for this patient is a trial of corticosteroids with clinical follow-up and reimaging to assess for resolution of the biliary stricture.

A resection procedure such as pancreaticoduodenectomy is not indicated for treatment of this autoimmune inflammatory disease.

KEY POINT

- Corticosteroids are the cornerstone of treatment for autoimmune pancreatitis.

Bibliography

Sugumar A, Chari ST. Diagnosis and treatment of autoimmune pancreatitis. Curr Opin Gastroenterol. 2010;26(5):513-518. [PMID: 20693897]

Item 36   Answer: B

Educational Objective: Evaluate obscure gastrointestinal bleeding.

The next diagnostic step is to repeat the upper endoscopy. The sources of gastrointestinal bleeding may not be readily identified at the time of the initial endoscopy for various reasons. Lesions may bleed intermittently. Volume contraction or a low hemoglobin concentration may alter the appearance of a bleeding source. In a patient with recurrent bleeding, endoscopy and/or colonoscopy should be repeated. Endoscopy also allows for treatment of the lesion if one is found. Approximately 30% to 50% of lesions can be detected on repeat endoscopy. If a repeat study is nondiagnostic, the next step depends upon the severity and suspected location of blood loss.

Wireless capsule endoscopy, single-balloon enteroscopy, and intraoperative endoscopy are reserved for patients in whom repeat endoscopy does not identify a diagnosis. Intraoperative endoscopy is not usually required for diagnosis because wireless capsule endoscopy and double-balloon enteroscopy have improved the ability to diagnose and treat small-bowel sources of bleeding. Nevertheless, intraoperative endoscopy may be required for ongoing life-threatening bleeding without an identified source. Push single-balloon enteroscopy consists of direct insertion of an endoscope longer than the standard upper endoscope. Push enteroscopy is most often performed for the evaluation of lesions detected on capsule endoscopy that are within the reach of the enteroscope. In wireless capsule endoscopy, a patient swallows a video capsule that passes through the stomach and into the small intestine. The video capsule transmits images to a recording device worn by the patient. The images are downloaded onto a computer where they can be reviewed. Capsule endoscopy has been shown to detect sources of bleeding in 50% to 75% of patients and is considered the test of choice to follow standard endoscopy in patients with obscure bleeding.

KEY POINT

- Patients with suspected obscure gastrointestinal bleeding should undergo repeat colonoscopy and/or upper endoscopy (depending on the suspected site of bleeding), as approximately 30% to 50% of lesions can be detected using this approach.

Bibliography

ASGE Standards of Practice Committee, Fisher L, Lee Krinsky M, Anderson MA, et al. The role of endoscopy in the management of obscure GI bleeding. Gastrointest Endosc. 2010;72(3):471-479. [PMID: 20801285]

Item 37   Answer: A

Educational Objective: Manage high-grade dysplasia in a patient with Barrett esophagus.

This patient should receive endoscopic ablation. Options for the management of high-grade dysplasia in patients with Barrett esophagus (BE) include esophagectomy and endoscopic therapy (combined mucosal resection and ablation of residual BE). However, esophagectomy is associated with a mortality rate of 2% to 8% and a morbidity rate of 30% to 40% in the immediate postoperative period; this patient has a significant medical comorbid condition and is a suboptimal candidate for esophagectomy. Endoscopic therapy is a reasonable alternative because of its lower morbidity rates, especially in patients with high surgical risk. Results of endoscopic therapy have been shown in cohort studies to be comparable with those of esophagectomy.

Fundoplication is recommended when uncontrolled gastroesophageal reflux symptoms persist despite maximal medical therapy; however, this patient's symptoms are well controlled with proton pump inhibitor therapy. Fundoplication has not been shown to reduce the risk of BE progression to dysplasia or cancer compared with medical therapy.

Repeat endoscopic evaluation would be recommended at intervals of no longer than 3 months because of the substantial risk of progression of high-grade dysplasia to adenocarcinoma (6% per year) and risk of coexisting neoplasia (10%-12%). If subsequent surveillance detects progression to adenocarcinoma, endoscopic therapy can be utilized at that time.

KEY POINT

- Endoscopic mucosal resection and ablative therapy have been shown in cohort studies to be effective in the management of patients with Barrett esophagus and high-grade dysplasia.

Bibliography

Wang KK, Sampliner RE; Practice Parameters Committee of the American College of Gastroenterology. Updated guidelines 2008 for the diagnosis, surveillance and therapy of Barrett's esophagus. Am J Gastroenterol. 2008;103(3):788-797. [PMID: 18341497]

Item 38   Answer: D

Educational Objective: Manage dysplasia surveillance in a patient with inflammatory bowel disease.

The most appropriate management strategy is colonoscopy in 10 years. Patients with inflammatory bowel disease (IBD), including ulcerative colitis and Crohn disease, are at increased risk for colorectal cancer. Established risk factors are longer IBD duration, greater anatomic extent of disease, concomitant diagnosis of primary sclerosing cholangitis (PSC), and family history of sporadic colorectal cancer. In the absence of PSC or a family history of colorectal cancer, screening colonoscopy should be performed approximately 8 to 10 years after the onset of IBD symptoms to rule out neoplasia (dysplasia or cancer). During the screening colonoscopy, IBD extent should also be evaluated with biopsies for histologic assessment. Patients who have features of ulcerative proctitis only (confined to the rectum) have little, if any, increase in colorectal cancer risk compared with the general population. Average-risk colorectal cancer prevention guidelines can be followed in this setting, which makes colonoscopy in 10 years the most appropriate management strategy for this patient.

For patients with extensive ulcerative colitis (proximal to the splenic flexure) or left-sided ulcerative colitis (in the descending colon up to but not beyond the splenic flexure), surveillance colonoscopy should be performed 1 to 2 years after the initial colorectal cancer screening examination.

Surveillance intervals of 3 years and 5 years pertain to patients at increased risk for sporadic colorectal cancer, rather than those with IBD-associated dysplasia.

KEY POINT

- Patients who have ulcerative proctitis (confined to the rectum) have little, if any, increase in colorectal cancer risk compared with the general population and should undergo colonoscopy for colorectal cancer surveillance every 10 years.

Bibliography

Farraye FA, Odze RD, Eaden J, Itzkowitz SH. AGA technical review on the diagnosis and management of colorectal neoplasia in inflammatory bowel disease. Gastroenterology. 2010;138(2):746-774. [PMID: 20141809]

Item 39   Answer: D

Educational Objective: Manage short-bowel syndrome with acid suppression therapy.

This patient should receive a proton pump inhibitor (PPI) such as omeprazole. In patients who have undergone massive resection of the small intestine and are left with short-bowel syndrome, there is a tremendous surge of gastric acid in the postoperative period. The increased acid can inactivate pancreatic lipase, leading to significant diarrhea and possible ulceration in the remaining bowel. Therefore, all patients who have undergone significant bowel resection should receive acid suppression therapy in the postoperative period with a PPI.

Decreasing the lipids in this patient's diet, rather than in his parenteral nutrition, may provide some clinical improvement, because oral long-chain triglycerides may not be handled well in the state of bile-salt deficiency and may result in diarrhea.

Although increasing the loperamide may help with diarrhea control, it will not target the underlying pathophysiology of the increased acid production and will not prevent small-bowel ulceration. Overlooking that point may lead to adverse consequences for this patient if his acid hypersecretion is not controlled.

Because this patient has had resection of such a large amount of small intestine, there is likely significant disruption of the enterohepatic circulation of bile with resulting bile salt deficiency. Giving this patient cholestyramine will bind the remaining bile salts that are present and worsen the diarrhea.

Stopping this patient's oral intake may lead to some improvement of his diarrhea; however, it is often not recommended if the patient is otherwise tolerating oral intake, because continued oral intake will allow for bowel adaptation over time.

KEY POINT

- Patients who have undergone significant bowel resection should receive acid suppression therapy in the postoperative period owing to the acid hypersecretion that occurs.

Bibliography

Donohoe CL, Reynolds JV. Short bowel syndrome. Surgeon. 2010;8(5):270-279. [PMID: 20709285]

Item 40   Answer: B

Educational Objective: Manage colorectal cancer screening based on family history.

The most appropriate management strategy is colonoscopy at age 40 years. Family history may contribute to approximately 30% to 35% of all colorectal cancer cases. Several well-recognized hereditary cancer syndromes, such as familial adenomatous polyposis and hereditary nonpolyposis colorectal cancer syndrome are associated with markedly increased risks for colorectal neoplasia and other malignancies. This patient has a nonsyndromic family history, which is also associated with increased colorectal cancer risk. In patients with one first-degree relative with colorectal cancer diagnosed at any age, the lifetime risk of developing colorectal cancer is elevated two- to threefold compared with the general population. When two first-degree relatives are affected, the cumulative risk is increased by three- to fourfold. Younger age at colorectal neoplasia diagnosis appears to potentiate the family history–based risk association. The 2012 American College of Physicians Guidance Statement on colorectal cancer screening recommends initiation of screening in high-risk patients at age 40 years, or 10 years younger than the earliest colon cancer diagnosis in the family, whichever is earlier. Therefore, in this patient, screening beginning at age 40 years is appropriate.

In the absence of gastrointestinal symptoms, there is no role for performing colonoscopy now because colon cancer screening can be safely postponed until age 40 years.

KEY POINT

- Guidelines recommend initiating screening for colorectal cancer with colonoscopy at age 40 years (or 10 years younger than the earliest diagnosis in the family, whichever comes first) for patients without an identifiable hereditary cancer syndrome but with a first-degree relative with a diagnosis of colon cancer.

Bibliography
Qaseem A, Denberg TD, Hopkins RH Jr, et al; for the Clinical Guidelines Committee of the American College of Physicians. Screening for Colorectal Cancer: A Guidance Statement From the American College of Physicians. Ann Intern Med. 2012;156(5):378-386. [PMID: 22393133]

Item 41   Answer: D
Educational Objective: Manage constipation in a patient with alarm features.

This patient should undergo colonoscopy. She has had a relatively sudden change in bowel habits without a good explanation, and she has also recently noted blood in her stool; the presence of either of these alarm features would warrant a colonoscopy. Other features of constipation that would warrant colonoscopy include weight loss, family history of colorectal cancer, or age at onset greater than 50 years.

Fiber supplementation is often the initial management for most patients with uncomplicated constipation without alarm features; it would not be recommended in this patient without further evaluation for her alarm symptoms.

Although this patient has a history of hypothyroidism, she is taking thyroid replacement therapy and has a thyroid-stimulating hormone level that is within normal limits, so it is unlikely that her constipation could be explained by thyroid dysfunction. Additionally, thyroid disease cannot account for the blood in her stool.

Anorectal manometry would be recommended for a patient with suspected pelvic floor dysfunction; however, this patient does not have any clinical features (digitation with defecation and sense of blockage in the anorectal region) or examination features (paradoxical contraction of the puborectalis or external anal sphincter) of pelvic floor dysfunction.

Because there was visible blood on the examination glove, performing a stool guaiac test would not add any information. Additionally, a negative stool guaiac test could provide false reassurance.

KEY POINT

- Patients with constipation who have alarm features (age of onset greater than 50 years, weight loss, rectal bleeding, sudden change in bowel habits, family history of colorectal cancer) should undergo colonoscopy.

Bibliography
Spiller RC, Thompson WG. Bowel disorders. Am J Gastroenterol. 2010;105(4):775-785. [PMID: 20372130]

Item 42   Answer: D
Educational Objective: Manage asymptomatic gallstones.

The most appropriate management is observation. Asymptomatic cholelithiasis is increasingly diagnosed mainly because of widespread use of abdominal ultrasonography for the evaluation of unrelated or vague abdominal symptoms. Approximately 10% to 20% of the population in most Western countries have gallstones, and among them 50% to 70% are asymptomatic at the time of diagnosis. Asymptomatic gallstone disease has a benign natural course, with the progression of asymptomatic to symptomatic disease ranging from 10% to 25%. The majority of patients rarely develop gallstone-related complications without first having at least one episode of biliary pain ("colic"). In the past, open cholecystectomy was generally performed for symptomatic disease. Despite the widespread availability of laparoscopic cholecystectomy, most experts agree that nearly all patients with asymptomatic gallstones should be managed with observation (expectant management). Selective cholecystectomy may be performed in patients undergoing surgical procedures that may predispose them to symptomatic biliary disease (such as bariatric surgery).

Given the absence of symptoms and absence of liver abnormalities on ultrasound, abdominal CT imaging is not indicated.

Bile-binding agents such as ursodeoxycholic acid are unlikely to be extremely effective in dissolving stones but may help prevent development of additional ones. However, because most patients with asymptomatic gallstones remain asymptomatic, there is no need to treat this patient. Additionally, treatment is usually reserved for patients with mildly symptomatic small cholesterol stones and good gallbladder function who are poor surgical candidates owing to comorbidities.

KEY POINT

- Asymptomatic gallstone disease has a benign natural course and can be managed with observation.

Bibliography
Sakorafas GH, Milingos D, Peros G. Asymptomatic cholelithiasis: is cholecystectomy really needed? A critical reappraisal 15 years after the introduction of laparoscopic cholecystectomy. Dig Dis Sci. 2007;52(5):1313-1325. [PMID: 17390223]

Item 43   Answer: D

Educational Objective: Treat a patient at risk for NSAID-induced gastrointestinal injury with proton pump inhibitor therapy.

The appropriate treatment is to initiate a proton pump inhibitor (PPI) such as omeprazole. Patients at highest risk for NSAID-related gastrointestinal toxicity are those with a history of complicated peptic ulcer disease (designated by bleeding or perforation) or with more than two of the following moderate risk factors: age greater than 65 years; high-dose NSAID therapy; concomitant use of aspirin, anticoagulants, or corticosteroids; or history of an uncomplicated peptic ulcer. Patients with one or two moderate risk factors are considered to have a moderate risk for NSAID-induced gastrointestinal toxicity; a low-risk patient has none of these risk factors. This patient has two risk factors (high-dose naproxen and aspirin use) and is therefore at moderate risk. He is also at high risk for cardiovascular events, as defined by his history of a myocardial infarction and need for aspirin. Therefore, if he continues to take naproxen, a gastroprotective strategy using a PPI is recommended. Another appropriate option would be misoprostol. Standard-dose misoprostol (200 micrograms four times daily) is very effective for prevention of NSAID-induced ulcers but is not well tolerated owing to the side effects of cramping and diarrhea. Lower doses of misoprostol (400-600 micrograms/d) are another option, because they are as effective as PPI therapy for prevention of NSAID-induced ulcers and have a side effect profile similar to placebo.

Enteric-coated aspirin is not effective in preventing NSAID-induced peptic ulcer disease.

Substitution of celecoxib for naproxen would be an incorrect choice because the patient wishes to continue taking naproxen. In addition, cyclooxygenase-2 (COX-2) inhibitors such as celecoxib are less likely to cause gastric ulcers compared with traditional NSAIDs, but this effect is negated when COX-2 inhibitors are taken with low-dose aspirin.

This patient had a previous myocardial infarction and requires ongoing daily aspirin for secondary prevention. Therefore, discontinuation of aspirin is not an appropriate option for this patient.

KEY POINT

- Standard-dose proton pump inhibitors are effective, have limited side effects, and are first-line therapy for prophylaxis of NSAID-related ulcers.

Bibliography

Lanza FL, Chan FK, Quigley EM; Practice Parameters Committee of the American College of Gastroenterology. Guidelines for prevention of NSAID-related ulcer complications. Am J Gastroenterol. 2009;104(3):728-738. [PMID: 19240698]

Item 44   Answer: B

Educational Objective: Treat constipation-predominant irritable bowel syndrome that is refractory to therapy with fiber and standard laxatives.

The correct choice for treatment of constipation in this patient with constipation-predominant irritable bowel syndrome (IBS-C) is lubiprostone. Lubiprostone is a C_2 chloride channel activator that causes secretion of salt water into the intestine and may improve colonic motility. It has been approved by the FDA for treatment of IBS-C in women at a dose of 8 micrograms twice daily and in all adults (>18 years) for idiopathic chronic constipation at a dose of 24 micrograms twice daily. Because this medication is pregnancy category C, a negative pregnancy test should be obtained in women of reproductive age before initiating lubiprostone. Lubiprostone is not a first-line agent in IBS-C, but it is appropriate for patients whose symptoms persist despite the use of fiber and standard laxatives.

Hyoscyamine is an oral medication used in IBS for its antispasmodic properties; it blocks the action of acetylcholine at parasympathetic sites in gastrointestinal smooth muscle. Although hyoscyamine and similar antispasmodic agents can be used to reduce abdominal discomfort in IBS, evidence to support their efficacy is weak. Furthermore, in patients with IBS-C, the anticholinergic effect can theoretically worsen constipation. For this reason, hyoscyamine would not be a good option for this patient.

Metoclopramide is a prokinetic agent that can be used in the treatment of gastroparesis; however, it does not have a role in the treatment of IBS.

Tricyclic antidepressants are used for symptomatic treatment of abdominal pain in IBS and have been found to be superior to placebo. However, because of their anticholinergic effects, this class of medication can exacerbate constipation and thus would not be the optimal choice for this patient.

KEY POINT

- Lubiprostone is not a first-line agent in constipation-predominant irritable bowel syndrome, but it is appropriate for patients whose symptoms persist despite the use of fiber and standard laxatives.

Bibliography

Drossman DA, Chey WD, Johanson JF, et al. Clinical trial: lubiprostone in patients with constipation-associated irritable bowel syndrome—results of two randomized, placebo-controlled studies. Aliment Pharmacol Ther. 2009;29(3):329-341. [PMID: 19006537]

Item 45   Answer: C

Educational Objective: Manage postpolypectomy surveillance.

The most appropriate management strategy is colonoscopy in 3 years. For patients with colorectal adenomas, surveillance colonoscopy is recommended to reduce the risk of subsequent colorectal cancer arising from metachronous neoplasia (or previously undetected lesions). Consensus guidelines have been established to decrease the cost, risk, and overuse of surveillance colonoscopy. Postpolypectomy surveillance recommendations are based largely on the size, number, and microscopic features of identified adenomas, although medical history and family history must also be factored into the decision-making process. Patients found to have any adenoma greater than 1 cm in diameter or with villous histology should undergo their next surveillance colonoscopy in 3 years, assuming complete resection was performed at the index polypectomy. Other indications for a 3-year surveillance interval include multiple (3-10) or histologically advanced (high-grade dysplasia) adenomas.

Repeat colonoscopy in 2 to 6 months should be advised for patients with sessile adenomas that are removed in piecemeal fashion. This is done to ensure complete removal.

Follow-up colonoscopy in 1 year may be appropriate when family history data meet criteria for a hereditary colorectal cancer syndrome or when other risk factors such as inflammatory bowel disease are present.

A surveillance interval ranging from 5 to 10 years can be considered for patients with one or two small (<1-cm) tubular adenomas with low-grade dysplasia.

KEY POINT

- Patients with high-risk adenomas (≥3 adenomas, ≥1 cm, villous morphology, or high-grade dysplasia) should undergo their next surveillance colonoscopy in 3 years, assuming complete inspection and resection was performed at the index colonoscopy.

Bibliography

Winawer SJ, Zauber AG, Fletcher RH, et al. Guidelines for colonoscopy surveillance after polypectomy: a consensus update by the US Multi-Society Task Force on Colorectal Cancer and the American Cancer Society. CA Cancer J Clin. 2006;56(3):143-159. [PMID: 16737947]

Item 46   Answer: A

Educational Objective: Diagnose Budd-Chiari syndrome.

The most likely diagnosis is Budd-Chiari syndrome (BCS). This patient's clinical presentation is consistent with hepatic venous thrombosis or BCS. In this case, the most likely underlying risk factor for BCS is this patient's polycythemia vera. Thrombotic disorders (erythromelalgia, transient ischemic attacks, myocardial infarction or stroke, deep venous thrombosis, and Budd-Chiari syndrome) are the most serious presenting signs of the disease and occur in about two thirds of patients with polycythemia vera. The most common symptoms of BCS are abdominal pain, hepatomegaly, and ascites. BCS is diagnosed by the finding of hepatic venous outflow tract obstruction on cross-sectional imaging. Based on widespread availability, it is recommended that Doppler ultrasonography be used initially to make the diagnosis of BCS. Initial treatment of BCS includes anticoagulation therapy for all patients regardless of whether an underlying prothrombotic disorder is discovered. Oral diuretics may be used for control of ascites. The treatment of underlying myeloproliferative diseases is also encouraged, and oral contraceptives are generally contraindicated in patients with BCS. Hepatic vein or inferior vena cava angioplasty with or without stenting is also recommended in patients with symptomatic BCS that is refractory to anticoagulation. Hepatic venography is needed for establishing a diagnosis of BCS in difficult cases or when precise delineation of venous stenoses is required. When disease is not fully controlled with medical management, the next step should be insertion of a transjugular intrahepatic portosystemic shunt (TIPS). For disease that is unresponsive to TIPS, liver transplantation is the only remaining therapeutic option.

Although the clinical presentation of constrictive pericarditis may be very similar to BCS, the absence of hepatic vein obstruction coupled with evidence of thickening of the pericardium by CT or MRI is suggestive of a diagnosis of constrictive pericarditis.

Fulminant hepatic failure may be associated with tender hepatomegaly and ascites, but this patient's liver chemistry tests are only mildly elevated and the INR is normal, excluding this diagnosis.

Splenic vein thrombosis may be associated with isolated gastric varices but not tender hepatomegaly or ascites. Furthermore, Doppler studies confirm absent blood flow in the hepatic veins, but the portal vein is patent.

KEY POINT

- Budd-Chiari syndrome is diagnosed by the finding of hepatic venous outflow tract obstruction on cross-sectional imaging; ultrasonography is recommended as the diagnostic test of choice based on its widespread availability.

Bibliography

Darwish Murad S, Plessier A, Hernandez-Guerra M, et al; EN-Vie (European Network for Vascular Disorders of the Liver). Etiology, management, and outcome of the Budd-Chiari syndrome. Ann Intern Med. 2009;151(3):167-175. [PMID: 19652186]

Item 47   Answer: D

Educational Objective: Diagnose an anastomotic leak that is a complication of bariatric surgery.

The most appropriate next step is an upper gastrointestinal oral contrast radiograph. This patient has clinical features suggestive of an anastomotic leak, and an upper gastrointestinal radiograph with water-soluble oral contrast will be helpful to document the presence and location of the

CONT.

leak and guide surgical management. The clinical presentation of an anastomotic leak can be subtle and may include fever, abdominal pain, or tachycardia. Although her laboratory studies and plain radiograph of the abdomen are unremarkable, she does have unexplained tachycardia, which may be the only clinical feature and should not be overlooked. Sustained tachycardia with a heart rate greater than 120/min is an indicator of an anastomotic leak after bariatric surgery in the absence of gastrointestinal bleeding. CT of the abdomen could also be used to identify an anastomotic leak in place of a water-soluble oral contrast radiograph.

CT angiography of the chest may be used to evaluate for a pulmonary embolism in the postoperative period, but the presence of abdominal pain and absence of chest pain, cough, dyspnea, or tachypnea make this diagnosis much less likely than a leak.

Although this patient would require surgical intervention if an anastomotic leak were found, emergent surgical exploration would not be required at this time because the patient is hemodynamically stable. This allows time for diagnostic testing, which will better direct the appropriate surgical approach. However, even if imaging of the abdomen does not reveal an anastomotic leak or other postoperative complication (such as an internal hernia) and the index of suspicion remains high, exploratory surgery should still be considered because the morbidity and mortality associated with missing these diagnoses are greater than that of a negative surgical exploration.

An upper endoscopy would be contraindicated if a perforation or anastomotic leak is being considered.

KEY POINT

- Sustained tachycardia with a heart rate greater than 120/min can be an indicator of an anastomotic leak after bariatric surgery in the absence of gastrointestinal bleeding.

Bibliography

Bellorin O, Abdemur A, Sucandy I, Szomstein S, Rosenthal RJ. Understanding the significance, reasons and patterns of abnormal vital signs after gastric bypass for morbid obesity. Obes Surg. 2011;21(6):707-713. [PMID: 20582574]

Item 48   Answer: A
Educational Objective: Diagnose an insulinoma with endoscopic ultrasound.

The patient has fasting hypoglycemia and an inappropriately elevated insulin level and should undergo endoscopic ultrasound (EUS). An insulin-secreting islet cell tumor, or insulinoma, is the most serious diagnosis in a patient with fasting hypoglycemia. The biochemical diagnosis of insulinoma is made when the fasting plasma glucose level falls below 45 mg/dL (2.5 mmol/L) and there are accompanying hypoglycemic symptoms and inappropriate hyperinsulinemia (insulin level >5-6 microunits/mL

[36-43 pmol/L]) after exogenous factors have been eliminated. After the diagnosis of insulinoma is confirmed biochemically, imaging studies of the pancreas are required, beginning with a CT of the abdomen. Although these lesions are missed on CT scans if they are smaller than 2 cm, this modality is essential to exclude larger lesions or those already metastatic to the liver. If there are no significant findings, further evaluation may include EUS of the pancreas, hepatic venous sampling with arterial calcium stimulation, or pancreatic arteriography. Of these tests, the least invasive is EUS, which has an approximately 90% detection rate for insulinomas.

MRI would not offer any diagnostic benefit over CT in this situation.

When preoperative localization has been unsuccessful, operative exploration by an experienced pancreatic surgeon should proceed, with the lesion detected by palpation or on intraoperative ultrasound. In patients who are not surgical candidates, medical therapy with diazoxide, octreotide, or corticosteroids (or some combination) can be attempted.

Pentetreotide scintigraphy (octreotide scanning) is not an effective diagnostic tool because insulinomas do not produce adequate numbers of somatostatin receptors to make scintigraphy accurate.

KEY POINT

- Endoscopic ultrasound has an approximately 90% detection rate for insulinomas.

Bibliography

Mathur A, Gorden P, Libutti SK. Insulinoma. Surg Clin North Am. 2009;89(5):1105-1121. [PMID: 19836487]

Item 49   Answer: B
Educational Objective: Manage a complex liver cyst with surgical resection.

The most appropriate management is surgical resection. Cystic lesions of the liver are among the most common incidental findings on abdominal imaging. The majority of cystic lesions are simple liver cysts that are benign and typically asymptomatic. However, complex cysts with septations or wall irregularity may represent cystic neoplasms such as hepatic cystadenomas or hepatic cystadenocarcinomas. Hepatic cystadenomas constitute less than 5% of all cystic lesions of the liver but have malignant potential. In this patient with abdominal discomfort and a complex cyst (septations and wall irregularity), the best available therapy is complete cyst resection.

Cyst aspiration can yield findings such as elevated cyst fluid levels of tumor markers such as CA 19-9 or carcinoembryonic antigen; however, the role of these findings in differentiating between simple hepatic cysts and cystadenomas is not defined. Treatment options such as cyst aspiration and partial resection do not eliminate the risk of malignant transformation.

Observation with repeat ultrasound is not appropriate for this patient because repeating abdominal imaging in 6 months will not yield data that will alter the need for operative resection of the hepatic lesion.

Reassurance is not appropriate because the malignant potential of a possible complex hepatic cyst should be taken seriously in a patient who is otherwise healthy and is a candidate for surgery.

KEY POINT

- Complex hepatic cysts (with septations or wall irregularity) carry a risk of malignant transformation and should be resected.

Bibliography

Choi HK, Lee JK, Lee KH, et al. Differential diagnosis for intrahepatic biliary cystadenoma and hepatic simple cyst: significance of cystic fluid analysis and radiologic findings. J Clin Gastroenterol. 2010;44(4):289-293. [PMID: 19770676]

Item 50   Answer: A

Educational Objective: Manage esophageal adenocarcinoma.

The most appropriate initial management of this patient is staging of the cancer with CT/PET and endoscopic ultrasonography. Squamous cell carcinoma often arises in the upper portions of the esophagus, whereas adenocarcinoma arises more distally; however, the presentation of the two variants is similar. Dysphagia for solids is the most common presenting symptom (70%) of esophageal cancer; odynophagia is less common and often is associated with ulceration of the lesion. Chest pain, anorexia, weight loss, gastrointestinal bleeding, and regurgitation are other presenting symptoms. The diagnosis is often made with direct endoscopic visualization and biopsy, as it was in this patient. Staging of the tumor with CT and PET scans (to detect distant metastatic disease) and endoscopic ultrasound (for tumor and lymph node staging) is important for guiding management. Accurate staging may incorporate cross-sectional imaging, endoscopic ultrasonography, PET, laparoscopy, and video-assisted thoracoscopy. The choice of these modalities depends on their availability and the expertise of the team caring for the patient. In patients discovered to have metastatic regional lymphadenopathy, neoadjuvant chemoradiotherapy followed by surgery has been shown to confer a modest survival benefit compared with surgery alone. Proceeding to surgery directly would not allow administration of neoadjuvant therapy if indicated.

In the absence of substantial ongoing weight loss and inability to sustain caloric intake, feeding tube placement would be premature. Loss of more than 10% of body weight, evidence of malnutrition on examination and laboratory evaluation, and inability to maintain caloric intake would be indications for alternative enteral nutrition with a nasojejunal tube or a percutaneous endoscopic gastrostomy tube.

Radiation therapy is a treatment option for patients with localized cancer who are poor surgical candidates or patients with clearly unresectable carcinoma. Radiation therapy is also used as palliative therapy in patients with severe pain due to metastases that is not controlled adequately with pain medications. None of these indications are currently applicable to this patient.

KEY POINT

- Following the diagnosis of esophageal adenocarcinoma, staging with CT/PET and endoscopic ultrasonography is important for guiding management.

Bibliography

Wang KK, Wongkeesong M, Buttar NS. American Gastroenterological Association technical review on the role of the gastroenterologist in the management of esophageal carcinoma. Gastroenterology. 2005;128(5):1471-1505. [PMID: 15887129]

Item 51   Answer: D

Educational Objective: Diagnose lactose malabsorption.

This patient likely has lactose malabsorption that developed as a result of her recent food-borne illness or gastroenteritis. This is not uncommon and is often self-limited. The patient has a stool osmotic gap of 170 mOsm/kg (170 mmol/kg). The stool osmotic gap calculation is:

$$290 - 2 \times [\text{stool sodium} + \text{stool potassium}]$$

A gap greater than 100 mOsm/kg (100 mmol/kg) indicates an osmotic cause of diarrhea. Lactose malabsorption is the most common cause of an osmotic gap in the stool. Reducing this patient's lactose intake to no more than 12 grams with each meal (equivalent to one glass of milk) will often result in symptom improvement. Lactose intake can slowly be increased as more time elapses after her acute illness.

Even though some patients may have an increase in stool frequency after cholecystectomy, her surgery was remote enough that it would not cause her current symptoms. In addition, it would not explain her osmotic gap, as bile-salt–induced diarrhea tends to cause a secretory diarrhea.

Both microscopic colitis and eosinophilic gastroenteritis cause diarrhea. However, microscopic colitis would present with a secretory diarrhea alone, and an osmotic gap should not be seen unless the patient had another concomitant condition like celiac disease. Eosinophilic gastroenteritis could cause both a secretory and osmotic diarrhea, but this diagnosis would be much less common compared with lactose malabsorption.

Features of irritable bowel syndrome (IBS) can develop after a bout of gastroenteritis. Although this patient may go on to have persistent symptoms due to IBS, an osmotic gap is not consistent with the diagnosis of IBS.

Bibliography

Shaukat A, Levitt MD, Taylor BC, et al. Systematic review: effective management strategies for lactose intolerance. Ann Intern Med. 2010;152(12):797-803. [PMID: 20404262]

Item 52   Answer: B
Educational Objective: Treat refractory gastroesophageal reflux disease with antireflux surgery.

This patient should be offered fundoplication. He continues to have persistent gastroesophageal reflux disease (GERD) manifested by esophagitis despite high-dose proton pump inhibitor (PPI) therapy. Patients with persistent symptoms despite PPI therapy should be assessed for adherence to medication regimens and correct administration (30 to 45 minutes before a meal). Patients should also be assessed for other symptoms that may indicate alternative diagnoses such as eosinophilic esophagitis, heart disease, or achalasia. The next step in evaluation should be endoscopy; if endoscopy is unrevealing, 24-hour ambulatory pH testing should be performed. In this patient, esophagitis on endoscopy indicates persistent uncontrolled GERD despite maximal medical therapy. The notable endoscopic findings make it unnecessary to perform an ambulatory reflux study. The best treatment is surgical fundoplication, which has been shown to be effective in controlling excessive distal esophageal acid exposure. The best outcomes are observed in patients whose symptoms respond to medical therapy and who have few comorbidities. Relief of symptoms with surgery is significant but not always long-lasting; more than half of patients who have surgery for GERD resume regular PPI therapy 10 to 15 years after surgery. Side effects of surgery, which include dysphagia, gas-bloat syndrome, and diarrhea, occur in approximately 25% of patients.

Increasing the dose of esomeprazole or adding sucralfate would not lead to long-term healing of esophagitis and symptom relief in this 50-year-old patient, given that doses of greater than 80 mg/d of esomeprazole do not lead to appreciably increasing acid suppression. Sucralfate is prescribed for short-term use as an adjunct to PPI therapy.

Endoscopic antireflux procedures such as radiofrequency ablation have not been shown to achieve significant long-term reduction in esophageal acid exposure and remain experimental at this time.

KEY POINT
- Fundoplication is a therapeutic option for confirmed gastroesophageal reflux disease that is refractory to proton pump inhibitor therapy.

Bibliography

Kahrilas PJ, Shaheen NJ, Vaezi MF, et al; American Gastroenterological Association. American Gastroenterological Association Medical Position Statement on the management of gastroesophageal reflux disease. Gastroenterology. 2008;135(4):1383-1391. [PMID: 18789939]

Item 53   Answer: C
Educational Objective: Treat fistulizing Crohn disease.

The most appropriate management is examination under anesthesia (EUA) and then initiation of infliximab. Fistulas are abnormal connections between the bowel and adjacent organs. Abscesses may form, and the fistula acts as a natural drainage mechanism, causing pus to emerge from the fistula. The fistula becomes symptomatic with drainage of fecal material around the anus, seepage of bowel contents through the skin, passage of feces through the vagina, and pneumaturia or recurrent urinary tract infections. EUA is performed to drain abscesses, and noncutting setons (drains that are threaded into the orifice of a fistula, through the fistula tract, and into the rectum) are placed through fistulas to allow for continued drainage and proper healing. Because this patient has active inflammatory bowel disease and is at risk for persistent luminal and perianal disease, starting a therapy known to be effective for fistulizing Crohn disease is warranted. Infliximab is FDA approved and is the most effective medical treatment for fistulizing Crohn disease. Before initiating infliximab therapy, however, perianal abscesses should be drained, and outcomes are improved by placement of a noncutting seton.

Ciprofloxacin or metronidazole can be used to treat simple fistulas (superficial, single opening, no abscess, no evidence of rectovaginal fistula, no anorectal stricture, no rectal inflammation), but these would not be appropriate on their own in this patient with a complex fistula (two openings and an associated abscess). Although antibiotics are commonly used in the treatment of fistulizing Crohn disease, there is no evidence from randomized trials that they are effective.

Corticosteroids have no effect on the healing rate of simple or complex fistulas and cannot be recommended.

KEY POINT
- Patients with a complex fistula resulting from perianal Crohn disease should receive surgical therapy (for drainage of abscesses and seton placement) and infliximab.

Bibliography

Regueiro M, Mardini H. Treatment of perianal fistulizing Crohn's disease with infliximab alone or as an adjunct to exam under anesthesia with seton placement. Inflamm Bowel Dis. 2003;9(2):98-103. [PMID: 12769443]

Item 54   Answer: B
Educational Objective: Evaluate the prognosis of a patient with acute pancreatitis.

The blood urea nitrogen (BUN) level most accurately reflects the prognosis. This patient has acute pancreatitis

CONT.

and has developed evidence of the systemic inflammatory response syndrome (temperature >38.0 °C [100.4 °F] or <36.0 °C [96.8 °F], leukocyte count >12,000/microliter [12×10^9/L] or <4000/microliter [4.0×10^9/L], respiration rate >20/min, and heart rate >90/min). In an observational study of patients admitted to 69 different hospitals with acute pancreatitis, serial BUN measurements were the most reliable routine laboratory test to predict mortality. For every 5 mg/dL (1.8 mmol/L) increase in BUN during the first 24 hours, the age- and gender-adjusted odds ratio for mortality increased by 2.2 (95% confidence limits, 1.8-2.7). Change in hemoglobin concentrations did not correlate with disease severity.

Amylase and lipase levels do not provide any value in terms of predicting the severity of acute pancreatitis. These tests should only be used to make the diagnosis of acute pancreatitis. In addition, they should not be used to follow the patient's progress while in the hospital because their levels generally do not correlate with clinical improvement or decline.

Most episodes of acute pancreatitis are of the mild interstitial form. Almost all associated morbidity and mortality occur in patients with necrotizing pancreatitis and particularly infected pancreatic necrosis, which has a mortality rate of 10% to 30%. Peripancreatic edema on CT imaging is not a marker of severity in acute pancreatitis.

An elevated temperature is not considered an independent marker of severity in acute pancreatitis.

> **KEY POINT**
> - Serial blood urea nitrogen measurements may be the most reliable routine laboratory test to predict severity of acute pancreatitis.

Bibliography
Wu BU, Johannes RS, Sun X, Conwell DL, Banks PA. Early changes in blood urea nitrogen predict mortality in acute pancreatitis. Gastroenterology. 2009;137(1):129-135. [PMID: 19344722]

Item 55   Answer: E

Educational Objective: Diagnose small intestinal bacterial overgrowth.

This patient has many features of small intestinal bacterial overgrowth (SIBO), including diarrhea, bloating, and weight loss. In addition, she appears to have macrocytic anemia secondary to vitamin B_{12} deficiency in association with an elevated serum folate level, which is a classic pattern seen in SIBO (bacteria consume vitamin B_{12} and also synthesize folate). Patients with systemic sclerosis may be particularly at risk for SIBO because of intestinal dysmotility or small-intestinal diverticula. Common risk factors for SIBO include altered gastric acid (achlorhydria, gastrectomy), structural abnormalities (strictures, small-bowel diverticula, blind loops or afferent limbs), and intestinal dysmotility (diabetes mellitus, neuromuscular disorders). The diagnosis of SIBO can be established with

hydrogen breath testing or upper endoscopy with small-intestinal cultures, if available.

Although celiac disease may cause diarrhea, weight loss, and bloating, this patient's normal tissue transglutaminase antibody and elevated serum folate level make this less likely than SIBO, especially given her risk factors for bacterial overgrowth.

Irritable bowel syndrome should not cause weight loss or nocturnal stools. These clinical findings represent alarm features in the evaluation of patients with diarrhea and abdominal pain or bloating, so it would be erroneous to diagnose irritable bowel syndrome with the presence of these findings.

Patients with lactose malabsorption in isolation should not have weight loss, so it would not explain this patient's clinical picture. Although patients with SIBO may have concomitant lactose intolerance, lactose restriction is discouraged before evaluating and treating the underlying problem, especially because this patient reports tolerance of lactose ingestion.

By definition, microscopic colitis is a disease with histologic changes limited to the colon, unless it occurs in the setting of celiac disease. Therefore, with a colonic disease, features of fat malabsorption and vitamin deficiencies should not be seen. Although patients with microscopic colitis may have mild degrees of weight loss due to volume depletion, this patient's weight loss is higher than what would typically be seen.

> **KEY POINT**
> - Small intestinal bacterial overgrowth should be considered in patients presenting with diarrhea, bloating, or weight loss; vitamin B_{12} deficiency or an elevated serum folate level can be laboratory clues to the diagnosis.

Bibliography
Bures J, Cyrany J, Kohoutova D, et al. Small intestinal bacterial overgrowth syndrome. World J Gastroenterol. 2010;16(24):2978-2990. [PMID: 20572300]

Item 56   Answer: C

Educational Objective: Manage hepatitis B virus infection in a patient in the immune-tolerant state.

The most appropriate management for this patient is observation with serial monitoring of aminotransferases every 3 to 6 months. Various subgroups of patients with hepatitis B virus (HBV) infection reflect the natural history of infection; these subgroups include the immune-tolerant patient, the patient in a phase of immune clearance, and the inactive carrier. This patient has chronic HBV infection in the immune-tolerant state, as identified by a high circulating viral level in the absence of markers of liver inflammation (normal hepatic aminotransferase levels). This is typically seen in patients born in a hepatitis B–endemic area such as Southeast Asia or Africa in whom HBV was likely acquired perinatally. As long as patients maintain normal hepatic aminotransferase levels, they are at low risk for progression of liver disease. As this patient ages, she is at increased risk for active hepatitis. Evidence of hepatic inflammation (persistently elevated hepatic aminotransferase levels) indicates active hepatitis; if significant inflammation is seen, liver biopsy should be considered and treatment should be initiated.

Immunization against HBV is not warranted because this patient has already been exposed to the virus, has significant replicating HBV, and has not developed immunity. Vaccination would not result in seroconversion to the antibody to hepatitis B surface antigen–positive state.

Liver biopsy is warranted only if liver chemistry tests become elevated. The presence of significant liver inflammation or fibrosis on biopsy indicates the need for antiviral therapy.

Initiation of antiviral therapy with tenofovir is not warranted in this patient with immune-tolerant HBV infection because she is unlikely to experience progression of liver disease if her hepatic aminotransferase levels are normal. In addition, antiviral therapy may potentially require life-long administration.

KEY POINT

- Monitoring of hepatic aminotransferases every 3 to 6 months is warranted in patients with immune-tolerant hepatitis B virus infection.

Bibliography
Lok AS, McMahon BJ. Chronic hepatitis B [erratum in Hepatology. 2007;45(6):1347]. Hepatology. 2007;45(2):507-539. [PMID: 17256718]

Item 57   Answer: D
Educational Objective: Manage noncardiac chest pain.

This patient should receive twice-daily proton pump inhibitor (PPI) therapy for 8 to 10 weeks. Pain associated with gastroesophageal reflux can mimic ischemic chest pain. A cardiac cause should be carefully assessed and excluded in all patients with chest pain. This patient has nonanginal chest pain, no additional risk factors, and a negative exercise stress test; the likelihood of a cardiac cause of chest pain is low. Randomized controlled trials have shown that a therapeutic trial of a twice-daily PPI is effective in 50% to 60% of patients with noncardiac chest pain, revealing gastroesophageal reflux disease as the underlying cause.

If the PPI trial is unsuccessful, further evaluation with endoscopy (to detect erosive esophagitis or achalasia), manometry (to detect esophageal motility disorders such as diffuse esophageal spasm), and ambulatory pH recording (to detect refractory reflux) would be reasonable.

Musculoskeletal chest pain has an insidious onset and may last for hours to weeks. It is most recognizable when sharp and localized to a specific area of the chest;

however, it can also be poorly localized. The pain may be worsened by turning, deep breathing, or arm movement. Chest pain may or may not be reproducible by chest palpation (pain reproduced by palpation does not exclude ischemic heart disease), and the cardiovascular examination is often normal. This patient does not have the typical features of musculoskeletal chest pain, and therefore treatment with an NSAID is not the most appropriate first step in management.

KEY POINT

- After cardiac causes have been excluded by comprehensive cardiac examination, an 8- to 10-week trial of proton pump inhibitor therapy is reasonable before further testing in patients with noncardiac chest pain who do not have alarm symptoms.

Bibliography
Kahrilas PJ, Shaheen NJ, Vaezi MF, et al; American Gastroenterological Association. American Gastroenterological Association Medical Position Statement on the management of gastroesophageal reflux disease. Gastroenterology. 2008;135(4):1383-1391. [PMID: 18789939]

Item 58   Answer: A
Educational Objective: Manage upper gastrointestinal bleeding and hemodynamic instability.

This patient should continue to receive fluid and erythrocyte resuscitation. She has experienced a large gastrointestinal hemorrhage with resultant hemodynamic instability. Her history of aspirin use suggests an upper gastrointestinal source of bleeding. Appropriate intravenous access has been obtained with normal saline fluid boluses and intravenous proton pump inhibitor infusion. Despite this, she remains unstable and has a hemoglobin level of 7.0 g/dL (70 g/L). The most important and urgent treatment for this patient is erythrocyte transfusion and intravenous crystalloid support to achieve hemodynamic stability. An intensive resuscitation strategy has been shown to improve mortality. Volume loss is estimated by pulse rate, blood pressure, and presence of orthostatic hypotension because changes in hemoglobin and hematocrit levels may not become evident immediately. An initial hemoglobin level of less than 8.0 g/dL (80 g/L) is concerning because re-equilibration in the 24 to 48 hours after the initial bleeding episode may reveal an even lower hemoglobin level.

Octreotide would be appropriate to use empirically in a patient with known or suspected liver disease, but this patient fits neither criterion. Octreotide is effective in variceal hemorrhage by decreasing portal venous inflow and consequently intravariceal pressure.

After further resuscitation with packed red blood cells and intravenous crystalloids, this patient will require an upper endoscopy within 24 hours of presentation. However, this is not appropriate at this time with ongoing instability

CONT.

in an incompletely resuscitated patient. Additionally, medications administered for moderate sedation during a standard upper endoscopy result in hypotension and would cause further hemodynamic insult.

Nasogastric tube placement can be helpful in selected patients in whom the location of bleeding is in question. However, there is a high enough false-negative rate (approximately 15%) and false-positive rate (due to nasogastric tube mucosal irritation) that this is not uniformly recommended and would not be the first priority in this patient. Furthermore, this patient has hematemesis, indicating significant upper gastrointestinal hemorrhage.

> **KEY POINT**
> - **Patients with upper gastrointestinal bleeding should be stabilized with fluid and erythrocyte resuscitation before diagnostic endoscopy is pursued.**

Bibliography

Barkun AN, Bardou M, Kuipers EJ, et al; International Consensus Upper Gastrointestinal Bleeding Conference Group. International consensus recommendations on the management of patients with nonvariceal upper gastrointestinal bleeding. Ann Intern Med. 2010;152(2):101-113. [PMID: 20083829]

Item 59   Answer: B

Educational Objective: Diagnose eosinophilic esophagitis.

Slowly progressive solid-food dysphagia in a young man who has allergic diseases is likely due to eosinophilic esophagitis. This patient's history (location of symptoms, absence of aspiration, and intact initiation of swallows) suggests esophageal dysphagia rather than oropharyngeal dysphagia. Patients with eosinophilic esophagitis can present with symptoms similar to those of gastroesophageal reflux disease, but young adults frequently present with extreme dysphagia and food impaction. There is a strong male predominance. The diagnosis is made by endoscopy, with mucosal biopsies showing marked infiltration with eosinophils (>15 eosinophils/hpf), and the exclusion of gastroesophageal reflux by either ambulatory pH testing or by nonresponse to a therapeutic trial of proton pump inhibitors for 6 weeks. Macroscopic findings at endoscopy are nonspecific and insensitive but proximal strictures are most consistently observed. Other findings include mucosal rings (sometimes multiple), mucosal furrowing, white specks, and mucosal friability. Some patients have evidence of a motility disorder, suggesting involvement of the muscular layers. Treatment with swallowed aerosolized topical corticosteroid preparations or systemic corticosteroids provides excellent short-term relief.

Slowly progressive solid-food dysphagia in the absence of dysphagia to liquids is more suggestive of an intraluminal mechanical cause (such as a stricture or ring) than a motility disturbance like achalasia, which usually presents with dysphagia to both solids and liquids and may be associated with chest pain and regurgitation.

Esophageal infections in immunocompetent persons are most common in patients who use swallowed aerosolized corticosteroids or in patients with disorders that cause stasis of esophageal contents. *Candida albicans* is the most common organism causing esophagitis in immunocompetent patients. Although esophageal candidiasis can present with dysphagia, the chronic nature of this patient's symptoms (lasting for years) and the absence of oropharyngeal candidiasis make esophageal candidiasis an unlikely cause.

Malignancy is an unlikely diagnosis because of this patient's young age, long duration of symptoms, and lack of weight loss despite prolonged symptoms.

Oropharyngeal dysphagia is characterized by difficulty in the initial phase of swallowing, in which the bolus is formed in the mouth and is transferred from the mouth through the pharynx to the esophagus. This patient is not experiencing difficulty swallowing.

> **KEY POINT**
> - **Slowly progressive solid-food dysphagia in a young man who has allergic diseases is likely due to eosinophilic esophagitis.**

Bibliography

Cook IJ. Diagnostic evaluation of dysphagia. Nat Clin Pract Gastroenterol Hepatol. 2008;5(7):393-403. [PMID: 18542115]

Item 60   Answer: C

Educational Objective: Evaluate for cholangiocarcinoma in a patient with primary sclerosing cholangitis.

The most appropriate next step in management is endoscopic retrograde cholangiography. This patient most likely has cholangiocarcinoma. Complications related to progressive duct destruction include recurrent cholangitis, bile duct stones, large strictures, and cholangiocarcinoma. The typical presentation of cholangiocarcinoma is that of biliary obstruction, resulting in the painless onset of jaundice. In most patients with primary sclerosing cholangitis, cholangiocarcinoma will develop within the first few years of their diagnosis. In this patient, the development of new jaundice and an obstructing lesion in the extrahepatic bile duct is most consistent with the development of cholangiocarcinoma. The best test to diagnose cholangiocarcinoma is endoscopic retrograde cholangiography, which provides the opportunity to obtain cytologic brushings and mucosal biopsies to evaluate for malignant changes.

Abdominal ultrasonography can show abnormalities of bile ducts and would be expected to demonstrate abnormal findings in this patient. In the setting of this patient's abnormal magnetic resonance cholangiopancreatography and concern for cholangiocarcinoma, abnormal findings on abdominal ultrasound do not provide any additional information to help guide therapy. Cytology specimens or tissue biopsy samples are needed to confirm the diagnosis, which cannot be supplied by ultrasonography.

CA 19-9 is a serologic test that is often elevated in the setting of cholangiocarcinoma but lacks the sensitivity and specificity necessary to establish the diagnosis of cholangiocarcinoma.

Patients with chronic liver disease often require serial monitoring of aminotransferase levels. However, cholangiocarcinoma is one of the most serious complications of primary sclerosing cholangitis and establishing this diagnosis by histologic evaluation is of primary importance at this time.

> **KEY POINT**
> • Patients with suspected cholangiocarcinoma should be referred for endoscopic retrograde cholangiography.

Bibliography

Blechacz BR, Gores GJ. Cholangiocarcinoma. Clin Liver Dis. 2008;12(1):131-150. [PMID: 18242501]

Item 61   Answer: A
Educational Objective: Treat hepatorenal syndrome.

The most appropriate treatment is intravenous albumin. Hepatorenal syndrome (HRS) occurs primarily in the setting of spontaneous bacterial peritonitis. Type 1 HRS is typically defined by at least a doubling of the initial serum creatinine to greater than 2.5 mg/dL (221 micromoles/L) in less than 2 weeks. Type 2 HRS is not as rapidly progressive but is a common cause of death in patients with refractory ascites. The major criteria for the diagnosis of HRS include cirrhosis with ascites; serum creatinine greater than 1.5 mg/dL (133 micromoles/L); no improvement of serum creatinine (improvement is defined by a decrease to ≤1.5 mg/dL [133 micromoles/L]) after at least 2 days of diuretic withdrawal and volume expansion with 1.5 L or more of albumin; absence of shock or hypotension; no current or recent treatment with nephrotoxic drugs; and the absence of parenchymal kidney disease (no significant proteinuria [<500 mg/d], hematuria, findings of acute tubular necrosis [pigmented granular casts on urinalysis], or evidence of obstruction on ultrasound). Systemic vasoconstrictor agents are recommended for the initial treatment of type 1 HRS. The most promising agent that reverses type 1 HRS is terlipressin; however, it is not currently available in the United States. The next most promising treatment is intravenous albumin, which has been shown in randomized trials to be associated with improvement in serum creatinine level and urine output in patients with type 1 HRS. Although reports exist supporting the use of octreotide with midodrine and intravenous albumin for type 1 HRS,

the uncertain status of midodrine availability potentially eliminates this regimen as a realistic option. Furthermore, there is no evidence demonstrating clinical benefit with octreotide monotherapy.

Studies investigating dopamine or low-dose vasopressin in combination with albumin for the treatment of type 1 HRS have not demonstrated significant clinical benefit.

> **KEY POINT**
> • In patients with suspected hepatorenal syndrome, volume expansion should be performed with intravenous albumin.

Bibliography

Runyon BA; AASLD Practice Guidelines Committee. Management of adult patients with ascites due to cirrhosis: an update. Hepatology. 2009;49(6):2087-2107. [PMID: 19475696]

Item 62   Answer: B
Educational Objective: Manage *Helicobacter pylori* testing in a patient with a bleeding peptic ulcer.

This patient should undergo *Helicobacter pylori* serology. Recent gastrointestinal bleeding can reduce the accuracy of certain methods to detect *H. pylori*, specifically the rapid urease test, histology, and culture. Therefore, in a patient with a bleeding peptic ulcer, a negative rapid urease test or histology is not sufficient to rule out *H. pylori* infection, and a second test is warranted. The sensitivity of the rapid urease test can be reduced up to 25% in patients who have taken a proton pump inhibitor (PPI) or bismuth within 2 weeks of testing or antibiotic therapy within 4 weeks. The sensitivity of the urea breath test and stool antigen test, like that of the rapid urease test, is reduced by medications that affect urease production. *H. pylori* serology is indicated in this patient because it is the only test that is not affected by recent gastrointestinal bleeding or use of PPIs.

Treatment with a PPI alone is incorrect because the finding of *H. pylori* infection has implications for treatment; eradication of *H. pylori* is superior to PPIs for healing and remission of duodenal ulcers. Therefore, a second form of testing for *H. pylori* is clinically important if the rapid urease test or histology is negative.

> **KEY POINT**
> • *Helicobacter pylori* serology is the only test that is not affected by recent gastrointestinal bleeding or use of proton pump inhibitors.

Bibliography

Chey WD, Wong BC; Practice Parameters Committee of the American College of Gastroenterology. American College of Gastroenterology guideline on the management of Helicobacter pylori infection. Am J Gastroenterol. 2007;102(8):1808-1825. [PMID: 17608775]

Item 63   Answer: A

Educational Objective: Manage dyspepsia without alarm features in a patient from a developing country.

The most appropriate management for this patient is stool antigen testing for *Helicobacter pylori*. Dyspepsia is chronic or recurrent discomfort in the upper midabdomen. The prevalence of dyspepsia is not well known because of the vagueness of its description by both patients and physicians. In addition to discomfort, affected patients may have mild nausea or bloating. The recommended approach for a patient younger than 50 years without alarm features (anemia; dysphagia; odynophagia; vomiting; weight loss; family history of upper gastrointestinal malignancy; personal history of peptic ulcer disease, gastric surgery, or gastrointestinal malignancy; and abdominal mass or lymphadenopathy on examination) is a test-and-treat strategy for *H. pylori* or empiric treatment with a proton pump inhibitor (PPI). The test-and-treat strategy for *H. pylori* is an appropriate first-line strategy when the patient is from an area where prevalence of *H. pylori* is high (such as developing countries); however, PPI is the most appropriate first-line strategy if the patient is from an area where prevalence of *H. pylori* is low. Patients such as this one from developing countries have a higher prevalence of *H. pylori* owing to likely fecal-oral transmission. Therefore, for this patient, a test-and-treat approach for *H. pylori* is preferred. If testing is positive, eradication of *H. pylori* may relieve symptoms, but it is important to note that randomized controlled trials provide conflicting results as to the efficacy of *H. pylori* eradication in improving symptoms of functional dyspepsia. If the patient does not test positive for *H. pylori*, a trial of a PPI is warranted.

PPIs are superior to H_2 blockers, so initiating an H_2 blocker would not be appropriate in this patient.

Empiric treatment for *H. pylori* is incorrect because the diagnosis of *H. pylori* should be determined before initiating treatment.

Endoscopy would be appropriate for patients whose symptoms do not respond to *H. pylori* treatment or PPI therapy. Patients older than 50 years or with alarm features should always be evaluated with upper endoscopy. In patients without alarm features, endoscopy as an initial management intervention would be unlikely to find gastritis, peptic ulcer disease, or esophagitis.

KEY POINT

- **For patients with dyspepsia who are younger than 50 years, have no alarm features, and are from areas with a high prevalence of *Helicobacter pylori*, a test-and-treat approach for *H. pylori* is reasonable and cost effective.**

Bibliography

Camilleri M, Tack JF. Current medical treatments of dyspepsia and irritable bowel syndrome. Gastroenterol Clin North Am. 2010;39(3):481-493. [PMID: 20951913]

Item 64   Answer: A

Educational Objective: Diagnose cannabinoid hyperemesis syndrome.

The most likely diagnosis is cannabinoid hyperemesis syndrome. The cannabinoid hyperemesis syndrome has become increasingly recognized in the last decade. Its hallmarks include episodic abdominal pain, nausea, and vomiting in a patient using marijuana. Symptoms are associated with compulsive washing. The syndrome is best treated with complete cessation of marijuana use. The putative mechanism includes buildup of metabolites in the central nervous system that act on central cannabinoid receptors or on gastrointestinal cannabinoid receptors that inhibit gastrointestinal transit; however, the exact mechanism has not yet been defined.

Chronic intestinal pseudo-obstruction (CIPO) usually presents with abdominal distention, abdominal pain, nausea, and sometimes vomiting that may be acute, chronic, or recurrent. CIPO is characterized radiologically by a dilated small bowel that may or may not include the large bowel in the absence of true obstruction. This disease can be caused by neuropathic disorders such as diabetes mellitus, amyloidosis, or paraneoplastic or myopathic processes. In a patient with characteristic clinical features and radiologic findings, the diagnosis can be made by gastric and small-bowel manometry. Abdominal radiographs are normal in this patient, so CIPO is an incorrect diagnosis.

This syndrome shares many features with the cyclic vomiting syndrome (CVS). CVS is characterized by stereotypical acute episodes of vomiting that last less than 1 week, three or more episodes in 1 year, and absence of nausea and vomiting between episodes in the absence of any alternative diagnosis. A personal or family history of migraine headache is a supportive criterion for CVS. The pathogenesis of CVS is unknown. However, this patient has a history of marijuana use, which makes the cannabinoid hyperemesis syndrome more likely.

Gastroparesis is incorrect because it most often (but not exclusively) occurs in the setting of long-standing diabetes, and patients are usually symptomatic on a daily basis.

KEY POINT

- **The cannabinoid hyperemesis syndrome is characterized by episodic abdominal pain, nausea, and vomiting in a patient using marijuana.**

Bibliography

Soriano-Co M, Batke M, Cappell MS. The cannabis hyperemesis syndrome characterized by persistent nausea and vomiting, abdominal pain, and compulsive bathing associated with chronic marijuana use: a report of eight cases in the United States. Dig Dis Sci. 2010;55(11):3113-3119. [PMID: 20130993]

Item 65   Answer: C

Educational Objective: Evaluate obscure gastrointestinal bleeding using the most sensitive test.

Nuclear scintigraphy should be performed next. This patient most likely has vascular ectasias (angiodysplasias) as the cause of her chronic, painless bleeding. Affected patients may present with iron deficiency anemia and occult gastrointestinal bleeding or with hematochezia that is indistinguishable from diverticular hemorrhage. The two primary types of nuclear scans are technetium-99m (^{99m}Tc) pertechnetate red blood cell and ^{99m}Tc sulfur colloid. Red blood cell scanning is positive in 45% of patients with an active bleed and has an overall accuracy of 78% for localizing the bleeding. It can detect ongoing bleeding occurring at a rate of 0.1 to 0.5 mL/min. This scan is more sensitive than angiography and is often the first radiologic test performed. Positive nuclear scintigraphy can sometimes direct angiography to allow for immediate therapy with arterial embolization.

Angiography can be an effective diagnostic and therapeutic modality for identifying and treating gastrointestinal bleeding, but it is not as sensitive as nuclear scintigraphy. It requires a bleeding rate greater than 1 mL/min. The patient's hemodynamic stability and 3-day hiatus before the hemoglobin level drops sufficiently to require a transfusion suggest a gastrointestinal bleed that is slower than 1 mL/min.

MR enterography and CT do not play much of a role in identifying active luminal gastrointestinal bleeding because they are insensitive, but they could be helpful if an extraintestinal bleeding site (for example, retroperitoneal hematoma) was being considered.

Small-bowel barium examination could be useful to identify a mass lesion or Crohn disease, but both of these are unlikely diagnoses in this patient.

KEY POINT

- Technetium-labeled nuclear scans provide the best sensitivity for actively bleeding lesions from an obscure source, requiring a flow rate of only 0.1 to 0.5 mL/min.

Bibliography

Barkun AN, Bardou M, Kuipers EJ, et al; International Consensus Upper Gastrointestinal Bleeding Conference Group. International consensus recommendations on the management of patients with nonvariceal upper gastrointestinal bleeding. Ann Intern Med. 2010;152(2):101-113. [PMID: 20083829]

Item 66   Answer: B

Educational Objective: Manage hereditary hemochromatosis.

The most appropriate management is liver biopsy. This patient has hereditary hemochromatosis, manifested as significant iron overload. Up to 50% of patients who are homozygous for the *C282Y* mutation will develop iron overload, but only 20% to 60% will develop hemochromatosis-related morbidity. The reasons for incomplete penetrance of hereditary hemochromatosis are not fully understood. It is important to determine if cirrhosis is present in patients with hemochromatosis, as cirrhosis portends a risk for hepatocellular cancer and portal hypertension. If cirrhosis is identified, the patient should be screened for complications of cirrhosis, including esophageal varices and hepatocellular carcinoma. Risk factors for cirrhosis include age greater than 40 years and serum ferritin level greater than 1000 ng/mL (1000 micrograms/L), and these are typically considered indications to consider liver biopsy. Because this patient is 45 years old and has evidence of significant iron overload (manifested by an elevated ferritin level), liver biopsy is warranted to ascertain whether cirrhosis or significant fibrosis of the liver is present.

Symptomatic patients or those with evidence of organ damage secondary to iron overload require treatment. The most efficient and effective treatment for hemochromatosis is phlebotomy. Iron chelation therapy will also remove iron but is usually unnecessary because phlebotomy is safe, inexpensive, and effective. In this patient, treatment for hemochromatosis is not indicated until the liver biopsy is performed, which will allow for estimation of liver iron accumulation and will indicate if there is liver damage that requires intervention.

Observation may be an appropriate course of action if the patient is asymptomatic, has a low (<50 ng/mL [50 micrograms/L]) ferritin level, and has no evidence of organ damage from iron accumulation. In these patients, the recommended follow-up is annual history and physical examination to monitor for signs and symptoms of organ dysfunction and measurements of serum iron, ferritin, and transferrin saturation levels. If a patient has genetic hemochromatosis and evidence of iron overload even without evidence of organ damage, phlebotomy may still be indicated, because maintaining lifelong low-normal iron levels will prevent the development of eventual organ damage.

KEY POINT

- Patients with hereditary hemochromatosis who are older than 40 years or have a serum ferritin level greater than 1000 ng/mL (1000 micrograms/L) are at risk for cirrhosis and should undergo liver biopsy.

Bibliography

Pietrangelo A. Hereditary hemochromatosis: pathogenesis, diagnosis, and treatment. Gastroenterology. 2010;139(2):393-408. [PMID: 20542038]

Item 67   Answer: D

Educational Objective: Manage thiamine deficiency following bariatric surgery.

The most appropriate next step is to administer intravenous thiamine. This patient has clinical features of thiamine deficiency manifesting as Wernicke encephalopathy (nystagmus, ophthalmoplegia, ataxia, and confusion), and administration of intravenous thiamine should occur promptly. Thiamine deficiency has been reported in patients

CONT.

who have undergone bariatric surgery and is caused by poor postoperative oral intake. Body stores of thiamine deplete quickly. Early recognition of thiamine deficiency is crucial before the patient develops irreversible neurologic and cognitive changes.

This patient has new-onset ataxia and ocular findings on examination, but these findings can be explained by a thiamine-deficient state. Therefore, a CT of the head would be unnecessary and could delay the urgently needed administration of appropriate treatment.

Although hypoglycemia could present with neurologic features, this patient's plasma glucose level was normal on admission. Glucose administration in a patient who is thiamine deficient may worsen the clinical course because thiamine is required as a cofactor in glucose metabolism.

Although naloxone can be helpful for reversal of opiate activity, the patient has not received opioids for several days, and opioid ingestion or withdrawal would not account for his neurologic changes.

Vitamin B_{12} deficiency can cause neurologic manifestations, typically beginning with paresthesias and ataxia associated with loss of vibration and position sense; however, it often takes months to years after vitamin intake or absorption is impaired for a deficient state to develop. This patient will be at risk for vitamin B_{12} deficiency if he does not take supplemental vitamin B_{12}, but deficiency would not have occurred within the 3 weeks since his surgery.

KEY POINT

- Patients who have recently undergone bariatric surgery may develop thiamine deficiency, which is characterized by confusion, ataxia, nystagmus, and ophthalmoplegia.

Bibliography
Aasheim ET. Wernicke encephalopathy after bariatric surgery: a systematic review. Ann Surg. 2008;248(5):714-720. [PMID: 18948797]

Item 68   Answer: D
Educational Objective: Diagnose rumination syndrome.

This patient has classic features of rumination syndrome, which is characterized by effortless regurgitation of undigested food and reswallowing of the contents. Rumination typically occurs within 30 minutes after a meal, may last 1 to 2 hours, and involves undigested and recognizable food that does not taste sour, which is then reswallowed or spit out depending on social circumstances. The Rome III diagnostic criteria are: (1) persistent or recurrent regurgitation of recently ingested food into the mouth with subsequent spitting or remastication and swallowing, (2) the regurgitation is not preceded by retching, and (3) these criteria are fulfilled for the last 3 months with symptom onset at least 6 months before diagnosis. Other supportive features of regurgitation events are absence of nausea and cessation of

the rumination when the regurgitated material tastes acidic. This condition has historically been seen most commonly in children with intellectual disability; however, rumination syndrome is now increasingly recognized in individuals of normal intellect. The treatment for rumination syndrome is postprandial diaphragmatic breathing exercises, which are typically taught by a psychologist. Using these deep breathing techniques after a meal prevents the patient from actively contracting the abdominal musculature, which initiates the regurgitation event.

Cannabinoid hyperemesis syndrome is not the correct diagnosis, because patients with this disorder have a history of using marijuana and develop recurrent nausea and vomiting, sometimes with abdominal pain. Symptoms improve with taking hot baths or marijuana cessation.

Cyclic vomiting syndrome is not present in this patient, because the patient does not describe vomiting and she has no interval periods of feeling well between episodes. The Rome III diagnostic criteria for cyclic vomiting syndrome are all of the following: (1) stereotypical episodes of acute nausea and vomiting lasting less than 1 week, (2) three or more discrete episodes in the past 12 months, and (3) absence of nausea and vomiting between episodes. A family history of migraine is a supportive criterion.

Clinical features of gastroparesis include nausea, vomiting, bloating, and postprandial fullness with early satiety. Abdominal discomfort is present in 50% to 90% of affected patients. The abdominal examination may show epigastric distention or tenderness, and there may be a succussion splash. Classically, most patients with diabetic gastroparesis have had diabetes for 10 years or more, which is not the case in this patient.

KEY POINT

- Rumination syndrome is characterized by effortless regurgitation of undigested food and reswallowing of the contents.

Bibliography
Tack J, Talley NJ. Gastroduodenal disorders. Am J Gastroenterol. 2010;105(4):757-763. [PMID: 20372127]

Item 69   Answer: D
Educational Objective: Manage gastroesophageal reflux disease with an empiric trial of proton pump inhibitor therapy.

This patient should receive proton pump inhibitor (PPI) therapy. Typical esophageal symptoms of gastroesophageal reflux (heartburn and acid regurgitation) have a reasonably high specificity and sensitivity (>75%-80%) for the diagnosis of gastroesophageal reflux disease (GERD). GERD is likely in this patient with typical, chronic, frequent symptoms and elevated BMI, especially with central obesity. Other risk factors include history of smoking and sleep apnea. Empiric therapy with a PPI is the most cost-effective management strategy. There are five PPIs available in the United States: omeprazole, esomeprazole, lansoprazole, pantoprazole, and rabeprazole; they all have approximately similar efficacy. PPI therapy is usually given once a day before meals, usually before breakfast. In patients who require twice-daily dosing for symptom control (for example, patients with noncardiac chest pain, extraesophageal manifestations, incomplete response to standard therapy, or Barrett esophagus), the second dose should be administered before dinner. Patients should be reassessed in 6 weeks; if symptoms respond, drug dosage can be decreased to the lowest effective dose. Long-term PPI therapy is considered generally safe for patients who require ongoing acid suppression. The risks and benefits of long-term PPI therapy should be considered in light of case-controlled studies that suggest an increased risk of enteric infections, pneumonia, and hip fractures with such use.

Ambulatory esophageal pH monitoring, which consists of inserting a pH monitor into the distal esophagus and recording the results over a period of usually 24 hours, is the most accurate means to confirm the diagnosis of GERD. The technique also allows determination of an association between symptoms and the amount and pattern of esophageal acid exposure. Ambulatory pH monitoring is useful to establish or exclude a diagnosis of GERD if the patient does not respond to a trial of PPIs.

In the absence of alarm symptoms such as dysphagia, weight loss, or gastrointestinal bleeding/anemia, endoscopy is not indicated. Patients with alarm symptoms, long-standing symptoms, or symptoms that are refractory to acid-suppression therapy should undergo further evaluation, including upper endoscopy.

Fundoplication is reserved for patients with intact esophageal peristalsis who have documented, uncontrolled reflux despite maximal medical therapy or intolerance of medications. It is premature to consider antireflux surgery prior to an empiric trial of a PPI in a patient with suspected GERD.

KEY POINT

- Empiric therapy with a proton pump inhibitor is the most cost-effective management strategy for suspected gastroesophageal reflux disease.

Bibliography

Kahrilas PJ, Shaheen NJ, Vaezi MF, et al; American Gastroenterological Association. American Gastroenterological Association Medical Position Statement on the management of gastroesophageal reflux disease. Gastroenterology. 2008;135(4):1383-1391. [PMID: 18789939]

Item 70   Answer: A
Educational Objective: Diagnose a biliary cyst.

The most likely diagnosis is a biliary cyst. Biliary cysts are often found incidentally when patients undergo imaging for nonspecific symptoms. The finding of fusiform dilatation of the common bile duct in the absence of obstruction or stones is characteristic of a type I biliary cyst. Intermittent chronic pain and episodic jaundice are the most common symptoms. Though biliary cysts are rare (1:10,000 to 1:15,000 births in the United States), recognition is important because a biliary cyst confers a risk for recurrent bouts of cholangitis and a high risk for biliary cancer (up to 75%). Extrahepatic dilatation of the common bile duct, as described in this patient, is the most common type of biliary cyst and is seen in 50% to 80% of cases.

Although cholelithiasis (gallstones) can result in obstruction of the bile ducts and subsequent dilatation of proximal bile ducts, this patient's abdominal imaging did not demonstrate findings of cholelithiasis.

The diagnosis of irritable bowel syndrome (IBS) is based solely on clinical grounds. Because no biochemical, radiographic, endoscopic, or histologic marker exists, several clinical indices have been published to aid in the diagnosis of IBS. IBS does not cause ascending cholangitis or fusiform dilatation of the common bile duct as seen in this patient.

Primary biliary cirrhosis (PBC) is a disease of the microscopic bile ducts that can result in jaundice, liver inflammation, and liver failure. However, the extrahepatic bile ducts are not dilated in PBC, and therefore this patient does not have PBC.

KEY POINT

- A biliary cyst should be suspected when dilatation of the bile duct is found without evidence of an obstructing lesion.

Bibliography

Singham J, Yoshida EM, Scudamore CH. Choledochal cysts: part 2 of 3: Diagnosis. Can J Surg. 2009;52(6):506-511. [PMID: 20011188]

Item 71   Answer: D
Educational Objective: Manage fulminant liver failure with referral to a liver transplantation center.

This patient should be referred for liver transplantation. Fulminant hepatic failure (FHF) is defined as hepatic encephalopathy in the setting of jaundice without preexisting liver disease. Liver failure is classified by the number of weeks after jaundice onset that encephalopathy appears; hyperacute liver failure is within 1 week, acute liver failure is between 1 and 4 weeks, and subacute liver failure is between 4 and 12 weeks. The most common causes of FHF are medications (especially acetaminophen) and viral infections; however, many cases are of indeterminate cause. Quick recognition of FHF is essential, because the mortality rate is as high as 85%. The survival rate with transplantation for FHF is 65% to 80%. Therefore, recognition is important so that affected patients can be transferred to a liver transplantation center.

An elevated INR reflects decreased hepatic synthesis of liver-derived factors of the clotting cascade. Although this increases the risk of bleeding complications in these patients, the administration of fresh frozen plasma to correct coagulopathy is not necessary in the absence of demonstrated bleeding or the need for an invasive procedure.

Cerebral edema is the most common cause of death in patients with FHF. Management of cerebral edema includes invasive monitoring for increased intracranial pressure, typically performed at a liver transplant center. Medical treatment of cerebral edema sometimes includes the use of mannitol, but mannitol therapy is contraindicated in a patient with kidney disease.

Endoscopic retrograde cholangiopancreatography (ERCP) is indicated for assessment and management of biliary obstruction; in the setting of acute liver failure without biliary dilatation on abdominal ultrasound, ERCP is not warranted.

KEY POINT

- The recognition of fulminant liver failure should prompt immediate referral to a liver transplantation center for intensive monitoring and consideration of liver transplantation.

Bibliography

Ichai P, Samuel D. Etiology and prognosis of fulminant hepatitis in adults. Liver Transpl. 2008;14(Suppl 2):S67-S79. [PMID: 18825677]

Item 72   Answer: B

Educational Objective: Diagnose diverticular bleeding.

The most likely diagnosis is diverticulosis. In patients with severe hematochezia, the most common site of bleeding is the colon (75%). Within the colon, the most likely cause of bleeding is diverticula, which constitute 33% of all colonic bleeding. Bleeding is arterial, resulting from medial thinning of the vasa recta as they drape over the dome of the diverticulum. Generally, patients do not have other symptoms. Physical examination is generally unremarkable unless large blood loss results in tachycardia, hypotension, and orthostasis. Colonoscopy may identify the bleeding diverticulum and permit endoscopic treatment with epinephrine and/or electrocautery; colonoscopy may also help identify other causes of bleeding such as vascular ectasias. Vascular ectasias or angiodysplasias (erroneously called arteriovenous malformations), account for up to 11% of episodes of lower gastrointestinal bleeding. They are painless dilated submucosal vessels that radiate from a central feeding vessel. Affected patients may present with iron deficiency anemia and occult gastrointestinal bleeding or with hematochezia that is indistinguishable from diverticular hemorrhage.

Colon cancer rarely, if ever, causes brisk arterial bleeding. Colon cancer typically causes chronic blood loss that is often occult; this is not compatible with this patient's findings.

The presence of melena (black, tarry stools) suggests an upper gastrointestinal tract source of bleeding (such as from a duodenal ulcer) but can be associated with loss of as

little as 150 to 200 mL of blood. Hematemesis of bright red blood is associated with ongoing upper gastrointestinal bleeding, whereas hematochezia secondary to an upper source is suggestive of brisk ongoing bleeding of at least 1000 mL of blood and is typically associated with hemodynamic instability, which is absent in this patient.

Ischemic colitis, which accounts for between 1% and 19% of episodes of lower gastrointestinal bleeding, results from a sudden temporary reduction in mesenteric blood flow. This hypoperfusion typically affects the "watershed" areas of the colon (that is, the splenic flexure and rectosigmoid junction). Patients may report dizziness but may not recall any such episodes. They present with the sudden onset of mild crampy abdominal pain and subsequent passage of bloody stool or bloody diarrhea.

KEY POINT

- The majority of patients with hematochezia have a colonic source of bleeding (75%); when bleeding is from the colon, the most frequent source is diverticula.

Bibliography

Wilkins T, Baird C, Pearson AN, Schade RR. Diverticular bleeding. Am Fam Physician. 2009;80(9):977-983. [PMID: 19873964]

Item 73   Answer: D

Educational Objective: Manage Barrett esophagus with appropriate surveillance.

This patient should undergo surveillance endoscopy in 1 year for follow-up on pathology findings consistent with Barrett esophagus (BE), which were detected on endoscopy to evaluate his changing reflux symptoms. BE is associated with an increased risk for esophageal adenocarcinoma. If BE is identified on histology, surveillance endoscopy with multiple biopsies should be performed at diagnosis and at 1 year to detect any prevalent dysplasia that was missed on the first endoscopy. If no dysplasia is found, further surveillance can be deferred for 3 years. The presence of low-grade or high-grade dysplasia requires further intensive assessment and management, including the possibility of esophagectomy. The increased risk for malignancy associated with BE has led to screening and surveillance programs, but there is no clear evidence that screening improves survival. Current standards for endoscopic screening in patients with gastroesophageal reflux disease are controversial, but there is some evidence that outcomes may be improved and that it may be cost effective.

Chemoprevention of malignancy with cyclooxygenase-2 (COX-2) inhibitors has been proposed for patients with BE based on studies suggesting an antiproliferative effect on BE-associated tumor cells. However, the effectiveness of this potential therapy has not been established.

Endoscopic ablation is currently not recommended in patients with nondysplastic BE, because the procedure carries risks, and the benefits of ablation do not appear to exceed the risk of progression to adenocarcinoma (0.5% per year). Ablative therapies that consist of removal of metaplastic epithelium can, when combined with intensive acid suppression therapy, lead to the regeneration of squamous mucosa. Concerns remain that areas of abnormal mucosa below the normal-appearing regenerated epithelium may still harbor cancer risk.

Surgical fundoplication is considered in patients with reflux symptoms refractory to medical therapy. However, it has not been shown to decrease the risk of cancer in patients with BE.

KEY POINT

- Patients with Barrett esophagus should undergo endoscopic surveillance to monitor for progression of dysplasia.

Bibliography

Wang KK, Sampliner RE; Practice Parameters Committee of the American College of Gastroenterology. Updated guidelines 2008 for the diagnosis, surveillance and therapy of Barrett's esophagus. Am J Gastroenterol. 2008;103(3):788-797. [PMID: 18341497]

Item 74   Answer: C

Educational Objective: Diagnose pancreatic cancer using endoscopic ultrasound.

This patient should undergo endoscopic ultrasonography (EUS). He most likely has pancreatic adenocarcinoma based on the CT scan findings. In elderly patients with painless jaundice and a focal cutoff sign of the bile and pancreas ducts with upstream dilation, pancreatic malignancy is the most likely differential diagnosis. EUS is as accurate as CT for detecting tumors and may be more sensitive for tumors smaller than 2 cm in diameter. EUS with fine-needle aspiration biopsy can provide specimens for histologic evaluation. MRI and CT are not as sensitive as EUS for detecting tumors less than 2 cm in diameter within the pancreas.

Serum concentration of CA 19-9 increases with pancreatic cancer, particularly in unresectable tumors, but the test has a low sensitivity and specificity and cannot be used as a screening or diagnostic tool for pancreatic cancer.

An MRI is unlikely to be any more successful in detecting a pancreatic tumor than was the CT scan.

Pancreaticoduodenectomy should not be performed because the definitive diagnosis has not yet been made.

KEY POINT

- Endoscopic ultrasonography is as accurate as CT scan for detecting pancreatic tumors and may be more sensitive for tumors smaller than 2 cm in diameter.

Bibliography

Gardner TB, Levy MJ, Takahashi N, Smyrk TC, Chari ST. Misdiagnosis of autoimmune pancreatitis: a caution to clinicians. Am J Gastroenterol. 2009;104(7):1620-1623. [PMID: 19574965]

Item 75   Answer: A

Educational Objective: Treat a patient with large esophageal varices and contraindication to β-blocker therapy.

The most appropriate treatment is endoscopic ligation. The lifetime risk for a first-time variceal bleed in the setting of cirrhosis is 30% and carries a mortality risk of 15% to 20%. Therefore, primary prophylaxis is crucial. Current practice guidelines recommend that all patients with cirrhosis undergo screening endoscopy to detect large esophageal varices. Small varices are usually less than 5 mm in diameter and easily flatten with air insufflation during endoscopy. Large varices are larger than 5 mm or persist despite air insufflation. The presence of red wale markings (longitudinal red streaks on varices) indicates an increased risk of rupture. When large varices are present, as in this patient, the next step in management is to offer nonselective β-blockers or endoscopic variceal ligation as primary prophylaxis to prevent variceal hemorrhage. Although no head-to-head trials have been performed between these treatments, each modality has a similar effect on preventing an index variceal bleed compared with placebo. However, patients with contraindications to β-blocker therapy such as asthma or resting bradycardia can be offered endoscopic ligation. Thus, propranolol would not be the preferred choice in this patient.

Because of adverse effects such as esophageal stricturing, endoscopic sclerotherapy has been replaced by variceal band ligation and is not recommended by major guidelines for primary prophylaxis of large varices.

In patients with active variceal hemorrhage in whom band ligation does not control primary bleeding, or if bleeding recurs or is due to gastric varices, balloon tamponade followed by portal decompression by placement of a transjugular intrahepatic portosystemic shunt (TIPS) can be performed. In the absence of recurrent or refractory variceal hemorrhage, there is no indication for TIPS.

KEY POINT

- Patients with large esophageal varices and contraindications to nonselective β-blockers should receive endoscopic variceal ligation as prophylactic treatment for variceal hemorrhage.

Bibliography

Garcia-Tsao G, Sanyal AJ, Grace ND, Carey W; Practice Guidelines Committee of the American Association for the Study of Liver Diseases; Practice Parameters Committee of the American College of Gastroenterology. Prevention and management of gastroesophageal varices and variceal hemorrhage in cirrhosis. Hepatology. 2007;46(3):922-938. [PMID: 17879356]

Item 76   Answer: B

Educational Objective: Treat erythema nodosum associated with ulcerative colitis.

The most effective treatment is to intensify this patient's therapy for ulcerative colitis. This patient has erythema nodosum (EN), which is a focal noninfectious panniculitis of subcutaneous tissue. The typical clinical presentation is the sudden onset of one or more tender, erythematous nodules on the anterior legs that are more easily palpated than visualized. The eruption is often preceded by a prodrome of fever, malaise, and/or arthralgia. At least half of EN cases are idiopathic. Causes of EN fall into three broad categories: infections, drugs, and systemic diseases (usually inflammatory disorders such as ulcerative colitis or sarcoidosis). EN is self-limited or resolves with treatment of the underlying disorder. Symptomatic treatment includes NSAIDs or potassium iodide. Systemic corticosteroids are rarely needed. Recurrent or chronic EN in the absence of an associated disorder may require therapy with corticosteroids and/or immunosuppressive agents.

Because EN is not an infectious disorder, treatment with an antibiotic is not indicated. Although EN can be a manifestation of an infection, most commonly a recent streptococcal infection, this patient has no history of such an infection.

NSAIDs are a reasonable treatment strategy for idiopathic EN, but they should be avoided in patients with inflammatory bowel disease owing to the risk of exacerbating a bowel-related flare.

While systemic corticosteroids can potentially treat both the patient's inflammatory bowel disease flare and the EN, there is no role for topical corticosteroid creams. Topical corticosteroids can treat local cutaneous processes, but they are not an effective treatment for this systemic manifestation of inflammatory bowel disease.

KEY POINT

- Erythema nodosum associated with ulcerative colitis typically resolves with treatment of the underlying inflammatory bowel disease.

Bibliography

Ardizzone S, Puttini PS, Cassinotti A, Porro GB. Extraintestinal manifestations of inflammatory bowel disease. Dig Liver Dis. 2008;40(Suppl 2):S253-S259. [PMID: 18598997]

Item 77   Answer: B

Educational Objective: Manage post–colorectal cancer surveillance.

The most appropriate management strategy is colonoscopy in 1 year. Patients with a personal history of colorectal cancer are at increased risk for both recurrent cancer and metachronous neoplasia in the remaining colorectum. Consensus guidelines have been established to clarify the appropriate utilization of surveillance colonoscopy among patients with stage I, II, III, or a subset of stage IV (distant metastases resected with curative intent) colorectal cancers. If possible, endoscopic and/or imaging studies should be used to identify and remove synchronous malignancies (present in 2% to 7% of patients with colorectal cancer) or other relevant lesions in the initial perioperative period.

Subsequently, surveillance colonoscopy is recommended in 1 year.

For patients with obstructing primary tumors that do not allow complete endoscopic evaluation during the preoperative evaluation, a postoperative "clearing" (detection and removal of synchronous polyps) colonoscopy is recommended 3 to 6 months after surgery, with surveillance colonoscopy again in 1 year. If the surveillance colonoscopy examination is normal, then future surveillance intervals can be extended.

KEY POINT

- Patients who are candidates for curative treatment of colon or rectal cancer should have a clearing colonoscopy prior to surgery (if not obstructed) and a surveillance colonoscopy 1 year after resection.

Bibliography

Rex DK, Kahi CJ, Levin B, et al. Guidelines for colonoscopy surveillance after cancer resection: a consensus update by the American Cancer Society and US Multi-Society Task Force on Colorectal Cancer. CA Cancer J Clin. 2006;56(3):160-167. [PMID: 16737948]

Item 78   Answer: A

Educational Objective: Manage an incidentally discovered high-risk gallbladder polyp.

The most appropriate management is cholecystectomy. Gallbladder cancer is the most common cancer of the biliary tree, but it is nonetheless quite uncommon, with an observed frequency of less than 1%. Risk factors for gallbladder cancer include cholelithiasis and family history of gallbladder cancer. Cholecystectomy is not generally recommended for asymptomatic gallstones. However, prophylactic cholecystectomy should be considered in patients with gallbladder polyps larger than 10 mm, gallstones larger than 3 cm, or porcelain gallbladder (calcified gallbladder) to prevent gallbladder cancer. Gallbladder polyps are typically found incidentally on gallbladder imaging, as in this patient. A polypoid lesion of the gallbladder that is larger than 10 mm has a 45% to 67% likelihood of cancer, and surgical resection of the gallbladder should be performed.

Endoscopic retrograde cholangiopancreatography is an excellent technique for imaging the bile ducts and gallbladder, but in this case it offers no diagnostic advantage to abdominal ultrasonography and offers no therapeutic options for resection of a polyp that has malignant potential.

Serial imaging is indicated for patients who have gallbladder polyps smaller than 10 mm. If polyps increase in size, there is a significant risk of malignancy. In this patient with a polyp larger than 10 mm, this strategy is not appropriate.

Ursodeoxycholic acid is effective for dissolving certain types of gallstones and is therefore a potential treatment for gallstones in a patient who is not a candidate for cholecystectomy. However, this therapy is not appropriate in this patient because she does not have primary gallstone disease; in addition, this treatment does not cause gallbladder polyps to regress or reduce their malignant potential.

KEY POINT

• A polypoid lesion of the gallbladder that is larger than 10 mm has a 45% to 67% likelihood of cancer, and surgical resection of the gallbladder should be performed.

Bibliography

Miyazaki M, Takada T, Miyakawa S, et al; Japanese Association of Biliary Surgery; Japanese Society of Hepato-Pancreatic Surgery; Japan Society of Clinical Oncology. Risk factors for biliary tract and ampullary carcinomas and prophylactic surgery for these factors. J Hepatobiliary Pancreat Surg. 2008;15(1):15-24. [PMID: 18274840]

Item 79   Answer: D
Educational Objective: Evaluate oropharyngeal dysphagia with videofluoroscopy.

This patient should undergo videofluoroscopy. Her history is characteristic of transfer or oropharyngeal dysphagia, with classic symptoms of aspiration (choking, coughing) while swallowing and an episode of pneumonia (presumedly aspiration pneumonia). Patients with amyotrophic lateral sclerosis (ALS) typically report progressive painless weakness, atrophy, and fasciculations beginning in an arm or leg. In addition to lower motoneuron signs of atrophy and fasciculations, upper motoneuron signs, such as hyperreflexia and extensor plantar responses, are also typically seen. Approximately 20% of patients have bulbar-onset ALS, characterized by slurred speech, oropharyngeal dysphagia, and emotional lability. These findings may also be a later manifestation of the disease. In this patient, videofluoroscopy can assess the oropharyngeal phase of swallowing with foods of different consistencies. Results of this test may be helpful in determining the consistency of food that may allow the patient to continue oral nutrition. If aspiration occurs with all consistencies of food, alternative feeding methods should be explored.

The patient's history is not suggestive of esophageal dysphagia (dysphagia to solids more than liquids) or an esophageal motility disorder (dysphagia to liquids and solids); therefore, an upper gastrointestinal (UGI) series, endoscopy, and esophageal manometry would not be as helpful as the initial diagnostic test for this patient. UGI series and endoscopy would be more helpful in assessing a suspected intraluminal esophageal cause of dysphagia, such as a stricture or ring (which would likely cause symptoms of esophageal dysphagia), whereas manometry would be

more useful in the evaluation of suspected motility disorders such as achalasia (dilated esophagus seen on endoscopy or UGI series).

KEY POINT

• The diagnostic test of choice for oropharyngeal dysphagia is videofluoroscopy, in which the oropharyngeal phase of swallowing is assessed with foods of different consistencies.

Bibliography

Cook IJ. Diagnostic evaluation of dysphagia. Nat Clin Pract Gastroenterol Hepatol. 2008;5(7):393-403. [PMID: 18542115]

Item 80   Answer: A
Educational Objective: Diagnose acalculous cholecystitis.

The most appropriate diagnostic test to perform next is abdominal ultrasound. Acute acalculous cholecystitis (AAC) accounts for approximately 10% of all cases of acute cholecystitis and occurs in about 0.2% of all critically ill patients, especially those with trauma, surgery, shock, burns, sepsis, total parenteral nutrition, and/or prolonged fasting. The disorder usually results from chronic stasis of bile in the gallbladder secondary to underlying disease, resulting in inflammation and distention of the gallbladder wall and ultimately infection. Perforation may occur in severe cases. Many of the clinical findings are nonspecific for AAC, including right upper quadrant pain, fever, leukocytosis, and abnormal liver chemistry tests. Early diagnosis of AAC is based on imaging. Although fever and a dilated gallbladder on CT imaging suggest the presence of AAC, the use of ultrasonography or cholescintigraphy (using technetium-99m [^{99m}Tc]–labeled hepatobiliary agents) has better diagnostic accuracy for AAC. The most studied and cited criteria for AAC are gallbladder wall thickness, sludge, and hydrops. In contrast, CT imaging is unable to provide data on wall thickness as reliably as ultrasound. It is generally agreed that cholecystectomy is the definitive therapy for AAC. However, sometimes percutaneous drainage may be necessary and life-saving in patients who cannot undergo cholecystectomy; it may be the only treatment needed.

Endoscopic ultrasound would have no clear role in this scenario, because a lymph node biopsy is unlikely to provide an explanation for the elevated liver chemistry tests, distended gallbladder, and fever.

In the absence of ultrasound features associated with AAC, an MRI with magnetic resonance cholangiopancreatography would be reasonable to rule out biliary tract pathology such as choledocholithiasis, biliary stricture, or extrinsic bile duct compression from porta hepatis lymphadenopathy. A negative MRI result could be followed by liver biopsy if serum liver chemistry tests remain elevated.

KEY POINT

- Acute acalculous cholecystitis is gallbladder inflammation in the absence of obstructive cholelithiasis; abdominal ultrasonography demonstrates significant gallbladder wall thickening and/or distention.

Bibliography

Huffman JL, Schenker S. Acute acalculous cholecystitis: a review. Clin Gastroenterol Hepatol. 2010;8(1):15-22. [PMID: 19747982]

Item 81   Answer: D

Educational Objective: Evaluate diarrhea in a patient who does not meet diagnostic criteria for irritable bowel syndrome.

This patient should undergo flexible sigmoidoscopy with random colon biopsies. She does not fulfill the simplified American Gastroenterological Association (AGA) clinical diagnostic criteria for irritable bowel syndrome diarrhea subtype (IBS-D) or the Rome III criteria for IBS. The AGA criteria require abdominal pain or discomfort as well as diarrhea for diagnosis of IBS-D. The Rome III criteria for IBS require recurrent abdominal pain or discomfort at least 3 days per month in the last 3 months associated with two or more of the following: (1) improvement with defecation, (2) onset associated with a change in frequency of stool, and (3) onset associated with a change in form of stool. Although these criteria have not been formally validated, they are the guidelines most frequently used in clinical practice to diagnose IBS. Because this patient has painless diarrhea and does not meet the IBS diagnostic criteria, further diagnostic testing is required. Although the differential diagnosis for chronic painless diarrhea is broad, microscopic colitis could be considered as a cause of painless, watery diarrhea in a 67-year-old woman. A recent normal colonoscopy does not exclude microscopic colitis, because this diagnosis requires random colon biopsies to look for a thickened subepithelial collagen band (collagenous colitis) or a subepithelial lymphocytic infiltrate (lymphocytic colitis).

Antispasmodic agents, including dicyclomine, hyoscyamine, and possibly peppermint oil, function as gastrointestinal smooth-muscle relaxants. Although these agents may reduce abdominal pain in the short term for patients with IBS, their efficacy is not well substantiated, and because their action is not specific to the gut, they may be associated with side effects that preclude their use. Furthermore, this patient does not have abdominal pain and does not meet clinical criteria for IBS.

In this patient with a normal tissue transglutaminase IgA level, celiac disease is unlikely, and additional testing for celiac disease is unnecessary. Furthermore, antigliadin antibody studies are less accurate than tissue transglutaminase antibody studies and have high false-positive test rates.

Initiating treatment for painless diarrhea in a 67-year-old woman without understanding the cause of diarrhea is not appropriate. Although loperamide can be part of the treatment approach for microscopic colitis, it would be most appropriate to diagnose first and initiate treatment thereafter.

KEY POINT

- Patients with painless diarrhea who do not meet American Gastroenterological Association or Rome III diagnostic criteria for irritable bowel syndrome should undergo further diagnostic testing.

Bibliography

American College of Gastroenterology Task Force on Irritable Bowel Syndrome, Brandt LJ, Chey WD, Foxx-Orenstein AE, et al. An evidence-based position statement on the management of irritable bowel syndrome. Am J Gastroenterol. 2009;104(Suppl 1):S1-S35. [PMID: 19521341]

Item 82   Answer: D

Educational Objective: Diagnose fulminant Wilson disease.

The most likely diagnosis is Wilson disease. A young patient who presents with acute liver failure should always be suspected of having Wilson disease. In this setting, with an associated hemolytic anemia characterized by a high reticulocyte count and large fraction of unconjugated hyperbilirubinemia, the most likely diagnosis is Wilson disease. Supporting evidence is a low alkaline phosphatase level. Zinc is a cofactor in the production of alkaline phosphatase, and excessive copper acts as a competitive inhibitor of zinc and results in diminished production of alkaline phosphatase. It is important to recognize acute Wilson disease, as the most appropriate management is referral for consideration of liver transplantation. In the setting of acute liver failure, patients with Wilson disease have a nearly 100% mortality rate without urgent liver transplantation; survival has rarely been obtained without liver transplantation.

Acetaminophen intoxication is determined by patient history and/or identification of acetaminophen metabolites on urine drug screen. This patient has not ingested acetaminophen and does not have acetaminophen metabolites in urine studies. Also, acetaminophen toxicity does not cause unconjugated hyperbilirubinemia or hemolytic anemia.

Acute viral hepatitis is unlikely because the most common causes of acute viral hepatitis (hepatitis A and hepatitis B viruses) have been ruled out by serologic evaluation. Antibody to hepatitis B surface antigen denotes immunity to hepatitis B and IgG antibody to hepatitis A virus denotes past infection with and immunity to hepatitis A.

Primary biliary cirrhosis (PBC) does not present as acute liver failure. The presentation of liver failure from PBC is always preceded by progressive clinical decline. In addition, the hyperbilirubinemia seen in PBC is conjugated bilirubinemia, and the alkaline phosphatase level is typically very elevated owing to the bile duct inflammation that characterizes PBC.

KEY POINT

- A young patient who presents with acute liver failure should always be suspected of having Wilson disease.

Bibliography

Moini M, Mistry P, Schilsky ML. Liver transplantation for inherited metabolic disorders of the liver. Curr Opin Organ Transplant. 2010;15(3):269-276. [PMID: 20489626]

Item 83   Answer: C

Educational Objective: Manage eosinophilic esophagitis.

This patient should receive a proton pump inhibitor (PPI) such as omeprazole and should be reassessed in 6 weeks. He presents with symptoms and findings suggestive of eosinophilic esophagitis. Esophageal eosinophilic inflammation can occur secondary to gastroesophageal reflux disease (GERD), but there are currently no accurate criteria to distinguish eosinophilic esophagitis from GERD. The first step in treatment of suspected eosinophilic esophagitis is exclusion of GERD by an ambulatory pH study (to detect excessive esophageal acid exposure) or a 6-week therapeutic trial of a high-dose PPI. If there is a substantial clinical response (which occurs in 30% to 40% of patients), PPI therapy can be continued indefinitely. If the response is poor, the appropriate therapy is 6 weeks of a swallowed aerosolized corticosteroid such as fluticasone (administered by metered dose inhaler without a spacer and without inhalation).

Empiric dilation without beginning medical therapy is not appropriate at this time. Patients with eosinophilic esophagitis have an increased risk of perforation and deep mucosal tears, because untreated inflammation leads to mucosal fragility. Endoscopic dilation is usually reserved for patients who are unresponsive to medical therapy.

Food allergy testing is not helpful in most adults with eosinophilic esophagitis because results do not correlate with response to food elimination diets based on the results of food allergy testing.

A swallowed aerosolized corticosteroid such as fluticasone would be appropriate in this patient if the PPI trial is unsuccessful.

KEY POINT

- The first step in treatment of suspected eosinophilic esophagitis is exclusion of gastroesophageal reflux disease by an ambulatory pH study or a 6-week therapeutic trial of a high-dose proton pump inhibitor.

Bibliography

Furuta GT, Liacouras CA, Collins MH, et al; First International Gastrointestinal Eosinophil Research Symposium (FIGERS) Subcommittees. Eosinophilic esophagitis in children and adults: a systematic review and consensus recommendations for diagnosis and treatment. Gastroenterology. 2007;133(4):1342-1363. [PMID: 17919504]

Item 84   Answer: C

Educational Objective: Manage fundic gland polyps identified on endoscopy.

The most appropriate management strategy is colonoscopy. Gastric fundic gland polyps account for about half of all stomach polyps and are reportedly detected in 1% to 2% of all endoscopies. Typically, these lesions are described as multiple, small (<1 cm), transparent-appearing, sessile polyps in the gastric body and fundus. Fundic gland polyps can occur sporadically, in association with proton pump inhibitor (PPI) therapy, or in the setting of familial adenomatous polyposis (FAP) syndrome. Sporadic fundic gland polyps and those associated with PPI use have low to no malignant potential; gastric fundic gland polyps in the setting of FAP are rarely malignant. Sporadic fundic gland polyps usually present with a lower total number (<10) than PPI-associated or FAP-associated lesions. Based on available data, management guidelines recommend that patients with numerous fundic gland polyps (with or without dysplasia) who are younger than 40 years should undergo colorectal evaluation for signs of possible FAP.

Discontinuing PPI therapy may lead to fundic gland polyp regression, but the effectiveness of this approach remains controversial and may require longer than 3 months to observe. The patient's symptoms and signs of gastroesophageal reflux disease would also discourage stopping PPI therapy.

APC gene testing can be used to screen for FAP or attenuated familial adenomatous polyposis in high-risk patients. For this patient, however, colonoscopy would still be indicated to assess for phenotypic expression regardless of a positive or negative gene testing result.

Because the risk of malignancy is low, extensive polypectomy is not indicated (and is often not feasible) for diminutive fundic gland polyps. However, endoscopic resection of large (>1 cm) fundic gland polyps should be considered.

KEY POINT

- Management guidelines recommend that patients with numerous gastric fundic gland polyps who are younger than 40 years of age should undergo colorectal evaluation for signs of possible familial adenomatous polyposis.

Bibliography

Goddard AF, Badreldin R, Pritchard DM, Walker MM, Warren B; British Society of Gastroenterology. The management of gastric polyps. Gut. 2010;59(9):1270-1276. [PMID: 20675692]

Item 85   Answer: B

Educational Objective: Diagnose acute cholangitis.

The most appropriate test is endoscopic retrograde cholangiopancreatography (ERCP). Acute cholangitis is a bacterial infection of the biliary tract that occurs in an obstructed

CONT.

system and leads to systemic signs of infection. Choledocholithiasis is the leading cause of acute cholangitis and is present in 10% to 20% of patients who present with symptomatic gallstone disease. The risk of symptomatic acute cholangitis for these patients has been reported to be 0.2%. In addition to choledocholithiasis, risk factors for acute cholangitis include age greater than 70 years and diabetes mellitus. The diagnosis of acute cholangitis is based on the Charcot triad of right upper quadrant pain, fever, and jaundice. The addition of septic shock and confusion to the Charcot triad is known as the Reynolds pentad, which may not be present in elderly patients. This patient has clinical features consistent with sepsis, and the absence of fever, leukocytosis, and/or abdominal pain is common among elderly patients with acute cholangitis. Empiric medical management requires prompt initiation of broad-spectrum antibiotics with coverage of enteric gram-negative bacteria such as *Escherichia coli* and *Klebsiella* species. Imaging studies such as ultrasound or CT may or may not identify bile duct dilatation and/or choledocholithiasis. In severely ill patients with hypotension, sepsis, and a high clinical suspicion for acute cholangitis with or without confirmatory imaging studies, the preferred next diagnostic test is ERCP. ERCP also provides immediate biliary decompression with stone extraction and/or stent placement if a biliary stricture is also found.

Based on this patient's age and hemodynamic parameters consistent with sepsis, the performance of cholecystectomy would not be recommended because of an increased risk of morbidity and mortality. However, it may be reasonable to perform in selected patients who are appropriate candidates for surgery after recovery from acute cholangitis.

A hepatobiliary iminodiacetic acid scan is typically used for the detection of acute cholecystitis and does not have a central role in the management of severe acute cholangitis.

MRI with magnetic resonance cholangiopancreatography is not indicated because of the clinical evidence for acute cholangitis and the need for a therapeutic intervention, which is provided by ERCP.

KEY POINT

- In severely ill patients with hypotension and sepsis and a high clinical suspicion for acute cholangitis with or without confirmatory imaging studies, the preferred next diagnostic test is endoscopic retrograde cholangiopancreatography.

Bibliography
Lee JG. Diagnosis and management of acute cholangitis. Nat Rev Gastroenterol Hepatol. 2009;6(9):533-541. [PMID: 19652653]

Item 86   Answer: A

Educational Objective: Manage severe acute pancreatitis.

The most appropriate treatment is aggressive hydration with intravenous fluids. This patient has acute necrotizing pancreatitis based on clinical symptoms, elevated amylase and lipase levels, and CT scan demonstrating hypoperfusion of the pancreas. Necrosis can be defined via CT only when there is hypoperfusion of the pancreas during a contrast-enhanced study. This patient's pancreatitis is likely alcohol induced. The most important initial intervention for this patient is aggressive fluid resuscitation because he has evidence of hypovolemia (tachycardia, hypotension, dry mucous membranes, and elevated hematocrit). Aggressive fluid resuscitation is one of the key initial measures to avoid organ failure in acute pancreatitis.

Broad-spectrum antibiotics are generally not used in acute pancreatitis, even if necrosis is present. Several randomized controlled trials have demonstrated no benefit of intravenous antibiotics as prophylaxis against infection in severe necrotic pancreatitis. In addition, the use of antibiotics without a documented infection may contribute to the development of intra-abdominal fungal infections. Patients with pancreatic necrosis and concern for infection should undergo percutaneous fine-needle aspiration for culture and Gram stain to evaluate for infected pancreatic necrosis. Patients should receive antibiotics only if infection of the pancreas is documented by tissue sampling.

Endoscopic retrograde cholangiopancreatography (ERCP) may cause a flare in pancreatitis, so it is performed rarely in acute pancreatitis. ERCP should be performed only if a patient with gallstone pancreatitis has worsening liver chemistry tests in the setting of clinical instability or has documented ascending cholangitis. This patient does not have evidence of cholangitis. Although the patient may have worsening of liver chemistry tests and clinical symptoms later in the course, ERCP is not advised at admission.

Nasogastric tube decompression is not advocated in the management of acute pancreatitis because it does not lead to improved outcomes and will interfere with early enteral feedings.

KEY POINT

- Aggressive fluid resuscitation is one of the key initial measures to avoid organ failure in acute pancreatitis.

Bibliography
Banks PA, Freeman ML; Practice Parameters Committee of the American College of Gastroenterology. Practice guidelines in acute pancreatitis. Am J Gastroenterol. 2006;101(10):2379-2400. [PMID: 17032204]

Item 87   Answer: C

Educational Objective: Manage achalasia.

This patient has achalasia, and the most appropriate management is laparoscopic myotomy. The goal of therapy for achalasia is to disrupt the lower esophageal sphincter and lower the resting pressure to the point where the sphincter no longer impedes the passage of food or water. Surgical myotomy can now be performed laparoscopically and leads to a shorter hospital stay, faster recovery, and similar results compared with open procedures. Antireflux procedures such as Nissen fundoplication are routinely performed after surgical myotomy to decrease postoperative reflux. Laparoscopic myotomy has been shown to have durable results in greater than 80% of patients 5 to 10 years following surgery. Laparoscopic myotomy is considered first-line therapy; this is the best therapeutic option for this patient, particularly because of her young age and her location in a remote rural area.

Endoscopic injection of botulinum toxin into the lower esophageal sphincter provides symptomatic relief; however, the effect is usually temporary (6-9 months). Injection of botulinum toxin is reserved for patients who are not candidates for surgery and cannot tolerate endoscopic dilatation with its attendant risk of perforation.

Endoscopic dilatation is an alternative method for disrupting the lower esophageal sphincter. However, it is associated with an approximately 5% risk of perforation and a shorter duration of response, which may necessitate repeated dilatations. It may be less successful in younger patients. For these reasons, it is not recommended for this patient.

Medications such as nitrates, calcium channel blockers (such as nifedipine), and nitric oxide donors do not lead to consistent results in patients with achalasia and are usually reserved for patients who cannot tolerate more invasive procedures. Additionally, medical therapy is frequently associated with tachyphylaxis and therefore is not recommended as first-line therapy.

> **KEY POINT**
> - Surgical release of the lower esophageal sphincter by laparoscopic myotomy is first-line therapy for achalasia.

Bibliography

Francis DL, Katzka DA. Achalasia: update on the disease and its treatment. Gastroenterology. 2010;139(2):369-374. [PMID: 20600038]

Item 88   Answer: C

Educational Objective: Diagnose celiac disease in a patient with iron-deficiency anemia.

This patient should have a repeat upper endoscopy with small-bowel biopsies. Although first described in infants, celiac disease often presents later in life, including adulthood. Celiac disease should be considered in all patients presenting with iron-deficiency anemia, especially after routine upper endoscopy and colonoscopy fail to reveal a source of gastrointestinal blood loss. Iron-deficiency anemia may be the only manifestation of celiac disease and should not be overlooked. Patients with Down syndrome have an increased risk of developing celiac disease (prevalence as high as 6% to 8%). Small-bowel biopsies should be obtained even if the tissue transglutaminase (tTG) antibody

is negative in patients in whom there is ongoing concern about the diagnosis based on the disease probability in a specific patient, because the sensitivity of tTG varies significantly among laboratories (69%-93%). Because this patient has both Down syndrome and unexplained iron-deficiency anemia, small-bowel biopsies should be obtained even with a negative tTG, because both of these findings are associated with celiac disease.

A Meckel diverticulum often presents with acute bleeding or features of obstruction; it would be unlikely to present in an occult fashion with iron-deficiency anemia alone.

Push enteroscopy would allow for deeper intubation of the small bowel and can be useful to evaluate for structural lesions or mucosal abnormalities that could not be reached by a standard endoscope. However, without biopsies, the diagnosis of celiac disease could be missed.

Capsule endoscopy can be used in the evaluation of occult bleeding, but it would be utilized only after more common causes of iron-deficiency anemia, such as celiac disease, have been evaluated.

An office-based stool guaiac examination would be unhelpful in this situation owing to the rate of false-positive and negative results. It also does not assess for disorders associated with iron malabsorption. A false-positive test may subject this patient to unnecessary invasive tests, and a negative test should not reassure the physician that no further evaluation is needed for the iron-deficiency anemia.

> **KEY POINT**
> - Celiac disease should be considered in all patients presenting with iron-deficiency anemia, especially after routine upper endoscopy and colonoscopy fail to reveal a source of gastrointestinal blood loss.

Bibliography

Tack GJ, Verbeek WH, Schreurs MW, Mulder CJ. The spectrum of celiac disease: epidemiology, clinical aspects and treatment. Nat Rev Gastroenterol Hepatol. 2010;7(4):204-213. [PMID: 20212505]

Item 89   Answer: E

Educational Objective: Treat a patient with microscopic colitis.

The most appropriate treatment is to stop lansoprazole. This patient has collagenous colitis, one of the two forms of microscopic colitis (the other is lymphocytic colitis). Microscopic colitis occurs most often after the age of 40 years and is more common in women. Symptoms include a chronic relapsing-remitting pattern of watery diarrhea that varies in severity and may be accompanied by weight loss, abdominal pain, fatigue, and nausea. Comorbid autoimmune diseases are common, including thyroid disorders, celiac disease, diabetes mellitus, and rheumatoid arthritis. The cause of microscopic colitis is probably multifactorial and likely represents an abnormal mucosal response to various luminal exposures, including infection and drugs. On colonoscopy, the bowel mucosa appears normal and the diagnosis is made by colonic biopsies. An increase in intraepithelial lymphocytes (>20 per 100 epithelial cells) is pathognomonic for lymphocytic colitis, and a subepithelial collagen band in the lamina propria greater than 10 micrometers (compared with the normal thickness of 5 to 7 micrometers) is diagnostic of collagenous colitis. Multiple medications have been implicated as a cause of microscopic colitis. Lansoprazole is one of the most highly associated medications; other common causative medications are NSAIDs, sertraline, ranitidine, ticlopidine, and acarbose. Although H_2 blockers have also been associated with microscopic colitis, cimetidine may be less strongly associated and may be a reasonable choice for this patient instead of a proton pump inhibitor. Supportive treatment with antidiarrheal agents, such as loperamide, bismuth subsalicylate, and diphenoxylate, may be necessary on a temporary basis.

Mesalamine and budesonide can be effective treatments for microscopic colitis, but the first step in treatment is to withdraw possible offending medications.

Patients who do not respond to drug withdrawal or standard medical therapy for microscopic colitis should be tested for coexisting celiac disease, as there is a clear association between these diseases. However, empirically starting a gluten-free diet would not be appropriate for this patient.

Prednisone is reserved for the most refractory cases of microscopic colitis and would not be appropriate as a first-line treatment for this patient.

> **KEY POINT**
> - The first step in treatment of a patient with microscopic colitis is to stop any potentially causative drugs; the most commonly implicated drugs are lansoprazole, NSAIDs, sertraline, ranitidine, ticlopidine, and acarbose.

Bibliography

Beaugerie L, Pardi DS. Review article: drug-induced microscopic colitis - proposal for a scoring system and review of the literature. Aliment Pharmacol Ther. 2005;22(4):277-284. [PMID: 16097993]

Item 90   Answer: A
Educational Objective: Manage opioid-induced constipation with methylnaltrexone.

The most appropriate management is addition of methylnaltrexone. In the setting of this patient's advanced pancreatic cancer, he has a legitimate reason for optimization of his analgesia program. A drawback of opioid analgesia is constipation, which can be compounded by poor intake of food and fluid. Methylnaltrexone, which is a micro-opioid–receptor antagonist, has been found to help with opioid-induced constipation without negating the beneficial effects of the analgesia.

Naloxone is a drug used in the treatment of opioid overdose to counteract the negative effects of respiratory and central nervous system depression, and it should not be mistaken for methylnaltrexone. Naloxone will cross the blood-brain barrier and cause opioid withdrawal, which would not be desired in this patient.

A diatrizoate sodium enema could help if this patient had obstipation that was not responsive to more conservative measures, but it is not currently required because he is still passing stool.

Although decreasing the morphine dose may help with this patient's constipation, it will leave him with inadequate pain control and is therefore not appropriate.

> **KEY POINT**
> - Methylnaltrexone has been found to help with opioid-induced constipation without negating the beneficial effects of the analgesia.

Bibliography

Thomas, J, Karver S, Cooney GA, et al. Methylnaltrexone for opioid-induced constipation in advanced illness. N Engl J Med. 2008;358(22):2332-2343. [PMID: 18509120]

Item 91   Answer: D
Educational Objective: Treat refractory hepatic encephalopathy.

Hepatic encephalopathy (HE) is a complex neuropsychiatric syndrome characterized by symptoms ranging from minimal neurologic changes to severe confusion or coma. HE is typically associated with cirrhosis and portal hypertension, but it may also occur in patients with severe acute liver failure. Oral lactulose has been considered standard medical therapy for the treatment and/or prevention of clinically significant HE. However, a number of patients will have recurrent hospitalizations for refractory HE in the absence of a known trigger for acute HE (such as bacterial infection, dehydration, electrolyte disturbances, gastrointestinal bleeding, constipation, and the use of sedative or narcotic agents). Therefore, several adjunctive medical therapies have been tried to prevent recurrent HE in susceptible patients. Multiple studies have demonstrated rifaximin to be of equal or superior efficacy compared with lactulose. A recent study found that rifaximin significantly reduced the annual risk of recurrent HE by 60%, including in patients who continued to use lactulose. Rifaximin is considered safe, and dose adjustments are not required in patients with liver or kidney dysfunction. Significant drug interactions have not been reported. Rifaximin was approved by the FDA in 2010 for the treatment of HE.

The efficacy of ciprofloxacin for treating HE has not been proved.

Metronidazole has also been used for the treatment of chronic HE, but it is associated with neurologic toxicity and is not recommended for patients with cirrhosis.

Protein restriction is not recommended for treating HE, because it results in malnutrition and increased predisposition to infections in patients with cirrhosis and HE.

Bibliography

Bass NM, Mullen KD, Sanyal A, et al. Rifaximin treatment in hepatic encephalopathy. N Engl J Med. 2010;362(12):1071-1081. [PMID: 20335583]

Item 92   Answer: B

Educational Objective: Evaluate possible mechanical obstruction in a patient with symptoms of achalasia.

The most appropriate next step in management is endoscopy. This patient's history (dysphagia to solids and liquids with intermittent chest pain) and evaluation (barium radiography showing a dilated esophagus with a smoothly tapering end [bird's beak]; esophageal manometry showing aperistalsis) are suggestive of achalasia. Achalasia, the best characterized of the esophageal motility disorders, consists of the failure of the lower esophageal sphincter to relax with swallowing. The resulting functional obstruction of the distal esophagus leads to dysphagia, chest pain, regurgitation of food, and weight loss. Achalasia is thought to be caused by degeneration of the myenteric plexus with resulting loss of inhibitory neurons in the lower esophageal sphincter, which remains tonically contracted. Owing to the relatively short history (6 months) and weight loss of 4.5 kg (10.0 lb), endoscopy should be performed to rule out a malignant mass at the gastroesophageal junction before considering therapeutic options. A malignant mass could be associated with nonrelaxation of the lower esophageal sphincter owing to direct malignant infiltration or a paraneoplastic syndrome (pseudoachalasia).

CT of the chest and abdomen might be indicated in a patient in whom a malignant mass is discovered at the gastroesophageal junction. Because most malignancies associated with pseudoachalasia are gastric adenocarcinomas, abdominal and chest CT examinations are usually performed for proper staging. Evidence of metastatic spread will spare the patient unnecessary surgery. However, it would be premature to pursue these diagnostic studies before endoscopy is performed.

Surgical disruption of the lower esophageal sphincter (myotomy) can be performed laparoscopically through the abdomen and is considered a first-line therapy for achalasia. However, performing the procedure before excluding the presence of tumor-related pseudoachalasia would be inappropriate.

Swallowed aerosolized corticosteroids would be indicated in the setting of eosinophilic esophagitis, which is unlikely in this patient owing to his barium radiograph and esophageal manometry findings.

Bibliography

Francis DL, Katzka DA. Achalasia: update on the disease and its treatment. Gastroenterology. 2010;139(2):369-374. [PMID: 20600038]

Item 93   Answer: D

Educational Objective: Treat primary biliary cirrhosis.

This patient has primary biliary cirrhosis (PBC) and the most appropriate treatment is ursodeoxycholic acid (UDCA). PBC is a slowly progressive autoimmune disease that mainly affects women older than 25 years. Because of increased awareness of the disease, more patients are being diagnosed while asymptomatic. Symptoms, when present, typically consist of fatigue, pruritus, and later jaundice. The diagnosis of PBC is confirmed by a cholestatic serum liver enzyme profile (serum alkaline phosphatase levels greater than 1.5 times the upper limit of normal; increases in serum alanine aminotransferase and aspartate aminotransferase levels less than 5 times the upper limit of normal) and a positive serum antimitochondrial antibody titer greater than 1:40. A liver biopsy is not needed to confirm the diagnosis in patients with a compatible clinical picture, but it may be done in some patients to stage the severity of disease. UDCA is the only therapy approved by the FDA for PBC. UDCA is associated with improved transplant-free survival and fewer complications from portal hypertension when compared with placebo. In addition, recent studies have demonstrated that patients with earlier stages of PBC who respond to UDCA have long-term survival rates comparable to the general population. Monitoring is performed with serum liver chemistry tests; a reduction in serum alkaline phosphatase by greater than or equal to 40% of baseline values is recognized as a treatment response parameter. Higher doses of UDCA have not been associated with greater clinical response rates. Cholestyramine or other bile acid–binding sequestrants should be administered separately from UDCA because they may interfere with drug absorption. Side effects are minimal but include weight gain, loose stools, and alopecia.

Azathioprine has not demonstrated clinical or survival benefits overall, even when combined with systemic corticosteroids.

Colchicine and methotrexate have been shown to improve clinical symptoms, serum liver enzyme values, and liver histology in PBC; however, no convincing survival benefit is observed with either drug.

KEY POINT

- The most appropriate drug therapy for primary biliary cirrhosis is ursodeoxycholic acid.

Bibliography

Lindor KD, Gershwin ME, Poupon R, Kaplan M, Bergasa NV, Heathcote EJ; American Association for the Study of Liver Diseases. Primary biliary cirrhosis. Hepatology. 2009;50(1):291-308. [PMID: 19554543]

Item 94   Answer: A

Educational Objective: Diagnose chronic mesenteric ischemia.

The most likely diagnosis is chronic mesenteric ischemia, which is also referred to as intestinal angina. This patient has the classic presentation of abdominal pain after eating that leads to weight loss. The weight loss is a result of decreased oral intake due to the fear of pain induced by eating (sitophobia). In contrast with acute mesenteric ischemia, which leads to a sudden and dramatic clinical picture, chronic mesenteric ischemia starts with mild pain with eating, then food intolerance, and eventually can progress to persistent abdominal pain even without eating. This patient's age and history of hypertension, hypercholesterolemia, and smoking are predisposing factors. Doppler ultrasonography can be used as a screening test, but it is insensitive; when there is a high enough suspicion, a more accurate test (such as MR or CT angiography) should be performed. Percutaneous angioplasty can be attempted, but definitive treatment typically requires surgical revascularization.

Patients with chronic pancreatitis may present with one or more of the following: pain, malabsorption, and new-onset diabetes mellitus. The pain of chronic pancreatitis affects at least 85% of patients, is usually chronic and constant, is localized to the midepigastrium, radiates to the back, and is often exacerbated by food.

Colonic ischemia, also called ischemic colitis, is much more common than acute or chronic mesenteric ischemia. The disorder is characterized by a wide spectrum of ischemic injury to the colon including reversible colonopathy, transient colitis, chronic colitis, stricture, gangrene, and fulminant universal colitis. Patients typically present with acute-onset left lower quadrant pain, urgent defecation, and red or maroon rectal bleeding.

Clinical features of gastroparesis include nausea, vomiting, bloating, and postprandial fullness with early satiety. Weight loss may occur because of inadequate nutritional intake. Abdominal discomfort is present in 50% to 90% of affected patients, and it may be the predominant symptom in patients with gastroparesis and

functional dyspepsia. The abdominal examination may show epigastric distention or tenderness, and there may be a succussion splash.

KEY POINT

- The classic presentation of chronic mesenteric ischemia is abdominal pain after eating that leads to weight loss.

Bibliography

Brandt LJ, Boley SJ. AGA technical review on intestinal ischemia. American Gastrointestinal Association. Gastroenterology. 2000;118(5):954-968. [PMID: 10784596]

Item 95   Answer: A

Educational Objective: Manage screening in a patient who has had inadequate bowel preparation for colonoscopy.

The most appropriate management strategy is to repeat colonoscopy now. Colorectal cancer screening and surveillance guidelines assume the performance of a high-quality baseline evaluation. Characteristics of a high-quality baseline colonoscopy evaluation are cecal intubation, well-visualized mucosa with minimal fecal debris, and withdrawal time greater than or equal to 6 minutes. As defined by the American Society for Gastrointestinal Endoscopy/American College of Gastroenterology task force on quality in endoscopy, an adequate preparation allows confidence that mass lesions other than small (<5 mm) polyps were generally not obscured by residual debris. If the bowel preparation is not adequate, as in this patient, the screening evaluation should be repeated before planning a long-term surveillance program.

After confirming a high-quality baseline evaluation, repeat colonoscopy in 3 years would be appropriate for patients with 3 to 10 adenomas (not hyperplastic polyps).

Repeat colonoscopy in 5 years should be recommended for patients with 1 or 2 small (<1 cm) tubular adenomas, with low-grade dysplasia as the most advanced histologic finding.

Repeat colonoscopy in 10 years is acceptable for patients with no colorectal polyps or small rectal hyperplastic polyps only.

KEY POINT

- If the bowel preparation is inadequate for a screening colonoscopy, the colonoscopy should be repeated before planning a long-term surveillance program.

Bibliography

Winawer SJ, Zauber AG, Fletcher RH, et al. Guidelines for colonoscopy surveillance after polypectomy: a consensus update by the US Multi-Society Task Force on Colorectal Cancer and the American Cancer Society. CA Cancer J Clin. 2006;56(3):143-159. [PMID: 16737947]

Item 96   Answer: B

Educational Objective: Treat *Helicobacter pylori* infection with second-line therapy after initial treatment failure.

The most appropriate treatment is quadruple therapy with bismuth, metronidazole, tetracycline, and a proton pump inhibitor (PPI) such as omeprazole. Treatment failure occurs in more than 20% of patients with *Helicobacter pylori* infection. Test of cure should be performed at least 4 weeks after treatment. Patients should stop taking PPIs 2 weeks prior to testing, and H_2 blockers should be stopped 24 to 48 hours prior to testing. Urea breath testing or *H. pylori* stool antigen testing can be used in this setting, but *H. pylori* serology should not be used because it will remain persistently positive despite treatment. The standard initial triple therapy with amoxicillin, clarithromycin, and a PPI was unsuccessful in this patient, and therefore quadruple therapy is the next best option. Quadruple therapy is also a valid first-line regimen, and it can be used for second-line therapy when standard triple therapy fails. Quadruple therapy may supplant the typical triple therapy as a first-line regimen based on a recent randomized controlled trial. Treatment failure can be caused by resistance to antimicrobial agents or nonadherence. The patient should be counseled about the importance of adhering to medical therapy.

This patient most likely has infection with a clarithromycin-resistant organism, because a clarithromycin-based regimen was previously unsuccessful. Therapy with amoxicillin, clarithromycin, and omeprazole is incorrect because repeating the same regimen will result in treatment failure. The most important general concept in *H. pylori* treatment failure is to avoid previously used antibiotics. This is especially true for clarithromycin, given the high resistance rates. In a patient with an *H. pylori*–positive duodenal ulcer in whom first-line treatment for *H. pylori* has been unsuccessful, it is imperative to provide a second treatment course for *H. pylori* to heal the duodenal ulcer and provide secondary prevention of future duodenal ulcers. Therefore, a PPI alone or observation would not provide adequate treatment.

KEY POINT

- **Failure to eradicate *Helicobacter pylori* infection mandates retreatment with a 14-day regimen of different antibiotics.**

Bibliography

Chey WD, Wong BC; Practice Parameters Committee of the American College of Gastroenterology. American College of Gastroenterology guideline on the management of Helicobacter pylori infection. Am J Gastroenterol. 2007;102(8):1808-1825. [PMID: 17608775]

Index

Note: Page numbers followed by f and t denote figures and tables, respectively. Test questions are indicated by Q.

A   **NAME AND ADDRESS (Please complete.)**

Last Name   First Name   Middle Initial

Address

Address cont.

City   State   ZIP Code

Country

Email address

ACP ®
AMERICAN COLLEGE OF PHYSICIANS
INTERNAL MEDICINE | Doctors for Adults

Medical Knowledge Self-Assessment Program® 16

TO EARN *AMA PRA CATEGORY 1 CREDITS*™ YOU MUST:

1. Answer all questions.
2. Score a minimum of 50% correct.

==

TO EARN *FREE* SAME-DAY *AMA PRA CATEGORY 1 CREDITS*™ ONLINE:

1. Answer all of your questions.
2. Go to **mksap.acponline.org** and access the appropriate answer sheet.
3. Transcribe your answers and submit for CME credits.
4. You can also enter your answers directly at **mksap.acponline.org** without first using this answer sheet.

To Submit Your Answer Sheet by Mail or FAX for a $10 Administrative Fee per Answer Sheet:

1. Answer all of your questions and calculate your score.
2. Complete boxes A–F.
3. Complete payment information.
4. Send the answer sheet and payment information to ACP, using the FAX number/address listed below.

B   **Order Number**

(Use the Order Number on your MKSAP materials packing slip.)

C   **ACP ID Number**

(Refer to packing slip in your MKSAP materials for your ACP ID Number.)

COMPLETE FORM BELOW ONLY IF YOU SUBMIT BY MAIL OR FAX

Last Name   First Name |MI

Payment Information. Must remit in US funds, drawn on a US bank.

The processing fee for each paper answer sheet is $10.

☐ Check, made payable to ACP, enclosed

Charge to   ☐ **VISA**   ☐ MasterCard   ☐ ▪   ☐ DISCOVER

Card Number _____

Expiration Date _____ / _____
            MM   YY

Security code (3 or 4 digit #s) _____

Signature _____

Fax to: 215-351-2799

Questions?
Go to **mskap.acponline.org** or email **custserv@acponline.org**

Mail to:
Member and Customer Service
American College of Physicians
190 N. Independence Mall West
Philadelphia, PA 19106-1572

1 Ⓐ Ⓑ Ⓒ Ⓓ Ⓔ   46 Ⓐ Ⓑ Ⓒ Ⓓ Ⓔ   91 Ⓐ Ⓑ Ⓒ Ⓓ Ⓔ   136 Ⓐ Ⓑ Ⓒ Ⓓ Ⓔ
2 Ⓐ Ⓑ Ⓒ Ⓓ Ⓔ   47 Ⓐ Ⓑ Ⓒ Ⓓ Ⓔ   92 Ⓐ Ⓑ Ⓒ Ⓓ Ⓔ   137 Ⓐ Ⓑ Ⓒ Ⓓ Ⓔ
3 Ⓐ Ⓑ Ⓒ Ⓓ Ⓔ   48 Ⓐ Ⓑ Ⓒ Ⓓ Ⓔ   93 Ⓐ Ⓑ Ⓒ Ⓓ Ⓔ   138 Ⓐ Ⓑ Ⓒ Ⓓ Ⓔ
4 Ⓐ Ⓑ Ⓒ Ⓓ Ⓔ   49 Ⓐ Ⓑ Ⓒ Ⓓ Ⓔ   94 Ⓐ Ⓑ Ⓒ Ⓓ Ⓔ   139 Ⓐ Ⓑ Ⓒ Ⓓ Ⓔ
5 Ⓐ Ⓑ Ⓒ Ⓓ Ⓔ   50 Ⓐ Ⓑ Ⓒ Ⓓ Ⓔ   95 Ⓐ Ⓑ Ⓒ Ⓓ Ⓔ   140 Ⓐ Ⓑ Ⓒ Ⓓ Ⓔ

6 Ⓐ Ⓑ Ⓒ Ⓓ Ⓔ   51 Ⓐ Ⓑ Ⓒ Ⓓ Ⓔ   96 Ⓐ Ⓑ Ⓒ Ⓓ Ⓔ   141 Ⓐ Ⓑ Ⓒ Ⓓ Ⓔ
7 Ⓐ Ⓑ Ⓒ Ⓓ Ⓔ   52 Ⓐ Ⓑ Ⓒ Ⓓ Ⓔ   97 Ⓐ Ⓑ Ⓒ Ⓓ Ⓔ   142 Ⓐ Ⓑ Ⓒ Ⓓ Ⓔ
8 Ⓐ Ⓑ Ⓒ Ⓓ Ⓔ   53 Ⓐ Ⓑ Ⓒ Ⓓ Ⓔ   98 Ⓐ Ⓑ Ⓒ Ⓓ Ⓔ   143 Ⓐ Ⓑ Ⓒ Ⓓ Ⓔ
9 Ⓐ Ⓑ Ⓒ Ⓓ Ⓔ   54 Ⓐ Ⓑ Ⓒ Ⓓ Ⓔ   99 Ⓐ Ⓑ Ⓒ Ⓓ Ⓔ   144 Ⓐ Ⓑ Ⓒ Ⓓ Ⓔ
10 Ⓐ Ⓑ Ⓒ Ⓓ Ⓔ   55 Ⓐ Ⓑ Ⓒ Ⓓ Ⓔ   100 Ⓐ Ⓑ Ⓒ Ⓓ Ⓔ   145 Ⓐ Ⓑ Ⓒ Ⓓ Ⓔ

11 Ⓐ Ⓑ Ⓒ Ⓓ Ⓔ   56 Ⓐ Ⓑ Ⓒ Ⓓ Ⓔ   101 Ⓐ Ⓑ Ⓒ Ⓓ Ⓔ   146 Ⓐ Ⓑ Ⓒ Ⓓ Ⓔ
12 Ⓐ Ⓑ Ⓒ Ⓓ Ⓔ   57 Ⓐ Ⓑ Ⓒ Ⓓ Ⓔ   102 Ⓐ Ⓑ Ⓒ Ⓓ Ⓔ   147 Ⓐ Ⓑ Ⓒ Ⓓ Ⓔ
13 Ⓐ Ⓑ Ⓒ Ⓓ Ⓔ   58 Ⓐ Ⓑ Ⓒ Ⓓ Ⓔ   103 Ⓐ Ⓑ Ⓒ Ⓓ Ⓔ   148 Ⓐ Ⓑ Ⓒ Ⓓ Ⓔ
14 Ⓐ Ⓑ Ⓒ Ⓓ Ⓔ   59 Ⓐ Ⓑ Ⓒ Ⓓ Ⓔ   104 Ⓐ Ⓑ Ⓒ Ⓓ Ⓔ   149 Ⓐ Ⓑ Ⓒ Ⓓ Ⓔ
15 Ⓐ Ⓑ Ⓒ Ⓓ Ⓔ   60 Ⓐ Ⓑ Ⓒ Ⓓ Ⓔ   105 Ⓐ Ⓑ Ⓒ Ⓓ Ⓔ   150 Ⓐ Ⓑ Ⓒ Ⓓ Ⓔ

16 Ⓐ Ⓑ Ⓒ Ⓓ Ⓔ   61 Ⓐ Ⓑ Ⓒ Ⓓ Ⓔ   106 Ⓐ Ⓑ Ⓒ Ⓓ Ⓔ   151 Ⓐ Ⓑ Ⓒ Ⓓ Ⓔ
17 Ⓐ Ⓑ Ⓒ Ⓓ Ⓔ   62 Ⓐ Ⓑ Ⓒ Ⓓ Ⓔ   107 Ⓐ Ⓑ Ⓒ Ⓓ Ⓔ   152 Ⓐ Ⓑ Ⓒ Ⓓ Ⓔ
18 Ⓐ Ⓑ Ⓒ Ⓓ Ⓔ   63 Ⓐ Ⓑ Ⓒ Ⓓ Ⓔ   108 Ⓐ Ⓑ Ⓒ Ⓓ Ⓔ   153 Ⓐ Ⓑ Ⓒ Ⓓ Ⓔ
19 Ⓐ Ⓑ Ⓒ Ⓓ Ⓔ   64 Ⓐ Ⓑ Ⓒ Ⓓ Ⓔ   109 Ⓐ Ⓑ Ⓒ Ⓓ Ⓔ   154 Ⓐ Ⓑ Ⓒ Ⓓ Ⓔ
20 Ⓐ Ⓑ Ⓒ Ⓓ Ⓔ   65 Ⓐ Ⓑ Ⓒ Ⓓ Ⓔ   110 Ⓐ Ⓑ Ⓒ Ⓓ Ⓔ   155 Ⓐ Ⓑ Ⓒ Ⓓ Ⓔ

21 Ⓐ Ⓑ Ⓒ Ⓓ Ⓔ   66 Ⓐ Ⓑ Ⓒ Ⓓ Ⓔ   111 Ⓐ Ⓑ Ⓒ Ⓓ Ⓔ   156 Ⓐ Ⓑ Ⓒ Ⓓ Ⓔ
22 Ⓐ Ⓑ Ⓒ Ⓓ Ⓔ   67 Ⓐ Ⓑ Ⓒ Ⓓ Ⓔ   112 Ⓐ Ⓑ Ⓒ Ⓓ Ⓔ   157 Ⓐ Ⓑ Ⓒ Ⓓ Ⓔ
23 Ⓐ Ⓑ Ⓒ Ⓓ Ⓔ   68 Ⓐ Ⓑ Ⓒ Ⓓ Ⓔ   113 Ⓐ Ⓑ Ⓒ Ⓓ Ⓔ   158 Ⓐ Ⓑ Ⓒ Ⓓ Ⓔ
24 Ⓐ Ⓑ Ⓒ Ⓓ Ⓔ   69 Ⓐ Ⓑ Ⓒ Ⓓ Ⓔ   114 Ⓐ Ⓑ Ⓒ Ⓓ Ⓔ   159 Ⓐ Ⓑ Ⓒ Ⓓ Ⓔ
25 Ⓐ Ⓑ Ⓒ Ⓓ Ⓔ   70 Ⓐ Ⓑ Ⓒ Ⓓ Ⓔ   115 Ⓐ Ⓑ Ⓒ Ⓓ Ⓔ   160 Ⓐ Ⓑ Ⓒ Ⓓ Ⓔ

26 Ⓐ Ⓑ Ⓒ Ⓓ Ⓔ   71 Ⓐ Ⓑ Ⓒ Ⓓ Ⓔ   116 Ⓐ Ⓑ Ⓒ Ⓓ Ⓔ   161 Ⓐ Ⓑ Ⓒ Ⓓ Ⓔ
27 Ⓐ Ⓑ Ⓒ Ⓓ Ⓔ   72 Ⓐ Ⓑ Ⓒ Ⓓ Ⓔ   117 Ⓐ Ⓑ Ⓒ Ⓓ Ⓔ   162 Ⓐ Ⓑ Ⓒ Ⓓ Ⓔ
28 Ⓐ Ⓑ Ⓒ Ⓓ Ⓔ   73 Ⓐ Ⓑ Ⓒ Ⓓ Ⓔ   118 Ⓐ Ⓑ Ⓒ Ⓓ Ⓔ   163 Ⓐ Ⓑ Ⓒ Ⓓ Ⓔ
29 Ⓐ Ⓑ Ⓒ Ⓓ Ⓔ   74 Ⓐ Ⓑ Ⓒ Ⓓ Ⓔ   119 Ⓐ Ⓑ Ⓒ Ⓓ Ⓔ   164 Ⓐ Ⓑ Ⓒ Ⓓ Ⓔ
30 Ⓐ Ⓑ Ⓒ Ⓓ Ⓔ   75 Ⓐ Ⓑ Ⓒ Ⓓ Ⓔ   120 Ⓐ Ⓑ Ⓒ Ⓓ Ⓔ   165 Ⓐ Ⓑ Ⓒ Ⓓ Ⓔ

31 Ⓐ Ⓑ Ⓒ Ⓓ Ⓔ   76 Ⓐ Ⓑ Ⓒ Ⓓ Ⓔ   121 Ⓐ Ⓑ Ⓒ Ⓓ Ⓔ   166 Ⓐ Ⓑ Ⓒ Ⓓ Ⓔ
32 Ⓐ Ⓑ Ⓒ Ⓓ Ⓔ   77 Ⓐ Ⓑ Ⓒ Ⓓ Ⓔ   122 Ⓐ Ⓑ Ⓒ Ⓓ Ⓔ   167 Ⓐ Ⓑ Ⓒ Ⓓ Ⓔ
33 Ⓐ Ⓑ Ⓒ Ⓓ Ⓔ   78 Ⓐ Ⓑ Ⓒ Ⓓ Ⓔ   123 Ⓐ Ⓑ Ⓒ Ⓓ Ⓔ   168 Ⓐ Ⓑ Ⓒ Ⓓ Ⓔ
34 Ⓐ Ⓑ Ⓒ Ⓓ Ⓔ   79 Ⓐ Ⓑ Ⓒ Ⓓ Ⓔ   124 Ⓐ Ⓑ Ⓒ Ⓓ Ⓔ   169 Ⓐ Ⓑ Ⓒ Ⓓ Ⓔ
35 Ⓐ Ⓑ Ⓒ Ⓓ Ⓔ   80 Ⓐ Ⓑ Ⓒ Ⓓ Ⓔ   125 Ⓐ Ⓑ Ⓒ Ⓓ Ⓔ   170 Ⓐ Ⓑ Ⓒ Ⓓ Ⓔ

36 Ⓐ Ⓑ Ⓒ Ⓓ Ⓔ   81 Ⓐ Ⓑ Ⓒ Ⓓ Ⓔ   126 Ⓐ Ⓑ Ⓒ Ⓓ Ⓔ   171 Ⓐ Ⓑ Ⓒ Ⓓ Ⓔ
37 Ⓐ Ⓑ Ⓒ Ⓓ Ⓔ   82 Ⓐ Ⓑ Ⓒ Ⓓ Ⓔ   127 Ⓐ Ⓑ Ⓒ Ⓓ Ⓔ   172 Ⓐ Ⓑ Ⓒ Ⓓ Ⓔ
38 Ⓐ Ⓑ Ⓒ Ⓓ Ⓔ   83 Ⓐ Ⓑ Ⓒ Ⓓ Ⓔ   128 Ⓐ Ⓑ Ⓒ Ⓓ Ⓔ   173 Ⓐ Ⓑ Ⓒ Ⓓ Ⓔ
39 Ⓐ Ⓑ Ⓒ Ⓓ Ⓔ   84 Ⓐ Ⓑ Ⓒ Ⓓ Ⓔ   129 Ⓐ Ⓑ Ⓒ Ⓓ Ⓔ   174 Ⓐ Ⓑ Ⓒ Ⓓ Ⓔ
40 Ⓐ Ⓑ Ⓒ Ⓓ Ⓔ   85 Ⓐ Ⓑ Ⓒ Ⓓ Ⓔ   130 Ⓐ Ⓑ Ⓒ Ⓓ Ⓔ   175 Ⓐ Ⓑ Ⓒ Ⓓ Ⓔ

41 Ⓐ Ⓑ Ⓒ Ⓓ Ⓔ   86 Ⓐ Ⓑ Ⓒ Ⓓ Ⓔ   131 Ⓐ Ⓑ Ⓒ Ⓓ Ⓔ   176 Ⓐ Ⓑ Ⓒ Ⓓ Ⓔ
42 Ⓐ Ⓑ Ⓒ Ⓓ Ⓔ   87 Ⓐ Ⓑ Ⓒ Ⓓ Ⓔ   132 Ⓐ Ⓑ Ⓒ Ⓓ Ⓔ   177 Ⓐ Ⓑ Ⓒ Ⓓ Ⓔ
43 Ⓐ Ⓑ Ⓒ Ⓓ Ⓔ   88 Ⓐ Ⓑ Ⓒ Ⓓ Ⓔ   133 Ⓐ Ⓑ Ⓒ Ⓓ Ⓔ   178 Ⓐ Ⓑ Ⓒ Ⓓ Ⓔ
44 Ⓐ Ⓑ Ⓒ Ⓓ Ⓔ   89 Ⓐ Ⓑ Ⓒ Ⓓ Ⓔ   134 Ⓐ Ⓑ Ⓒ Ⓓ Ⓔ   179 Ⓐ Ⓑ Ⓒ Ⓓ Ⓔ
45 Ⓐ Ⓑ Ⓒ Ⓓ Ⓔ   90 Ⓐ Ⓑ Ⓒ Ⓓ Ⓔ   135 Ⓐ Ⓑ Ⓒ Ⓓ Ⓔ   180 Ⓐ Ⓑ Ⓒ Ⓓ Ⓔ